HEINEMANN

DENTAL DICTIONARY

FOURTH EDITION

HEINEMANN DENTAL DICTIONARY

FOURTH EDITION

Jenifer E H Fairpo
BA, DipLib (Lond)
and
C Gavin Fairpo
BDS, MChD

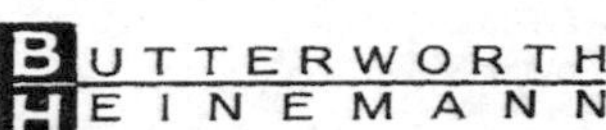

OXFORD AUCKLAND BOSTON JOHANNESBURG MELBOURNE NEW DELHI

Butterworth-Heinemann
Robert Stevenson House,
1-3 Baxter's Place,
Leith Walk,
Edinburgh EH1 3AF

First published as *Heinemann Modern Dictionary for Dental Students* 1962
Second edition 1973
First published as a paperback 1985
Reprinted 1986
Third edition 1987
Fourth edition 1997
Reprinted 2000, 2001, 2002

British Library Cataloguing in Publication Data
Fairpo, Jenifer E. H. (Jenifer Elizbeth Hawkes)
Heinemann dental dictionary – 4th ed.
1. Dentistry – Dictionaries
I. Title II. Fairpo, C. Gavin (Charles Gavin) III. Dental dictionary
617.6′003

ISBN 0 7506 2208 3

Library of Congress Cataloging in Publication Data
Fairpo, Jenifer E. H.
Heinemann dental dictionary/Jenifer E. H. Fairpo and C. Gavin Fairpo. – 4th ed.
p. cm.
Includes bibliographical references.
ISBN 0 7506 2208 3
1. Dentistry – Dictionaries. I. Fairpo, C. Gavin. II. Title.
[DNLM: 1. Dictionaries, Dental. 2. Head – anatomy & histology – terminology. 3. Neck – anatomy & histology – terminology. WU13F172h 1997]
RK27.F35 1997
617.6′003–dc21 96–52669 CIP

Typeset by Latimer Trend & Company Ltd, Plymouth
Printed and bound in Great Britain by Biddles Ltd, *www.Biddles.co.uk*

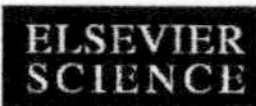

Contents

Preface to the First Edition

This dictionary has been compiled primarily to meet the needs of the dental student, but it is hoped that it may also prove useful to dental nurses, technicians, secretaries and other workers in the field of dentistry. In view of this the definitions have been kept as simple as possible. Many American terms are included, since the majority of books and periodical articles in dentistry today are published in the United States. A number of obsolete terms have been defined to aid those reading the early literature. Such medical terms have been included as are specifically relevant to dentistry, but it is not, of course, possible to produce an exhaustive list in a work of this size. For the benefit of foreign students particular attention has been paid to pronunciation.

At the end of the dictionary will be found three appendices: anatomical tables of the head and neck, the terminology of which is that approved by the Seventh International Congress of Anatomists, New York, 1960, published in *Nomina Anatomica*, 2nd edition (Amsterdam, etc., *Excerpta Medica Foundation*, 1961); an appendix of drugs used in dentistry, which has been prepared by Dr J.B. Roberts, of Liverpool University, to whom I should like to express my gratitude for the trouble he has taken over it; and a list of dental journals, with their country of origin, frequency, and the official abbreviation according to the International Standard ISO R4, as used in *World Medical Periodicals*, 2nd edition (London, *British Medical Association*, 1957), which it is hoped may prove of value to all concerned with the publication of dental material.

As would be expected in a work of this nature medical and dental dictionaries and many reference books have been consulted and I wish to express my indebtedness to all concerned, and especially to the Medico-Dental Publishing Company for permission to reproduce the Classification of tooth cavities from *Operative Dentistry*, 8th edition (1947), by G.V. Black.

I should like to thank most sincerely all those people who have so kindly helped me during the compilation of this work, especially Mr G. Wreakes, Registrar, Dental Hospital, Leeds, for reading the typescript and for many useful suggestions; Dr W.J.K. Walls, Reader in Anatomy, University of Leeds, for his careful scrutiny of the anatomical tables; and all members of staff of the Dental School of the University of Leeds, who have solved so many of my problems for me. I should also like to acknowledge with gratitude the interest and encouragement which I have received from Mr B.S. Page, the University Librarian.

My thanks are also due to Mr Frank Price for his effective line drawings, and to the Dental Manufacturing Company for the loan of the blocks illustrating various dental instruments; to Miss Jean Kershaw, formerly Librarian, British Dental Association, for her assistance on various matters, and for hospitality in the Association's Library; to Mr L.T. Morton, who persuaded me to undertake the work in the first instance, and to Mr Owen R. Evans, of William Heinemann Medical Books, for all his patience and help throughout.

Leeds, *January*, 1962. J.E.H.F.

Preface to the Fourth Edition

When Owen Evans, of Heinemann Medical Books, first approached me in 1959 to compile a small, pocket dictionary for dental students I never thought that almost forty years later we should be working on a fourth edition. Many of the original features of the first edition have now been dropped to allow for the expansion in the vocabulary. The use of computer technology has completely changed the approach to revision and to content. Because of the free availability to all dental students and practitioners of a current edition of the *Dental Practitioners' Formulary*, and also of the *British National Formulary*, the drug appendix was omitted from the third edition. Certain drugs and drug types are, however, still included in the main text.

Clinical terminology in this edition has been based on the British Standard BS EN 21942:1992 - 21942-4: 1994, - ISO 1942-1-4:1989/Amd.1:1992 (E/F) *Dental vocabulary*, parts 1-4 and BS EN ISO 1942-5: 1995: *Dental vocabulary*, part 5. The ISO designation system for teeth and areas of the oral cavity is taken from ISO 3950-1984(E). Cross-references have, once again, been provided from older terminology to what have become the preferred terms. Bacteriological nomenclature is based on *Bergey's Manual of systematic bacteriology*. Editor in Chief: John G. Holt. 4 vols. (Baltimore, *Williams & Wilkins*, 1984-1989). The terminology for the anatomical tables has been adjusted to conform with the revisions made at the Twelfth International Congress of Anatomists, London, 1985, published in *Nomina Anatomica*, 5th edition (Edinburgh, *Churchill Livingstone*, 1989).

In the periodicals section there has been, yet again, an enormous increase in the number of new titles as well as title changes. Because the list of titles indexed by the *Index to Dental Literature* now seems to change every year the indication of those journals covered by the *Index* has no longer been included. Those titles no longer in existence when the last edition was prepared have now been omitted altogether.

We should once again like to thank our colleagues at the Leeds Dental Institute for their ready assistance, and in particular Dr Chris Watson for his help with the material relating to implants and implant dentures and Mr Paul Cook for sorting out knotty orthodontic problems. Our thanks are also due to Mrs Anne Collins and the staff of the Medical and Dental Library of the University of Leeds, and to the staff of the National Lending Library at Boston Spa for their hospitality and assistance throughout the work of revision.

Abbreviations

List of commonly used initial abbreviations for dental institutions, degrees, etc. As most of these now omit full stops between letters, this convention has been followed here. Information on dental degrees, diplomas and other qualifications has been checked against the current issue of *The Dentist's Register*.
(* indicates that the qualification is no longer awarded.)

AACD American Academy of Cosmetic Dentistry.

AADE American Association of Dental Editors; American Association of Dental Examiners.

AADGP American Academy of Dental Group Practice.

AADP American Academy of Dental Prosthetics.

AADPA American Academy of Dental Practice Administration.

AADR American Academy of Dental Radiology.

AADS American Association of Dental Schools.

AAE American Association of Endodontists.

AAGFO American Academy of Gold Foil Operators.

AAGO American Academy of Gnathologic Orthopedics.

AAHD American Academy of the History of Dentistry; American Association of Hospital Dentists.

AAID American Academy of Implant Dentistry.

AAMP American Academy of Maxillofacial Prosthetics.

AAO American Association of Orthodontists.

AAOGP American Academy of Orthodontics for the General Practitioner.

AAOM American Academy of Oral Medicine.

AAOMS American Association of Oral and Maxillofacial Surgeons.

AAOP American Academy of Oral Pathology.

AAP American Academy of Periodontology; American Academy of Pedodontics.

AAPD American Academy of Pediatric Dentistry.

AAPHD American Association of Public Health Dentistry.

ABDSA Association of British Dental Surgery Assistants.

ABESP Associação Brasileira de Endodontia, secção São Paulo.

ABO American Board of Orthodontics; Associação Brasiliera de Odontologia.

ABOMS American Board of Oral and Maxillofacial Surgery.

ABOP American Board of Oral Pathology.

ABP American Board of Pedodontics; American Board of Periodontics; American Board of Prosthodontics.

ACD American College of Dentists.

ACP American College of Prosthodontists.

ACPA American Cleft Palate Association.

ADA American Dental Association; Association of Dental Anaesthetists; Australian Dental Association.

ADAA American Dental Assistants Association.

ADH Academy of Dentistry for the Handicapped; Association of Dental Hospitals.

ADHA American Dental Hygienists' Association.

ADHUK Association of Dental Hospitals of the United Kingdom.

ADI Association of Dental Implantology.

ADM Academy of Dental Materials; Asociación Dental Mexicana.

ADP Academy of Denture Prosthetics; Association for Denture Prosthesis.

ADS American Denture Society; Army Dental Services.

ADSA American Dental Students Association.

ADTA American Dental Trade Association.

AIDS Association of Industrial Dental Surgeons.

ALAFO Asociación Latinoamericana de Facultades de Odontología.

AMDI Associazione Medici Dentisti Italiani.

AOD Academy of Operative Dentistry.

APS American Prosthodontic Society.

ARPA International Association for Research in Paradentosis.

ASAAD American Society for the Advancement of Anesthesia in Dentistry.

ASAASD Australian Society for the Advancement of Anaesthesia and Sedation in Dentistry.

ASDA American Society for Dental Aesthetics; American Student Dental Association.

ASDC American Society of Dentistry for Children.

ASDR American Society of Dental Radiographers.

ASGD American Society of Geriatric Dentistry.

ASO American Society of Orthodontists.

ASOS American Society of Oral Surgeons.

ASP American Society of Periodontists (*now called* American Academy of Periodontology).

ATDT Association of Teachers of Dental Technology.

BADT British Association of Dental Therapists.

BAFO British Association for Forensic Odontology.

BAO British Association of Orthodontists.

BAOMS British Association of Oral and Maxillofacial Surgeons.

BASCD British Association for the Study of Community Dentistry.

BChD Baccalaureus Chirurgiae Dentalis.
University of Leeds.

BDA British Dental Association.

BDEF British Dental Editors Forum.

BDHA British Dental Hygienists' Association.

BDHF British Dental Health Foundation.

BDS Bachelor of Dental Surgery.
Universities of Birmingham, Bristol, Durham, Liverpool, London, Manchester, Newcastle upon Tyne, Sheffield, Dundee, Edinburgh, Glasgow, St Andrew's*, University of Wales – Cardiff, Queen's University, Belfast, National University of Ireland – Dublin and Cork.*

BDSA British Dental Students Association.

BDentSc Bachelor in Dental Science.
University of Dublin – Trinity College.

BDTA British Dental Trade Association.

BES British Endodontic Society.

BFS British Fluoridation Society (*now called* Fluoridation Society).

BIST British Institute of Surgical Technicians.

BNA Basle Nomina Anatomica.
A list of Latin anatomical terms, adopted as a standard at a conference in Basle in 1895, and since modified.

BPS British Paedodontic Society.

BSDH British Society of Dentistry for the Handicapped.

BSDMR British Society of Dental and Maxillofacial Radiology.

BSDR British Society for Dental Research.

BSI British Standards Institution.
Items approved by the Institution are identified by a BS number.

BSMDH British Society of Medical and Dental Hypnosis.

BSOM British Society for Oral Medicine.

BSP British Society of Periodontology.

BSPD British Society of Paediatric Dentistry.

BSRD British Society for Restorative Dentistry.

BSSO British Society for the Study of Orthodontics.

BSSPD British Society for the Study of Prosthetic Dentistry.

BTEC Business and Technical Education Council

CCHADT Central Council for Health Authority Dental Technology.

CNSD Confédération Nationale des Syndicats Dentaires. This is the French equivalent of the British Dental Association.

CPSM Council for Professions Supplementary to Medicine.

DCDH Diploma in Child Dental Health.
Queen's University, Belfast.

DChD Doctor Chirurgiae Dentalis.
University of Wales – Cardiff.

DDH Diploma in Dental Health.
University of Birmingham.*

DDO Diploma in Dental Orthopaedics.
Royal Faculty of Physicians and Surgeons, Glasgow.*

DDOrth Diploma in Dental Orthopaedics.
Royal College of Physicians and Surgeons, Glasgow.

DDPH Diploma in Dental Public Health.
Royal College of Surgeons of England.

DDR Diploma in Dental Radiology.
Royal College of Radiologists.

DDS Doctor of Dental Surgery.
Universities of Birmingham, Manchester, Edinburgh, Glasgow.

DDSc Doctor of Dental Science.
Universities of Leeds, Durham, Newcastle upon Tyne, Dundee, Glasgow*, St Andrew's*.*

DEAC Dental Education Advisory Council.

DGDP (UK) Diploma in General Dental Practice.
Royal College of Surgeons of England, Faculty of General Dental Practitioners (UK).

Dip.Odont Diploma in Odontology.
University of Dundee.

DLA Dental Laboratories Association.

DMD Doctor of Dental Medicine (Medicinae Dentalis).

DOrth Diploma in Orthodontics.
Royal College of Surgeons of England, Royal College of Surgeons of Edinburgh.

DPD Diploma in Public Dentistry.
*University of Dundee and St Andrew's**.

DPDS Diploma in Postgraduate Dental Studies.
University of Bristol.

DRD Diploma in Restorative Dentistry.
Royal College of Surgeons of Edinburgh.

DSA Dental Surgery Assistant.

DSASTAB Dental Surgery Assistants Standards and Training Advisory Board.

DTETAB Dental Technicians Education and Training Advisory Board.

EAMFS European Association for Maxillo-Facial Surgery.

EDS European Dental Society.

EOS European Orthodontic Society.

EPA European Prosthodontic Society.

FACD Fellow of the American College of Dentists.

FDI Fédération Dentaire International: International Dental Federation.

FDS Fellowship in Dental Surgery.
Royal College of Surgeons of England, Royal College of Physicians and Surgeons, Glasgow, Royal College of Surgeons of Edinburgh.

FFD Fellow in the Faculty of Dentistry.
Royal College of Surgeons in Ireland.

FICD Fellow of the Institute of Canadian Dentists; Fellow of the International College of Dentists.

FOA Federation of Orthodontic Associations.

FRACDS Fellow of the Royal Australasian College of Dental Surgery.

FS Fluoridation Society (*formerly* British Fluoridation Society).

GDC General Dental Council.

GDPA General Dental Practitioners' Association.

GIRSSO Groupement International pour la Recherche Scientifique en Stomatologie et Odontologie.

HDD Higher Dental Diploma.
Royal Faculty (now *College*) *of Physicians and Surgeons, Glasgow**.

IADC International Association of Dentistry for Children.

IADH International Association of Dentistry for the Handicapped.

IADMFR International Association of Dento-Maxillo-Facial Radiology.

IADP Irish Association for Dental Prosthesis.

IADR International Association for Dental Research.

IADS International Association of Dental Students.

IAG International Academy of Gnathology.

IAOMS International Association of Oral and Maxillofacial Surgeons.

IAOP International Association of Oral Pathologists.

IAOS International Association of Oral Surgeons.

IAPD International Association of Paediatric Dentistry.

IFDAS International Federation of Dental Anesthesiology Societies.

IMFT Institute of Maxillo-Facial Technology.

ISDC International Society for Dental Ceramics.

ISO International Standards Organization.

LDS Licentiate in Dental Surgery.
Used to be granted by all those universities granting dental degrees; also granted by the *Royal College of Surgeons of England, Royal College*

(formerly *Faculty) of Physicians and Surgeons, Glasgow, Royal College of Surgeons of Edinburgh, Royal College of Surgeons in Ireland.*

LDentSc Licentiate in Dental Science.
*University of Dublin**.

MCCD Diploma of Membership in Clinical Community Dentistry.
Royal College of Surgeons of England, Royal College of Physicians and Surgeons, Glasgow.

MCDH Master of Community Dental Health.
University of Birmingham.

MChD Magister Chirurgiae Dentalis (Master of Dental Surgery).
University of Leeds, University of Wales—Cardiff*.*

MDD Doctor of Dental Medicine (Medicinae Dentalis Doctor).

MDO Membership in Dental Orthopaedics.
Royal College of Physicians and Surgeons, Glasgow.

MDS Master of Dental Surgery.
Universities of Birmingham, Bristol, Durham, Leeds, Liverpool, London, Manchester, Newcastle upon Tyne, Sheffield, Dundee*, Edinburgh*, Glasgow*, St Andrew's*, Queen's University, Belfast, National University of Ireland – Dublin and Cork.*

MDSc Master of Dental Science.
Universities of Leeds, Liverpool, Dundee.*

MDentSc Master in Dental Science.
University of Dublin – Trinity College.

MDentSc Master of Dental Science.
University of Birmingham.

MDentSci Master of Dental Science.
University of Liverpool.

MGDS Membership in General Dental Surgery.
Royal College of Surgeons of England, Royal College of Physicians and Surgeons, Glasgow, Royal College of Surgeons of Edinburgh, Royal College of Surgeons in Ireland.

MMScDent Master of Medical Science (in Paediatric and Preventive Dentistry).
Queen's University, Belfast.

MOrth Membership in Orthodontics.
Royal College of Surgeons of England, Royal College of Surgeons of Edinburgh.

MRD Membership in Restorative Dentistry.
Royal College of Surgeons of England, Royal College of Surgeons of Edinburgh.*

MS(Dent) Master of Surgery (Dental Surgery).
*University of London**.

MSc Master of Science.
This degree is awarded by all British universities.

MScD (*formerly* **MScDent**) Magister Scientiae Dentalis (Master of Dental Science).
University of Wales—Cardiff.

NDA National Dental Association.

NDHEG National Dental Health Education Group.

NDTA National Dental Technicians' Association.

NHSTA National Health Service Training Authority.

NIDR National Institute for Dental Research.

NSDP National Society of Dental Prosthetists.

NZDA New Zealand Dental Association.

ORCA Organisme Européen de Coordination des Recherches sur la Fluor et la Prophylaxie de la Carie Dentaire: European Organization for Research on Fluorine and Dental Caries.

OTA Orthodontic Technicians Association.

PhD Philosophiae Doctor.

This degree is awarded by all British universities.

PNA Paris Nomina Anatomica.

The Latin anatomical terminology approved by the Sixth International Congress of Anatomists, Paris, 1955.

RCPS Royal College of Physicians and Surgeons, Glasgow (*formerly* Royal Faculty of Physicians and Surgeons, Glasgow).

RCSEd Royal College of Surgeons of Edinburgh.

RCSEng Royal College of Surgeons of England.

RCSI Royal College of Surgeons in Ireland.

RFPS Royal Faculty of Physicians and Surgeons, Glasgow (*now called* Royal College of Physicians and Surgeons, Glasgow).

SAAD Society for the Advancement of Anaesthesia in Dentistry.

SFOD Société Française d'Orthopédie Dentofaciale.

SGDS Society of General Dental Surgery.

SOLAIAT Sociedad Odontológico Latino-Americano de Implantes Aloplásticos y Transplantes.

SUDI Society of University Dental Instructors.

WHO World Health Organization.

Signs

The following signs have been used used throughout the text:

* before a word is used to direct a reader to the preferred term where a descriptive definition may be found. A superscript number following a starred term indicates which of several definitions is the one referred to.

See is used for an alternative, preferred, spelling or where the term is included in a wider definition.

fl. in biographical details given for eponyms indicates that the person is known to have been alive at that date.

pl. indicates the plural of a singular noun where this may not be easily recognizable as such.

A

a-, an- Prefix signifying *without, not.*

āā Abbreviation for *ana*—of each; used in prescription writing.

āāā Amalgam.

ABC Axiobuccocervical.

ABG Axiobuccogingival.

ABL Axiobuccolingual.

abs.feb. Abbreviation for *absente febre*—with fever absent, without fever.

AC Axiocervical.

a.c. Abbreviation for *ante cibum*—before meals; used in prescription writing.

ACE Alcohol:Chloroform:Ether; an anaesthetic mixture containing these substances.

ACTH Adrenocorticotrophic hormone.

AD Axiodistal.

ad. Abbreviation for *adde*—add; used in prescription writing.

ad hib. Latin for *ad hibendus*: to be administered; used in prescription writing.

ad lib. Abbreviation for *ad libitum*—to the desired amount; used in prescription writing.

ADC Axiodistocervical.

ADG Axiodistogingival.

ADI Axiodistoincisal.

ADO Axiodisto-occlusal.

aeq. Abbreviation for *aequales*—equal; used in prescription writing.

aet. Abbreviation for *aetas*—age; used in prescription writing.

AG Axiogingival.

Ag Chemical symbol for silver.

AHG Antihaemophilic globulin.

AI Axioincisal.

AIDS Acquired immune deficiency syndrome: a viral disease, often sexually transmitted, in which changes in infected lymphocytes lead to immune deficiency which predisposes to severe, usually fatal, secondary infections; oral manifestations include candidosis, 'hairy' leukoplakia and Kaposi's sarcoma.

AL Axiolingual.

Al Chemical symbol for aluminium.

ALa Axiolabial.

ALaG Axiolabiogingival.

ALaL Axiolabiolingual.

ALC Axiolinguocervical.

ALG Axiolinguogingival.

ALO Axiolinguo-occlusal.

alt. dieb. Abbreviation for *alternis diebus*—every other day; used in prescription writing.

alt. hor. Abbreviation for *alternis horis*—every other hour; used in prescription writing.

AMC Axiomesiocervical.

AMD Axiomesiodistal.

AMG Axiomesiogingival.

AMI Axiomesioincisal.

AMO Axiomesio-occlusal.

AO Axio-occlusal.

AP Axiopulpal.

APF Acidulated phosphate fluoride, a form of fluoride used for topical application.

aq. Abbreviation for *aqua*—water.

aq. ad Abbreviation for *aquam ad*—water up to; used in prescription writing.

aq. dest. Abbreviation for *aqua destillata*—distilled water; used in prescription writing.

aq. pur. Abbreviation for *aqua pura*—pure water; used in prescription writing.

Au Chemical symbol for gold.

'A' point *Subspinale.

ab- Prefix signifying *away from*.

abacterial Free from bacteria.

abapical Away from the apex.

abarthrosis Synovial *joint.

abarticulation 1. Dislocation of a joint. 2. Synovial *joint.

abate To decrease or to lessen; applied to symptoms, pain, etc.

abatement A decrease or a lessening in severity.

abaxial Situated away from the axis.

abducens oris M. levator anguli oris. *See* Table of Muscles.

abducent Drawing away from the axis, or separating.

abducent nerve Supplies the lateral rectus muscle of the eye. *See* Table of Nerves—abducens.

abduction A drawing or leading away from the axis.

aberrant Deviating from the normal form or course.

aberration 1. Variation from the normal form or course. 2. *In biology*, an abnormal part.

abirritant 1. Relieving irritation; soothing. 2. Any agent that relieves irritation.

ablation Removal of a part by excision or amputation.

ablepharous Having no eyelids.

ablephary Congenital partial or total absence of the eyelids, or of the palpebral fissure.

abluent 1. Cleansing or washing. 2. A cleansing agent or a detergent.

ablution The act of cleansing or washing.

abnormal Not normal, deviating in some way from the usual structure, position or state.

abnormality Not the normal or usual growth or development.

abocclusion Condition where the maxillary and mandibular teeth are not in contact.

aborad Situated or leading away from the mouth.

aboral Relating to areas away from or opposite to the mouth.

abradant An abrasive agent.

abrade To wear away by friction.

abrasio dentium Wearing away of the teeth.

abrasion 1. The wearing away of a structure or substance by mechanical means, such as scrubbing or grinding—for example, toothbrushing. 2. The wearing away of structure or substance because of a pathological condition—in dentistry, for example, bruxism. 3. A patch on the body surface which has been denuded of skin or mucous membrane, a graze.

abrasive 1. Containing a substance that tends to erode a surface. 2. The actual substance that wears away the surface.

abscess A collection of pus in a cavity formed by disintegration of tissue as a result of infection.
acute a. One having a short but severe course, producing painful local inflammation, and some fever.
alveolar a. An abscess affecting the alveolar bone.
apical a. An abscess occurring at the apex of a tooth root.
bicameral a. One containing two chambers.
blind a. One having no fistulous opening.

caseous a. An abscess containing cheese-like matter.
chronic a. Any abscess of long duration and slow development; it may be a cold abscess, or one resulting from the incomplete resolution of a pre-existing acute abscess, or from the presence of pyogenic organisms of low virulence. There is pus formation, but little inflammation.
circumtonsillar a. Peritonsillar *abscess.
cold a. A slow-developing tuberculous abscess, generally about a bone or joint, and with little inflammation.
collar-stud a. A superficial abscess connected by a sinuous tract to a larger, deep abscess.
congestive a. An abscess forming at a distance from the inflammation, because resistance from the tissues prevents it gathering.
dental a. Any abscess connected with a tooth.
dento-alveolar a. One affecting the tissues round the apex of a non-vital tooth root.
dry a. An abscess that disperses without bursting or coming to a head.
encysted a. An abscess in which the pus is contained within a serous cavity.
gingival a. An abscess occurring in a periodontal pocket and affecting the adjacent gingiva.
hypostatic a. A wandering *abscess which has reached its position as a result of the effect of gravity.
interradicular a. One in which the pus collects between the roots of a tooth.
lateral a., lateral alveolar a. Periodontal *abscess.
migrating a. Wandering *abscess.
miliary a. One of a group of many small abscesses.
palatal a. An apical abscess, usually of the maxillary lateral incisors or the palatal roots of the maxillary posterior teeth, pointing towards the palate.
parietal a. A periodontal abscess occurring at any site away from the apex of a tooth root.
parodontal a. An abscess arising in the periodontal membrane.
periapical a. An abscess erupting around the apex of a tooth root.
pericemental a. A parodontal abscess not arising from a diseased pulp or as an extension of a periodontal pocket.
pericoronal a. An abscess arising about the crown of an unerupted tooth.
peridental a. Periodontal *abscess.
periodontal a. An abscess in the periodontal tissues as a result of the extension of infection from a periodontal pocket into the supporting tissue.
peritonsillar a. An extension of acute suppurative tonsillitis, resulting in an abscess within the connective tissue capsule of the tonsil; *also called* quinsy.
phoenix a. An acute exacerbation of a chronic or suppurative apical periodontitis.
primary a. An abscess that develops at the point of infection.
pulp a., pulpal a. Acute or chronic inflammation of the tooth pulp associated with an area of necrotic tissue and pus; it may occur in the early stage of acute pulpitis.
radicular a. An apical *granuloma.
residual a. An abscess that develops near the remains of earlier inflammation.
root a. An apical *granuloma.
satellite a. A secondary abscess arising from and situated near to a primary abscess.

secondary a. One that develops as a result of infection from an existing abscess.
septal a. An abscess forming on the approximal surface of a tooth root.
sterile a. An abscess containing no micro-organisms.
superficial a. One situated near the surface.
sympathetic a. A secondary abscess arising at some distance from the original focus of infection.
wandering a. An abscess that tracks through the tissues and finally comes to a point some distance from the original site.

abscission Removal by cutting.

abscopal Relating to the effect on non-irradiated tissue of irradiation of other tissue.

absorbable Capable of being absorbed; used of materials which can be absorbed into the body.

absorbefacient An agent that promotes absorption.

absorbent 1. Capable of sucking up or drawing in. 2. Any drug or agent that promotes absorption.

absorptance The ratio of the amount of radiation absorbed by a surface to the amount incident upon it.

absorption 1. The taking up of one substance, or of a fluid, by another substance. 2. *Resorption.

absorption lacuna Resorption *lacuna.

abstraction *of the jaws* A form of malocclusion in which the jaws are abnormally distant.

abut To adjoin and touch; to be in contact with.

abutment 1. A supporting structure. 2. A tooth or tooth root used to support a fixed or removable appliance or partial denture. 3. A plate or implant used for this purpose.
auxiliary a. Secondary *abutment.
implant a. That part of an alveolar implant which protrudes through the gingiva into the mouth, and on which a crown or bridge is supported; *also called* transmucosal component.
intermediate a. A tooth or tooth root standing alone, used for support in addition to terminal abutments.
isolated a. A form of intermediate abutment, generally one used to support a removable partial denture.
multiple a. An abutment constructed by fixed splinting of two or more adjacent natural teeth, used in the support of a partial denture.
pier a. Intermediate *abutment.
primary a. A tooth used for direct support or retention for a denture or an appliance.
secondary a. A tooth used as an additional support for a denture or appliance.
terminal a. A tooth used to provide retention or support at one end of a denture or appliance.

abutment tooth A tooth used as support for a false tooth or for one end of a bridge.

acanthion A craniometric point on the base of the anterior nasal spine.

acanthoameloblastoma A form of ameloblastoma containing squamous cells.

acanthoid Spinous, spine-like.

acantholysis The pathological separation of epidermal or epithelial cells by breakdown of desmosomes, leading to blistering as in pemphigus.

accessory Auxiliary or supplementary; applied to minor organs that supply major ones.

accessory meningeal artery A. pterygomeningea. *See* Table of Arteries.

accessory nerve Supplies the striated muscles of the pharynx and larynx, and the sternocleidomastoid and trapezius muscles. *See* Table of Nerves—accessorius.

accrementition Increase or growth by the addition of similar tissue.

accretion 1. Normal increase in size. 2. A deposit of foreign matter adhering to a surface or accumulating in a cavity; in dentistry, for example, plaque or materia alba.

accretion lines Incremental *lines.

acellular Without, free from, cells.

ache 1. A continuous, dull fixed pain. 2. To suffer such a pain.

acheilia Congenital absence of a lip or lips.

acheilous Without lips.

achondroplasia A congenital disease affecting skeletal development and resulting in dwarfism.

acid 1. A chemical compound of hydrogen with one or more other elements: tastes sour, turns blue litmus red. 2. Sour-tasting. 3. Having the properties of an acid.

acid etching The use of an acid solution over a selected area of a tooth surface to demineralize the enamel partially and so provide a key for the retention of certain types of filling material.

acidic Relating to acid; with a pH of less than 7.

acidogenic Acid-forming.

acidulated Having been made acid.

acidulous Somewhat acid.

acinic cell tumour An epithelial tumour of the salivary glands made up of cells resembling the serous cells of those glands.

acinus (*pl.* acini) One of the minute sacs, with a narrow lumen, which form the lobules of a compound gland.

aclusion The condition of having the teeth parted; as opposed to *occlusion*.

acoustic nerve N. vestibulocochlearis. *See* Table of Nerves.

acquired Relating to something not of genetic origin but resulting from outside influences.

acrid Pungent and irritating, either in smell or taste.

acrocephalic Having a highly arched or pointed skull.

acrodont Having teeth attached directly to the jaw-bone and not set in sockets; as seen, for example, in lizards.

acromegaly Gigantism: associated with hyperfunction of the pituitary gland and characterized by enlargement of the bones and soft tissue of the head and the extremities.

acropis An old term for faulty articulation due to some defect of the tongue.

acrylic, acrylic resin Acrylic *polymer.

acrylic mould A stent used in oral plastic surgery to secure an intraoral skin graft.

actinic Relating to rays and radiation beyond the violet end of the spectrum.

actino- Prefix signifying *ray, ray-shaped*, or *radiation*.

Actinomyces A genus of bacteria, non-sporing and non-motile vegetable parasites, facultatively anaerobic, Gram-positive, and seen as filamentous rosettes with clubbing of the filaments. They are no longer considered part of the family Actinomycetaceae.

A. dentocariosus *Rothia dentocariosa.

Actinomycetales An order of bacterial fungi; mould-like organisms with a tendency to branch, found in soil and in fresh water; some forms occur normally in the human oral cavity.

actinomycosis A chronic infection caused by *Actinomyces israelii*, frequently commensal in the mouth, trauma allowing ingress of the organism; it is characterized by chronic inflammation, formation of granulation tissue, and suppuration discharging through multiple sinuses, the pus containing 'sulphur' granules. It mainly affects the jaw and neck, but may also affect the chest and abdomen.

activator 1. Any agent necessary to activate another substance. 2. *In orthodontics*, a myofunctional *appliance.

bow a. A type of myofunctional *appliance, the two halves being connected by a wire bow or hoop; used to open the bite anteriorly; *also called* Schwarz activator or Schwarz appliance.

acu- Prefix signifying *needle*.

acusection *Electrosection.

acute 1. Sharp. 2. Of rapid, severe onset and short duration; as opposed to *chronic*.

acutenaculum A surgical needle-holder.

ad Latin for *to, up to*; used in prescription writing to indicate the amount of a substance, usually a diluent, which should be added.

ad- Prefix signifying *to, in the direction of*.

-ad Suffix signifying *towards*.

ad hibenus Latin for *to be administered*; used in prescription writing, and abbreviated *ad hib*.

ad libitum Latin for *to the desired amount*; used in prescription writing, and abbreviated *ad lib*.

adamantine Relating to tooth enamel.

adamantinocarcinoma A malignant form of ameloblastoma.

adamantinoma *Ameloblastoma.

adamantoblast *Ameloblast.

adamantoblastoma *Ameloblastoma.

adamantoma *Ameloblastoma.

adamas dentis Tooth *enamel.

Adams clasp (C.P. Adams, contemporary British orthodontist). A modified form of arrowhead *clasp.

adaptation *In dentistry:* 1. The correct fitting of a denture. 2. The adjustment of bands to the teeth. 3. The correct packing of filling material into a prepared cavity.

adapter A device used to connect parts of an instrument or apparatus.

band a. An orthodontic tool used to fit an orthodontic band on to a tooth.

adde Latin for *add*; used in prescription writing, and abbreviated *ad*.

Addison's disease (Sir T. Addison, 1793-1860. English physician). Primary adrenocortical insufficiency, characterized by weight loss, general weakness, fatigue, hypotension and abnormal pigmentation. Pigmentation of the skin on the face and of the mucosa is an early sign of the disease; the pigmented areas are blue-black in colour, involving most commonly the mucous membrane of the cheek, but the lips, tongue, palate and gingiva may also be affected.

adduction A drawing in towards the centre, or to the median line; as opposed to *abduction*.

aden-, adeno- Prefix signifying *gland*.

adenalgia Pain affecting a gland.

adenectomy 1. Surgical removal of a gland. 2. *Adenoidectomy.

adenitis Inflammation of a gland.

adeno-ameloblastoma Adenomatoid odontogenic *tumour.

adenocarcinoma A malignant tumour derived from glandular tissue and to some extent resembling the organ of its origin.

adenocele *Cystadenoma.

adenocyst A glandular cyst.

adenocystoma *Cystadenoma.

adenofibroma A tumour composed of fibrous and glandular tissue.

adenoid 1. Like a gland. 2. (*pl.*) The adenoid tissue in the nasopharynx.

adenoidectomy Surgical excision of the adenoids.

adenoiditis Inflammation of the adenoids.

adenolymphoma 1. A benign cystic tumour of the salivary glands, most frequently the parotid gland, containing epithelial and lymphoid tissue; *also called* papillary cystadenoma lymphomatosum. 2. A benign epithelial tumour occurring in the lymph glands.

adenoma A benign epithelial tumour of glandular origin; adenomas may be described as *pleomorphic (mixed)* or *monomorphic*, depending on their histological make-up.
acidophilic a. *Oncocytoma.
oncocytic a. *Oncocytoma.
oxyphilic a. *Oncocytoma.

adenomatoid Like, resembling, an adenoma.

adenomatome A surgical instrument used for excision of the adenoids.

adenomatosis A condition characterized by multiple adenomas.

adenomatosis oris Swelling of the mucous glands of the lip, with no inflammation or secretion.

adenotome *See* adenomatome.

adhere To stick, cling, or become fastened together.

adherent Holding fast; attached to; sticking to.

adhesion 1. The sticking or fastening together of two adjacent surfaces. 2. *In surgery*, the abnormal joining of two separate parts by a band of new tissue. 3. The tissue that creates this union. 4. *In dentistry*, the force that retains a full upper denture in place without the use of vacuum cups.
palatopharyngeal a. Congenital bonding of the posterior part of the soft palate and the pharynx; may also be the result of scar tissue formation.
sublabial a. Abnormal bonding of the mucous membrane of the maxillary labial sulcus to the alveolar process; seen in cleft lip.

adhesive 1. Sticking closely. 2. Characterized by adhesion. 3. A substance used for sticking together.

adhesiveness The quality of being adhesive.

adipose Fat, fatty.

adjustment *In dentistry*, modification of a denture or appliance after it has been fitted in the mouth.
occlusal a. Occlusal *equilibration.
post-retention a. Minor movement of teeth after the completion of orthodontic treatment.

adjuvant An additive which assists the action of a drug.

adnasal Relating to, or situated near, the nose.

adolescent 1. Relating to the period from the onset of puberty to the end of somatic development. 2. A person during this period of life.

adoral Near to, in the direction of, the mouth.

adrenodontia Morphological indications of over-activity of adrenal glands, characterized by large, pointed canines, and teeth whose occlusal surfaces show a brown discoloration.

adsorption The property possessed by certain substances of sucking up fluids.

adult 1. Fully developed or mature. 2. One who is fully developed or mature.

adulteration The addition of inferior or unnecessary material to debase a substance; usually a fraudulent process.

adventitious 1. Acquired or accidental ; as opposed to *natural* or *hereditary*. 2. Found in an abnormal or unusual position.

Aeby's muscle (C.T. Aeby, 1835-85. German anatomist). *Krause's muscle.

aequales Latin for *equal*; used in prescription writing, and abbreviated *aeq.*

aer-, aero- Prefix signifying *air* or *gas.*

aerobe A micro-organism requiring air or free oxygen to live and grow.

aerobic Requiring air or free oxygen to live and grow.

aerocele A type of tumour caused by the development of an adventitious sac filled with air or gas.

aerodontalgia Toothache caused by high-altitude flying.

aerodontia, aerodontics That branch of dentistry concerned with the care and treatment of dental conditions caused by high-altitude flying.

aerodontodynia *Aerodontalgia.

aerophilic *Aerobic.

aetiologic, aetiological Relating to aetiology.

aetiology The study of the causes of disease.

afebrile Without fever.

affection Any pathologic condition or diseased state.

afferent Carrying to the centre, centripetal; as opposed to *efferent.*

afferent nerve Any nerve transmitting impulses from the periphery to the centre.

afibrillar Containing no fibrils.

afibrinogenaemia A blood-clotting disorder, caused by absence of fibrinogen; it may cause spontaneous gingival haemorrhage and post-extraction bleeding.

agar Extract of seaweed of the genus *Gelideum*, used in the preparation of bacteriological culture media.

agenesis Non-development or defective development.

agent Any substance or power that produces change in the body.
bleaching a. Any substance used to whiten or to remove discoloration.
disclosing a. A staining agent, which, when applied to the tooth surface either as a tablet to be chewed or in a mouthwash, attaches to the plaque and other surface deposits and shows them up in some distinct colour against the normal clean enamel.

ageusia Loss or absence of a sense of taste.

agger nasi The anterior portion of the ethmoidal crest on the maxilla.

agglutination 1. The grouping together into clumps of particles suspended in fluid. 2. A joining together, as in the physiological process of repair of a wound.

agglutinin An antibody capable of causing the cells of its specific antigen to become grouped together in clumps.

aglossia Congenital absence of the tongue.

aglossostomia Congenital absence of the tongue and of the mouth opening.

aglutition *Dysphagia.

agmatology The science and study of fractures.

agnathia Complete failure of development of the mandible or of the maxilla.

-agogue Suffix signifying *agent leading or inducing* some reaction.

agomphiasis 1. Looseness of the teeth. 2. Complete absence of teeth.

agomphious Having no teeth.

agomphosis *Agomphiasis.

-agra Suffix signifying *acute pain.*

agranular Containing no granules.

agranulocytosis The disease state arising from leukopenia, in which there is typically oral, gingival and pharyngeal ulceration.

ague A chill or fever, especially of malarial origin.

ailment Any disorder or disease; usually used of a mild or slight occurrence.

Ainsworth's punch (G.C. Ainsworth, 1852-1948. American dentist). Rubber-dam *punch.

air chamber A depression in the palatal portion of an upper denture, once thought to assist in its retention; *also called* a vacuum chamber.

air motor An air-driven motor, separate from the handpiece but which can be directly coupled to it.

air rotor Turbine *handpiece.

air sinus *Sinus^3.

air syringe A syringe by means of which compressed air may be blown into a cavity or root canal to dry it or to remove loose debris.

airbrasive An instrument used to cut tooth cavities by means of a mixture of sand and aluminium oxide ejected in a stream of gas under pressure.

airway 1. The passage by which air is breathed into and from the lungs. 2. The tube used to ensure the free passage of air during recovery after general anaesthesia.

akanthion *See* acanthion.

ala (*pl.* alae) A wing-like bone process.

ala-tragal line The line from the lower border of the ala of the nose to the upper border of the tragus of the ear.

alar Relating to an ala.

alar cartilage The U-shaped cartilage which forms the tip of the nose.

alate Having wings.

albation The bleaching or whitening of teeth or other discoloured matter.

Albers-Schönberg disease (H.E. Albers-Schönberg, 1865-1921. German radiologist). *Osteopetrosis.

Albinus' muscle (B.A. Albinus, 1697-1770. German anatomist and surgeon). M. risorius. *See* Table of Muscles.

Albrecht's bone (K.M.P. Albrecht, 1851-1894. German anatomist). An ossicle between the basisphenoid and the basi-occipital bones.

alcohol Colourless liquid, C_2H_5OH, obtained by distillation from fermented sugar, starch, grain or fruits. Used medicinally as an antiseptic and as a solvent. *Also called* ethanol or ethyl alcohol.

Alexander gold (C.L. Alexander, fl. 1923. American dentist). Gold mixed with a wax substance to make it plastic; used for certain types of gold filling.

Alexander's crown (C.L. Alexander, fl. 1923. American dentist). A metal cap crown used as a bridge abutment.

alg-, algi-, algo- Prefix signifying *pain.*

algesia Sensitivity to pain.

algesic Painful.

algesthesia, algesthesis 1. The sense of pain. 2. Any sensation of pain.

algetic Painful.

-algia Suffix signifying *pain.*

alginate Any salt of alginic acid; an irreversible colloid used as dental impression material.

algophobia Morbid irrational fear of pain.

aliform Wing-shaped.

align 1. To arrange in a line. 2. To correct the teeth by bringing them back into the normal arch. 3. To set up teeth in a normal arch for a denture.

aline *See* align.

alkali Any of the class of compounds that form soluble carbonates, and soaps with fats, and that turn litmus blue.

alkaline Relating to or having the character of an alkali.

alkalinity The quality of being alkaline.

alkaloid Any one of a large group of basic nitrogenous organic substances found in plants; used as drugs they have a powerful action and many are highly toxic, even in small doses.

all-, allo- Prefix signifying *variant, reversed,* or *referring to another.*

allel-, allelo- Prefix signifying *relating to another.*

allelograft A graft using materials not derived from a donor or from animal sources; e.g., synthetic resins, stainless steel alloy.

Allen's cement (J. Allen, 1810-1892. American dentist). A fusible siliceous cement used to attach porcelain teeth to a plate.

Allen's root pliers (A.B. Allen, 1862-1943. American dentist). Special pliers designed to remove small pieces of tooth root broken off during extraction.

allergenic Capable of inducing an allergy.

allergic Relating to or characterized by allergy.

allergy Hypersensitivity to any normally harmless substance, resulting in an exaggerated or abnormal reaction.

allograft A graft derived from a donor of the same species but genetically dissimilar.

alloplast A synthetic biomaterial that is relatively inert; it may be ceramic, metal or a polymer.

alloplastic Relating to an alloplast.

allotri-, allotrio- Prefix signifying *foreign, strange.*

allotriodontia 1. *Transplantation of teeth. 2. The presence of a tooth in an abnormal place, as in a cyst or tumour.

alloy The substance produced by the fusion of two or more metals.
amalgam a. Shavings or filings of a metal alloy to be mixed with mercury to form an amalgam.
cobalt-chromium casting a. A hard and corrosion-resistant alloy of cobalt and chromium, used in the construction of partial dentures.
contour a. One suitable for fillings that can be anatomically contoured.
eutectic a. One in which the fusion temperature of the alloy is lower than that of its constituent metals; such alloys are usually brittle, and corrode or tarnish easily. *In dentistry* eutectic alloys may be used to reduce the fusion temperature of solders.

submarine a. One used in cavities that cannot be kept free from moisture.

alloyage The process of making an alloy.

alternis diebus Latin for *every other day*; used in prescription writing and abbreviated *alt.dieb.*

alternis horis Latin for *every other hour*; used in prescription writing and abbreviated *alt.hor.*

aluminium A white, light and ductile metal, chemical symbol: Al; formerly used as a denture base.

alundum 1. A special form of aluminium used for apparatus in which heat has to be resisted. 2. Trade name for a carborundum-type abrasive.

alvealgia, alveolalgia Dry *socket; more specifically, the pain associated with this condition.

alveolar Relating to the alveolus.

alveolar artery Supplies blood to the mandibular teeth, floor of the mouth, and buccal mucous membrane (*inferior*), maxillary teeth and antral mucous membrane (*superior*). *Also called* dental artery (British terminology). *See* Table of Arteries—alveolaris.

alveolar line *In craniometry*, a line from the prosthion to the nasion.

alveolar nerves Supply the teeth and alveolar processes. *Also called* dental nerves (British terminology). *See* Table of Nerves—alveolaris.

alveolar point *Prosthion.

alveolare *Prosthion.

alveolectomy Surgical correction of bone deformity and removal of bone in the alveolar process.

alveolingual Relating to the alveolar process and the tongue.

alveolitis Inflammation of an alveolus, as of a tooth socket, or of the alveolar process.

a. sicca dolorosa Dry *socket.

alveoloclasia The breakdown of the alveolar process by disintegration or absorption, causing loosening of the teeth.

alveolocondylar, alveolocondylean Relating to the alveolus and the condyle.

alveolodental Relating to the alveolar process and the teeth.

alveololabial Relating to the alveolar process and the lips.

alveololabialis Buccinator muscle. *See* Table of Muscles.

alveololingual *Alveolingual.

alveolomaxillary Relating to the maxilla and the alveolar process.

alveolomaxillary muscle Buccinator muscle. *See* Table of Muscles.

alveolomerotomy Surgical removal of part of the alveolar process; alveolectomy.

alveolonasal Craniometric term relating to the alveolar point and the nasion.

alveolopalatal Relating to the alveolar process and the palate.

alveoloplasty Surgical alteration and improvement of the alveolar ridges for denture construction.

alveolosubnasal Craniometric term relating to the alveolar point and the acanthion.

alveolotomy Surgical incision of an alveolus or of the alveolar process.

alveolus (*pl.* alveoli) *In dentistry,* the bony socket in which the tooth is held.

alveolysis Resorption of the alveolar bone.

amalgam 1. An alloy of mercury with another metal or metals. 2. Any plastic alloy.

binary a. An amalgam containing mercury and one other metal.
copper a. An amalgam alloy containing mainly copper and mercury.
dental a. Any amalgam used for filling teeth; it usually contains silver, tin and mercury.
quaternary a. An amalgam containing mercury and three other metals; *also called* Black's amalgam.
quinary a. An amalgam containing mercury and four other metals.
retrograde a. Retrograde root *filling.
silver a. A type of dental amalgam which contains a high proportion of silver.

amalgam alloy Shavings or filings of a metal alloy to be mixed with mercury to form an amalgam.

amalgam carrier A syringe-like instrument used to transfer small quantities of amalgam to a prepared cavity in a tooth.

amalgam carver A specially designed type of carver with a sharp blade used for contouring amalgam restorations.

amalgam condenser An instrument used to condense amalgam in a cavity.

amalgam die A model cast in amalgam from an impression, and from which inlays or crowns may be fabricated.

amalgam gun *Amalgam carrier.

amalgam manipulator An instrument used to contour an amalgam filling.

amalgam matrix Matrix *band.

amalgam plugger *Amalgam condenser.

amalgam tattoo An area of pigmentation of the oral tissues as a result of the implantation of amalgam restorative materials; it may be black or brown in colour.

amalgamation The formation of an amalgam.

amasesis Inability to chew.

amb-, ambo- Prefix signifying *both*, or *on both sides*.

amel-, amelo- Prefix signifying *enamel*.

amelification *Amelogenesis.

ameloblast One of the germ cells developed from the epithelium, from which the enamel organ is formed.

ameloblastic process A projection of cytoplasm from an enamel cell, about which mineralization occurs.

ameloblastoma A locally malignant tumour of the jaw, most common in the mandibular molar region, and derived from odontogenic epithelium; it may be described as follicular, plexiform, acanthomatous, basal cell or granular cell, depending on the histological pattern.

ameloblastosarcoma A malignant tumour arising from the epithelial odontogenic tissues.

amelocemental *Cemento-enamel.

amelodentinal Relating to both the enamel and the dentine of a tooth.

amelogenesis The formation of enamel.

amelogenesis imperfecta An hereditary defect in enamel formation characterized by a brown colouring of the teeth.

amelogenic Enamel-forming.

amelogenins Young enamel *proteins.

amnion The innermost of the foetal membranes forming the fluid-filled sac enclosing the foetus and also a sheath for the umbilical cord.

amniotic Relating to the amnion.

Amoeba buccalis, Amoeba gingivalis **Entamoeba gingivalis*.

amorphous Shapeless; without form.

amphiarthrosis Old term for cartilaginous *joint.

amphicone The outer, buccal cusp on triangular maxillary molar teeth in primitive mammals; a term used in palaeontology and comparative dental anatomy.

amphidiarthrosis A joint that is both ginglymoid and arthrodial, such as the temporomandibular joint.

ampoule, ampule A small glass container which can be hermetically sealed, used to hold sterile drug preparations.

ampullary nerve Supplies the ampullae of the semicircular ducts. *See* Table of Nerves—ampullaris.

amputation The surgical removal of a limb or part of a limb, or of any other projecting part.
periosteoplastic a. Subperiosteal *amputation.
pulp a. *Pulpotomy.
root a. Surgical excision of the apical portion of a tooth root.
subperiosteal a. Amputation in which the stump of bone is covered by a periosteal flap.

amygdala 1. An almond. 2. A tonsil.

amyl-, amylo- Prefix signifying *starch.*

amylogenic Starch-producing.

amyloid 1. Starch-like. 2. A white, insoluble protein found in the tissues as an abnormal deposit.

amylolytic Relating to or causing the digestion of starch.

amylosis The digestion of starch or its conversion to glucose.

amyxorrhoea Deficiency of mucous secretion.

an- Prefix signifying *without, not.*

anabolic Relating to anabolism.

anabolism The process of assimilation of nutriment and its conversion to living tissue.

anachoresis The attraction of micro-organisms towards a local tissue lesion, associated with increased immunity to infections other than that of the lesion.

anaemia A deficiency in the blood, either qualitative or quantitative.

anaemic Relating to or affected with anaemia.

anaerobe A micro-organism that can live and grow without air or free oxygen.

anaerobic Capable of living and growing without air or free oxygen.

anaesthesia Loss of sensation or feeling.
block a. Regional *anaesthesia.
conduction a. Regional *anaesthesia.
facial a. Loss of sensation in an area of the face as a result of trauma or of a pathological process affecting either the central nervous system or the sensory nerves supplying the area.
general a. Anaesthesia of the whole body.
infiltration a. Local anaesthesia produced by the infiltration of an anaesthetic agent into the surrounding tissue.
inhalation a. General anaesthesia induced by the inhaling of gaseous or volatile liquid anaesthetic agents.
intra-oral a. Local anaesthesia produced by an injection into the oral tissues from within the mouth.
intraosseous a. Anaesthesia of a tooth produced by introducing the anaesthetic agent directly into the alveolar bone in the region of the tooth apex.
intrapulpal a. Local anaesthesia produced by introducing the anaesthetic agent directly into the dental pulp.

intravenous a. General anaesthesia induced by the introduction of an anaesthetic agent into the blood stream by injection into a vein.
local a. Anaesthesia of a circumscribed area of the body.
regional a. The injection of an anaesthetic agent into or around a major nerve.
surface a. Topical *anaesthesia.
topical a. Local anaesthesia produced by the application of an agent externally before injection or some other operation liable to cause pain.

anaesthesiology The study of anaesthesia and anaesthetics.

anaesthetic 1. Relating to, or marked by, anaesthesia. 2. Any drug that produces anaesthesia.

analeptic 1. Stimulating to the central nervous system. 2. Any agent that acts in this way; used of the restorative or strengthening property of certain drugs.

analgesia 1. Insensibility to pain. 2. Relief of pain.
conduction a. Regional *anaesthesia.
local a. Local *anaesthesia.
relative a. A sedation technique using a nitrous oxide—oxygen mixture but maintaining vocal contact with the patient.
surface a. Topical *anaesthesia.
topical a. Topical *anaesthesia.

analgesic 1. Not sensitive to pain. 2. Pain-relieving. 3. Any agent that relieves pain.

analysis 1. The separation and identification of the various constituents in a compound body or substance. 2. The application of accepted statistical tests to numeric data.

anamnesis 1. Memory. 2. A case history.

anaphylaxis An antigen—antibody reaction produced by the parenteral injection of an antigen, causing hypersensitivity.

anaplasia *of tooth enamel.* Defective development of the tooth enamel extending from the incisal edge or cuspal tip to the cemento-enamel junction.

anaraxia *Malocclusion.

anastomosis 1. A communication between two vessels. 2. A communication between two normally separate hollow parts or organs, either caused by disease or created by surgery.

anastomotic Relating to an anastomosis.

anatomic, anatomical Relating to anatomy.

anatomy The study of the body structure of any organism.

anchor band A band placed on one tooth to serve as anchorage for the movement of another during orthodontic treatment.

anchorage 1. The means of retention of a filling. 2. The means of retention of a bridge or artificial crown. 3. The structures or other means used to provide support and resistance with an orthodontic regulating appliance.
cervical a. Orthodontic anchorage obtained by a strap round the neck.
extra-oral a. Orthodontic anchorage obtained outside the mouth, usually from the head or neck.
intermaxillary a. A form of orthodontic anchorage in which the anchor points in one jaw provide resistance for tooth movement in the other.
intra-oral a. Orthodontic anchorage provided by structures within the mouth.

maxillomandibular a. Intermaxillary *anchorage.
multiple a. A form of orthodontic anchorage in which more than one type of support or resistance is used.
occipital a. Orthodontic anchorage provided by headgear, with heavy elastic bands attached to the teeth.
reciprocal a. Mutual support of two teeth or groups of teeth during orthodontic treatment.
reinforced a. Multiple *anchorage.
simple a. Orthodontic anchorage using larger teeth or groups of teeth to assist in the tipping of smaller teeth.
stationary a. Orthodontic anchorage which provides resistance because the form of attachment is rigid.

anchylosis *See* ankylosis.

ancillary Subsidiary, supplementary, auxiliary.

Andersch's ganglion (C.S. Andersch, 1732-77. German anatomist). The inferior ganglion on the glossopharyngeal nerve.

Andresen appliance (V. Andresen, 20th century Danish orthodontist). Myofunctional *appliance.

anemia *See* anaemia.

anesthesia *See* anaesthesia.

aneurysm A circumscribed dilatation of an artery wall, forming a pulsating, blood-containing swelling.

angeitis *Angiitis.

angi-, angio- Prefix signifying *blood vessel* or *lymph vessel.*

angiitis Inflammation affecting either a blood or a lymph vessel.

angina 1. Old term for peritonsillar *abscess. 2. Any condition characterized by painful spasm or cramp; now used almost exclusively to refer to angina pectoris.
pseudomembranous a. Necrotizing ulcerative *gingivostomatitis.

angina, Plaut's Necrotizing ulcerative *gingivostomatitis.

angina, Vincent's Acute ulcerative *tonsillitis.

angiofibroma A fibroma containing blood vessels or lymph vessels.

angiology The study of blood vessels and lymphatics.

angioma A tumour composed of blood or lymphatic vessels.

angiosarcoma A highly malignant tumour arising from the vascular endothelium.

angle 1. The inclination of one line or plane to another, expressed in degrees or radians. 2. The point of meeting of two lines or the line of intersection of two planes.
alveolar a. In craniometry, the angle between a line running through a point below the nasal spine and the most prominent point on the lower edge of the maxilla, and the cephalic horizontal line from the opisthocranion to the glabella.
alveolar profile a. The angle formed where the line joining the nasospinale to the prosthion meets the Frankfort plane; it is a measure of the degree of inclination of the upper facial skeleton.
buccal a. In dentistry, any angle formed by the junction of a buccal tooth surface or cavity wall, in a posterior tooth, with any other tooth surface or cavity wall.
cavity a. The angle formed by the walls of a tooth cavity, named according to the walls that form it.
cavosurface a. The angle formed between a cavity wall and the surface of a tooth.
craniofacial a. In craniometry, the angle between the basicranial and basifacial axes at the sphenoethmoid suture.

cusp a. The angle of incline of the sides of a cusp made with a perpendicular line bisecting the cusp, measured mesiodistally or buccolingually.
distal a. In dentistry, any angle formed by the junction of a distal tooth surface or cavity wall with any other tooth surface or cavity wall.
facial a. In craniometry, the angle between a line joining the nasion and the prosthion and one passing through the orbital opening and the auricular point; it indicates the degree of protrusion of the chin.
genial a. The angle formed between the ramus and the body of the mandible.
gonial a. *Gonion.
incisal a. In dentistry, any angle formed by the junction of an incisal edge or cavity wall, in an anterior tooth, with any other tooth surface or cavity wall.
labial a. In dentistry, any angle formed by the junction of a labial tooth surface or cavity wall, in an anterior tooth, with any other tooth surface or cavity wall.
line a. An angle formed at the junction of two tooth surfaces or of two cavity walls; line angles are named according to the surfaces of walls that form them.
lingual a. In dentistry, any angle formed by the junction of a lingual tooth surface or cavity wall with any other tooth surface or cavity wall.
mandibular a. The angle of the jaw; the angle between the base of the body of the mandible and the ramus, on either side.
maxillary a. The angle formed at the point of contact of the central incisors by the intersection of lines from the ophryon and the most prominent point of the mandible; *also called* Camper's angle.
mesial a. In dentistry, any angle formed by the junction of a mesial tooth surface or cavity wall with any other tooth surface or cavity wall.
nasal profile a. The angle formed where the line joining the nasospinale to the nasion meets the Frankfort plane; it is used as a measure of the degree of protrusion of the jaws.
occipital a. The angle formed at the junction of lines connecting the lambda and the point of the external protuberance with the point on the sagittal curvature of the occipital bone; *also called* Daubenton's angle.
occlusal a. In dentistry, any angle formed by the junction of an occlusal surface or cavity wall with any other tooth surface or cavity wall.
orifacial a. In craniometry, the angle formed by the facial line with the upper occlusal plane.
parietal a. The angle formed at the junction of lines connecting the bregma and the lambda to the highest point on the sagittal curvature above the horizontal plane passing through them; *also called* Quatrefages' angle.
point a. An angle formed at the junction of three tooth surfaces or cavity walls; point angles are named according to the surfaces or walls that form them.
tooth a. The angle formed by the surfaces of the tooth, named according to the surfaces that form it.
total profile a. The angle formed where the line joining the nasion to the prosthion meets the Frankfort plane; it is used to assess the degree of protrusion of the jaws.

uranal a. The angle formed at the junction of lines connecting the highest point on the sagittal curvature of the palate with the premaxillary point and with the posterior nasal spine.

For eponymous angles *see* under the name of the person by which the angle is known.

angle *of the mouth* The angle at the junction of the upper and lower lips on either side of the mouth.

Angle band (E.H. Angle, 1835-1930. American orthodontist). An orthodontic clamp band, having the clamp on the lingual side.

Angle's chin retractor (E.H. Angle, 1835-1930. American orthodontist). A metal chin-cup connected by elastic bands to a headcap.

Angle's classification of malocclusion (E.H. Angle, 1835-1930. American orthodontist). *See under* malocclusion.

Angle's fracture bands; Angle's splint (E.H. Angle, 1835-1930. American orthodontist). Anchor bands that have provision for the attachment of wires or elastic bands for intermaxillary fixation in jaw fracture.

angular artery Supplies the inferior portion of M. orbicularis palpebrum and the lacrimal sac. *See* Table of Arteries—angularis.

angulis oris The angle of the mouth.

anionic Relating to negatively charged particles or molecules, which are attracted to a positive electrode.

anis-, aniso- Prefix signifying *unequal, uneven.*

anisodont 1. Having unequal and irregular teeth. 2. One with unequal and irregular teeth; applied to certain reptiles.

anisognathous Having the upper jaw of much greater width than the lower.

ankyl-, ankylo- Prefix signifying 1. *fixed, stiff;* 2. *tied, fused.*

ankylocheilia Adhesion of the lips.

ankyloglossia Restricted movement of the tongue. It may be caused by fusion of the tongue with the floor of the mouth (*complete*) or by abnormal shortness of the lingual frenum, resulting in limited movement of the tongue (*partial*). *Also called* tongue-tie.

ankylosis 1. Abnormal stiffness or immobility of a joint. 2. *In dentistry,* the type of tooth attachment where the tooth is directly connected to the bone, with no intervening soft tissue; *sometimes called* dental ankylosis.

bony a. Complete joint fixation through bone fusion.

dental a. *Ankylosis[2].

false a. 1. Restricted mouth opening, actually caused by trismus, but suggestive of temporomandibular joint fixation. 2. Fibrous *ankylosis.

fibrous a. Stiffness due to fibrous adhesions or fibrosis of the joints.

glossopalatine a. A condition in which the tip of the tongue is attached to the hard palate.

ligamentous a. A form of fibrous ankylosis caused by rigidity of the ligaments.

spurious a. Fibrous *ankylosis.

true a. Bony *ankylosis.

ankylotic Relating to or affected by ankylosis.

ankylotomy An operation for releasing tongue-tie.

anlage The primary collection of cells from which any distinct organ or part of the embryo is developed.

anneal To soften a metal by heat and cooling, rendering it more malleable and ductile, and less brittle.

annular In the shape of a ring.

anodontia, anodontism Absence of teeth; where only a few teeth are missing the condition may be described as *partial*, and where no teeth are present as *total* anodontia.

anodyne 1. Pain-relieving. 2. Any drug used to ease pain.

anomalous Relating to an anomaly; irregular.

anomaly Deviation or irregularity compared with the normal.
developmental a. An anomaly due to defective development.

anomodont An extinct reptile, of the order Anomodontia, having long canines, a horny beak in place of incisors, and irregular molars.

anonymous vein V. brachiocephalica. *See* Table of Veins.

anorexia Lack of appetite.
a. nervosa An eating disorder, occurring predominantly in females, generally in adolescence, and characterized by a fear of obesity and an inability to maintain a minimal body weight because of a refusal to eat.

anosmia Absence of sense of smell.

anostosis Defective bone development.

anoxia Lack of oxygen either in the tissues or the blood.

anoxic Relating to anoxia.

ansa (*pl.* ansae) Anatomical term denoting a loop or loop-like structure.

ansa cervicalis A loop of nerves which supplies omohyoid, sternohyoid and sternothyroid muscles. *See* Table of Nerves.

ansa hypoglossi Ansa cervicalis, radix anterior. *See* Table of Nerves.

ant-, anti- Prefix signifying *opposed to*.

antagonist 1. Any muscle that acts against or in opposition to another muscle. 2. Any drug that counteracts or interferes with the action of another drug administered at the same time. 3. The tooth of one jaw that occludes with one in the other jaw.

ante- Prefix signifying *before*, in either place or time.

ante cibum Latin for *before meals*; used in prescription writing and abbreviated *a.c.*

antealveolism A condition in which the alveolar process is positioned anterior to the base of the jaw; it may be *maxillary* or *mandibular*.

antegenia A condition in which the chin is too far forward in relation to the rest of the facial skeleton.

antelabium The *procheilon.

antemandibulism A condition in which the body of the mandible is positioned anteriorly.

antemaxillism A condition in which the maxilla is positioned anteriorly.

antenatal Before birth; relating to anything occurring before birth.

anterior In front; as opposed to *posterior*.

anterior facial vein Facial vein. *See* Table of Veins—facialis.

anterocclusion A form of malocclusion in which the mandibular teeth are forward of their normal position in the arch.

anthracosis linguae Black *tongue.

anthrax A bacterial disease of sheep and cattle, caused by *Bacillus anthracis*, which may be transmitted to man; oral manifestations include swelling, bone destruction and bright red pustules on the mucous membrane.

anti- Prefix signifying *opposed to*.

antibiosis An antagonistic association between two micro-organisms, to the detriment of one of them.

antibiotic 1. Relating to antibiosis. 2. Destructive of life; applied to certain agents, such as penicillin, used against infections caused by micro-organisms.

antibody Any one of a class of substances produced in the body as a reaction to a specific antigen, and with which it reacts in some observable way to produce a specific effect such as inactivation, agglutination, flocculation, etc.

anticalculous Inhibiting the formation or deposition of calculus.

anticariogenic Relating to anything that prevents or delays the onset of caries.

anticarious Inhibiting dental caries.

anticoagulant 1. Preventing or delaying the coagulation of the blood. 2. An agent used to do this.

antidote An agent used to counteract or prevent the action of a poison.

antiflux A material used in soldering to limit the area of flow of the solder.

antigen Any substance that, when introduced into the body, excites the formation of specific antibodies.

antihistamine Any agent used to inhibit or reduce the effects of histamine.

antineoplastic 1. Preventing or delaying the development of neoplasms. 2. An agent used for this purpose.

antiodontalgic Counteracting toothache, or any agent that relieves toothache.

antiphlogistic 1. Counteracting inflammation and fever. 2. An agent used to allay inflammation and fever.

antipyretic 1. Fever-reducing. 2. Any substance or form of treatment that reduces fever.

antisepsis The prevention of sepsis by the destruction or inhibition of growth of pathogenic micro-organisms.

antiseptic 1. Relating to antisepsis. 2. Any substance that produces antisepsis.

antisialagogue 1. Saliva-inhibiting. 2. Any agent that inhibits excessive flow of saliva.

antisialic 1. Checking the flow of saliva. 2. Any agent that checks salivary secretion.

antitoxin A substance produced in the body, or which may be injected into it, that is antagonistic to a specific toxin and will neutralize it.

antitrismus Muscular spasm preventing the closing of the mouth.

antodontalgic *Antiodontalgic.

antr-, antro- Prefix signifying relationship to *an antrum* or *sinus*; often referring specifically to the *maxillary sinus*.

antracele *Antrocele.

antral Relating to an antrum.

antritis Inflammation of the maxillary sinus (or antrum).

antrobuccal Relating to the maxillary sinus (or antrum) and the buccal cavity.

antrocele An accumulation of fluid in the maxillary sinus (or antrum).

antrolith A concretion or calculus in the maxillary sinus (or antrum).

antronasal Relating to the maxillary sinus (or antrum) and the nose.

antro-oral Relating to the maxillary sinus (or antrum) and the mouth.

antroscope An instrument for inspecting the maxillary sinus (or antrum).

antrostomy The surgical opening up of the maxillary sinus (or antrum) by perforation of one of its walls.

antrotome An instrument used to cut open an antrum.

antrotomy Surgical opening of the maxillary sinus (or antrum) for drainage.

antrum An air cavity, generally in bone; *also called* a *sinus[3].
maxillary a. Maxillary *sinus.

antrum of Highmore (N. Highmore, 1613-1685. English anatomist). The maxillary *sinus.

anvil 1. An iron block, steel faced, on which, in a dental laboratory, metals may be hammered or forged. 2. The incus, one of the small bones in the ear, shaped like an anvil.

anxiolytic 1. Able to prevent or reduce anxiety. 2. Any agent used for this purpose.

apertognathia *In oral surgery,* a condition in which the anterior or the posterior teeth of the mandible cannot be brought into occlusion with those of the maxilla because of a fracture of the mandible, dislocation of the temporomandibular joint, or deformity of either the mandible or the maxilla. *Also called* open bite.

aperture An opening.
orbital a. One of the openings in the facial bones which contain the eyeballs.
piriform a. The pear-shaped nasal opening in the skull.

apex (*pl.* apices). 1. The point or tip of an object. 2. *In dentistry,* the extreme tip of a tooth root.

apexification A method aimed at inducing development of the apex of a tooth root in an immature pulpless tooth by the formation of osteodentine to narrow the canal or obtain apical closure.

apexogenesis The development and formation of the root apex in a tooth.

aphonia Hoarseness, loss of voice.

aphtha (*pl.* aphthae) 1. Any small ulcer. 2. An irregular whitish ulcer occurring in the mouth.
recurring scarring aphthae *Periadenitis mucosa necrotica recurrens.

aphthae For eponymous aphthae *see under* the personal name by which the aphthae are known.

aphthoid *Aphthous.

aphthosis Any condition characterized by the formation of aphthae.

aphthous Relating to or characterized by aphthae.

apical Relating to or affecting the apex of a tooth root.

apicectomy Surgical removal of the apex of a tooth root.

apico- Prefix signifying *apex.*

apicoectomy *Apicectomy.

apicolocator An instrument used to locate the apex of a tooth root.

apicostomy Surgical drainage achieved by the exposure of the apex of a tooth through the cortical bone and soft tissue.

aplasia Failure of, or defect in the development of, an organ or tissue; agenesis.

aplastic Relating to or affected by aplasia.

apnoea 1. Cessation of breathing, for whatever reason. 2. *Asphyxia.

apo- Prefix signifying *from.*

aponeurosis A flat tendon investing or serving as attachment to muscles.
epicranial a. The scalpal aponeurosis; *galea aponeurotica.

palatine a. The fibrous extension of the tensor palati muscles forming the anterior part of the soft palate and to which are attached the other palatal muscles.

apophysis An outgrowth or projection, used especially of a bone process.

apostema An *abscess.

apoxemena The material removed from periodontal pockets in the treatment of periodontitis; an obsolete term.

apoxesis *Curettage; old term.

apparatus *In anatomy,* a complex of structures associated by a common origin or function.

attachment a. The supporting tissues of a tooth, including the alveolar bone, periodontal ligament and gingiva.

masticatory a. All the organs and structures that are involved in mastication, including the teeth, tongue, lips, oral mucosa, jaws, temporomandibular joints, masticatory muscles and their associated nervous system.

appliance Any device used in the mouth to move or to immobilize the teeth in order to correct or prevent malocclusion, or to supply missing teeth or to serve as an obturator.

craniofacial a. A form of splint used either externally or internally to immobilize midfacial or mandibular fractures.

edgewise a. A form of fixed, multiunit orthodontic appliance, using rectangular section archwire, attached to brackets or bands on individual teeth, the archwire being inserted with the long cross-section horizontal.

fixed a. An orthodontic regulating appliance which is attached to the supporting teeth so that it cannot be removed by the wearer.

functional a. Myofunctional *appliance.

labiolingual a. An orthodontic appliance used for intermaxillary treatment, having a labial maxillary archwire and a lingual mandibular archwire attached to first molars and supporting springs.

multibanded a. A form of fixed orthodontic appliance in which several or even all teeth in one arch are banded.

myofunctional a. An orthodontic appliance that utilizes muscular force to effect treatment. It is used mainly for the treatment of Class II, div.1 malocclusion, and occasionally for the treatment of Class III malocclusion. It does not fit firmly to but lies in contact with all or parts of the teeth in both arches, and produces its effect by activating the muscles in and around the mouth and transmitting their force to the teeth and alveolar process. *Also called* the Andresen appliance, Norwegian appliance, activator, functional appliance or monobloc.

Norwegian a. Myofunctional *appliance.

orthodontic a. Any device, fixed or removable, used in orthodontic treatment to move teeth to or to retain them in the desired position and relationship.

overlay a. A form of overlay, covering the occlusal surfaces of several teeth, used to correct closed bite in prosthetic dentistry, or to splint natural teeth in the treatment of periodontal disease, and in bruxism.

permanent a. Fixed *appliance.

pin and tube a. *Herbst appliance.

removable a. Any orthodontic or prosthetic appliance that can be easily removed by the wearer.

ribbon a., ribbon arch a. An orthodontic appliance of flattened wire conforming to the dental arch, used for anchorage in the movement of teeth; a type of expansion arch.

twin wire a. *Johnson twin wire arch.

universal a. A fixed orthodontic appliance combining ribbon arch and edgewise techniques to give precise control of individual teeth, using brackets and/or bands for all teeth in both arches.

For eponymous appliances *see* under the personal name by which the appliance is known.

applicator Any instrument used for making local applications of a medicament.

apposition The contact between two opposed surfaces, and their fitting together.

approximal Near to, adjacent.

approximal surfaces *of the teeth* Those surfaces that adjoin each other in the same dental arch.

approximate Only roughly calculated, not precise and accurate.

approximate 1. To bring into close contact. 2. Situated close together, used of adjoining tooth surfaces.

aptyalism *Hyposalivation.

apyetous Not pus-producing.

apyogenous Not produced by or because of pus.

apyous *Apyetous.

apyrexia Absence or temporary reduction of fever.

aqua Latin for *water*; abbreviated *aq.*

aqua destillata Latin for *distilled water*; abbreviated *aq. dest.*

aqua pura Latin for *pure water*; abbreviated *aq. pur.*

aquam ad Latin for *water to, up to*; used in prescription writing to indicate the required volume up to which water is to be added; abbreviated *aq. ad.*

aqueduct of Fallopius Facial *canal.

aqueous Relating to or mixed with water.

arch 1. A curved or bow-shaped structure. 2. A form of orthodontic appliance.

alveolar a. The bow shape of the alveolar process of either the maxilla or the mandible.

branchial a's. A series of bars of mesenchymal tissue lying between the pharynx and the cervical ectoderm in the embryo, and from which arise the musculo-skeletal structures of the head and neck.

dental a. The bow-shaped arrangement of the teeth in the mandible and the maxilla.

expansion a. An orthodontic appliance used to assist in the lateral movement of teeth.

glossopalatine a. Palatoglossal *arch.

lingual a. An orthodontic wire appliance conforming to the lingual aspect of the mandibular teeth from first molar to first molar; it is used in the mixed dentition to maintain maximum molar anchorage.

mandibular a. 1. The first branchial arch, from which the jaws and parts of the face develop. 2. The dental arch of the mandible.

maxillary a. 1. Palatal *arch. 2. The dental *arch of the maxilla.

palatal a. The roof of the mouth.

palatine a., anterior: Palatoglossal *arch; *posterior:* Palatopharyngeal *arch.

palatoglossal a. The anterior pillar of the fauces.

palatopharyngeal a. The posterior pillar of the fauces.

ribbon a. Ribbon *appliance

superciliary a. The slight bulge over the medial part of the supra-orbital margin of the frontal bone.

transpalatal a. An orthodontic appliance, either fixed or removable, constructed from wire and extending from one maxillary first molar across the palate to the first molar on the opposite side; used in the mixed dentition to prevent mesial drift for the first molars and maintain space for the second premolars, and as an active appliance.
zygomatic a. The arch formed by the zygomatic bone and the zygomatic process of the maxilla and the temporal bone.

arch bar An orthodontic appliance consisting of a wire extending round the dental arch, to which the intervening teeth may be attached.

arch bridge Fixed *bridge.

archwire In an orthodontic appliance, any wire that follows closely the lingual or labial outline of the dental arch.

arciform Shaped like a bow.

arctation Narrowing or contracture of a canal or other opening.

arcuate 1. Shaped like a bow. 2. Arranged in arches.

areola (*pl.* areolae) A small space or interstice in tissue.

areolar Relating to areolae.

argyria, argyrosis A condition seen in those using silver-containing drugs or ointments, or working in the silver industry; it is characterized by blue-grey discoloration of the skin and mucous membranes, with pigmentation, and it may be localized or general.

ariboflavinosis Deficiency of riboflavin, one of the vitamin B complex, producing cheilosis, scaly seborrhoeic desquamation, glossitis, etc.

Arkansas stone A specially hard stone used to sharpen the cutting edges of dental instruments.

Arkovy's mixture (J. Arkovy, fl. 1923. Hungarian dentist). A preparation containing 8g phenol, 4g camphor and 4ml eucalyptus oil, used in the treatment of putrescent root canals.

arm
bracing a. That part of a partial denture which is designed to resist lateral movement or displacement.

armamentarium The instruments, books and appliances, and other equipment possessed by a medical or dental practitioner for use in his or her profession.

Arnold's ganglion (P.F. Arnold, 1803-90. German anatomist). Otic *ganglion.

Arnold's nerve (P.F. Arnold, 1803-90. German anatomist). N. auricularis. *See* Table of Nerves.

artefact An artificial product. Used in histology to mean a defect or distortion produced by some artificial means, resulting in a misleading appearance.

arteria auditiva A. labyrinthi. *See* Table of Arteries.

arterial Relating to an artery.

arteriole A minute branch of an artery.

arteriorrhexis Rupture of an artery.

arteriosclerosis A condition characterized by loss of elasticity and thickening of the artery walls.

arteriostenosis The narrowing of the calibre of an artery.

arteriostosis Arterial ossification.

artery One of the blood vessels carrying oxygenated blood from the heart.
pulmonary a. The artery conveying deoxygenated blood from the heart to the lungs.

artery of the pterygoid canal Supplies palatine muscles, pharyngotympanic tube and upper portion of pharynx. *See* Table of Arteries—canalis pterygoidei.

arthr-, arthro- Prefix signifying *joint* or *joints*.

arthral Relating to a joint.

arthralgia Pain affecting a joint.

arthritis Inflammation of a joint.
dental a. Inflammation affecting the periodontal membrane.

arthrochondritis Inflammation of joint cartilage.

arthrodia Plane *joint.

arthrodial Resembling an arthrodia or plane joint.

arthrodynia Pain affecting a joint; arthralgia.

arthrolith A calcareous deposit in a joint.

arthrology The study of joints.

arthropathy Any joint disease.

arthroplasty 1. Plastic surgery of a joint. 2. The construction of an artificial joint.

arthrosis 1. Any joint. 2. A joint disease.

arthrosteitis Inflammation affecting the bony structures of a joint.

arthrosynovitis Inflammation affecting the synovial membrane of a joint.

arthrotomy Surgical opening or incision into a joint.

articular Relating to a joint.

articular bone The lower jaw in non-mammalian vertebrates.

articular disc A fibrous plate between articulating bone surfaces in a joint.

articulare The point of intersection of the contours of the posterior edge of the mandible and the temporal bone; a cephalometric landmark.

articulating paper Carbon paper which, when bitten on, records the contact points of the teeth.

articulation 1. A *joint[1]. 2. The jointed movement of the upper and lower teeth in contact. 3. The arrangement of artificial teeth to fit the mouth and function like the natural dentition. 4. The production of sounds in speech.

articulator *In dentistry,* an instrument to which models are attached in order to simulate the relationship between the upper and lower jaws in centric relation and, to a varying extent, in opening and closing movements, in protrusion and in lateral excursion.
adjustable a. An articulator that can be adjusted for multiple records of positions or movements of the mandible in relation to the maxilla.
anatomical a. An articulator in which an attempt is made to reproduce the relationships of the upper and lower jaws in all positions and movements.
hinge a. One having only a hinged joint for opening and closing.

articulomachelian bar Embryonic cartilage from which the mandible develops.

artifact *See* artefact.

artifactual Relating to or caused by an artefact.

artificial Made by art; as opposed to *natural*.

aryepiglotticus muscle Inconstant fascicle of oblique arytenoid muscle. *See* Table of Muscles—aryepiglotticus.

arytenoid muscles Close inlet of larynx and approximate arytenoid cartilages. *See* Table of Muscles—arytenoideus.

asbestos A fibrous calcium or magnesium silicate, non-combustible. *In dentistry* it is used, mixed with plaster, as an investment material in soldering.

-ase Suffix signifying *enzyme.*

asepsis Absence of infection or of putrefaction.

aseptic Relating to asepsis; free from infection.

Ash's dowel crown A crown made of porcelain baked on to a platinum tube, and held in position by a fluted dowel.

asialia, asialorrhoea *Hyposalivation.

aspecific *Non-specific.

asphyxia Suffocation; deprivation of oxygen causing anoxia and the accumulation of carbon monoxide in the blood, with resultant coma.

aspirate 1. To suck up or to breathe in. 2. To remove fluid or gas from a body cavity by suction.

aspirating needle A long, hollow needle used to withdraw fluid from a cavity.

aspiration 1. The act of breathing in. 2. The removal of gas or liquid from a cavity by means of suction.

aspirator An appliance used to suck debris, saliva or blood from the mouth at high velocity during operative dentistry.

asporous Having no spores.

Assezat's triangle (J. Assezat, 1832-76. French anthropologist). A craniometric triangle bounded by lines joining the basion, the alveolar point and the nasion; the facial triangle.

assimilable Capable of assimilation.

assimilate To absorb and change into body tissue.

assimilation The processes whereby food is absorbed and changed into body tissue.

asterion The point on the skull surface at which the temporal, occipital and parietal bones meet; a craniometric landmark.

asthenic Lacking in strength and vigour; weak.

astringent 1. Capable of causing contraction, or of drawing together. 2. An agent producing organic contraction, or arresting discharge.

asymmetrical Relating to asymmetry; not symmetrical.

asymmetry Dissimilarity or irregularity of normally similar or corresponding parts; lack of symmetry.

asymphytous Not fused together; separate or distinct.

asymptomatic Without any symptoms.

asynovial Lacking synovial secretion.

ataxia Lack of muscular co-ordination.

atelo- Prefix signifying *faulty development*, or *incomplete development*.

atelocheilia Defective development of the lip.

ateloglossia Congenital defect of the tongue.

atelognathia Congenital defect of the jaw.

ateloprosopia Faulty or incomplete development of the facial processes.

atelostomia Deficient or faulty development of the mouth.

atlantoaxial Relating to the atlas and the axis.

atlantoepistrophic *Atlantoaxial.

atlas The first cervical vertebra.

atomizer An instrument for ejecting a liquid as a fine spray.

atonic Lacking in normal tone, slack or relaxed; used particularly of muscles.

atoxic Non-poisonous.

atretostomia Having no mouth, no normal opening into the oral cavity.

atrophic Affected by, or relating to, atrophy.

atrophy A reduction in size of tissue or of an organ due to a decrease in the size or number of its constituent cells; it may be physiological or pathological.
pulp a. A degenerative process seen in old age and characterized by a shrinking of the dental pulp and a decrease in the number of cells.

attachment 1. The means by which one thing is fastened to another. 2. Any clasp, hook or cap used to fasten a partial denture or an appliance to a natural tooth.
bar a. A bar linking two or more teeth or tooth roots to support and retain a denture.
epithelial a. The epithelium at the base of the gingival crevice or periodontal pocket, lying in close proximity to the tooth surface and 'attaching' the gingiva to the tooth. It is thought to originate from the cells of the reduced enamel epithelium.
extracoronal a. A form of precision attachment in which the retention device lies outside the clinical crown of the tooth.
friction a. Intracoronal *attachment.
internal a. Intracoronal *attachment.
intracoronal a. A form of precision attachment slotted into a restoration or artificial crown and retained either by friction or by some locking device.
parallel a. Intracoronal *attachment.
precision a. A prefabricated form of attachment for the retention of a bridge or partial denture; it consists of a male and a female portion, one being incorporated in the prosthesis and the other in the retainer cemented to the supporting tooth or root.
resilient a. One used with a combined tooth-borne/tissue-borne prosthesis, designed to allow slight movement to compensate for mucosal movements without stress to the abutments.
slotted a. Intracoronal *attachment.

attraction *of the jaws* A form of malocclusion in which the jaws are abnormally close together.

attrition Rubbing or wearing away; *in dentistry*, applied to the mechanical wearing down of the tooth surface in mastication.

atypical Not typical, irregular, not corresponding to the accepted norm.

audio-analgesia A method of producing insensibility to pain by means of music and background sounds to which the patient listens through earphones.

auditory Relating to hearing or to the organs of hearing.

auditory artery A. labyrinthi. *See* Table of Arteries.

auditory canal *Auditory meatus.

auditory meatus *external:* The external auditory canal from the concha to the tympanic membrane in the ear. *internal:* The canal from the tympanic membrane through the petrous bone, giving passage to the facial and auditory nerves and the internal auditory artery.

auditory nerve N. vestibulocochlearis. *See* Table of Nerves.

auditory ossicles The stapes, malleus and incus, in the middle ear.

auditory tube External *auditory meatus.

augmentation In implant surgery, the correction of bony defects with autogenous or alloplastic material.
augnathus A foetus having a double lower jaw; a rare anomaly.

aural Relating to the ear and hearing.

auric Relating to or containing gold.

auricle 1. One of the two upper chambers of the heart. 2. The pinna, or external ear.

auricular Relating to the auricle.

auricular artery Supplies digastric and other muscles, parotid gland, external auditory meatus, mastoid cells, etc.; three branches: posterior, anterior, deep. *See* Table of Arteries—auricularis.

auricular muscles Draw auricle or pinna forward or back, or raise it. *See* Table of Muscles—auricularis.

auricular nerves Supply auricle and external auditory meatus. *See* Table of Nerves—auricularis.

auriculare The central point of the external auditory meatus.

auriculo-infraorbital plane *Frankfort plane.

auriculonasal plane *Camper's plane.

auriculo-orbital plane *Frankfort plane.

auriculotemporal nerve Supplies skin over temple and scalp. *See* Table of Nerves— auriculotemporalis.

aurinasal Relating to the ear and the nose.

auto- Prefix signifying *self*.

autoclave A high-pressure steam type of sterilizer.

autogenous Produced within the body itself; self-generated.

autograft A graft taken from one area of the patient's body and transplanted to another part in the same individual.

autologous *Autogenous.

automallet Mechanical *condenser.

automatic Spontaneous, involuntary.
autonomic 1. Independent in function. 2. Spontaneous.

autonomic nerve Any nerve of the autonomic nervous system.

autoplast *Autograft.

autopolymer A plastic substance that polymerizes without the use of external heat, by the addition of a catalyst and an activator.

autotransplant *Autograft.

autotrophic Relating to micro-organisms that can obtain nourishment from carbon dioxide in an inorganic environment; as opposed to *heterotrophic*.

auxiliary 1. Aiding, supporting. 2. A person or thing providing help or support.
dental a. Dental *therapist.

auxometry Measurement of the rate of growth.

avascular Without vessels, more specifically without blood vessels.

avulsion Complete detachment of a tooth from its socket through trauma.

axial Relating to, or in relation to, an axis.

axial wall That wall lying nearest the pulp in cavities on an axial surface.

axio- Prefix signifying *axis*, especially the long axis of a tooth.

axiobuccal *Buccoaxial.

axiobuccocervical *Gingivobuccoaxial.

axiobuccogingival *Gingivobuccoaxial.

axiobuccolingual Relating to the buccal and lingual surfaces and the long axis of a molar or premolar tooth.

axiocclusal *Axio-occlusal.

axiocervical *Axiogingival.

axiodistal Relating to the axial and distal walls of a buccal or lingual cavity in a molar or premolar.
a. angle The angle formed at the junction of these walls; a *line* angle.

axiodistocclusal *Axiodisto-occlusal.

axiodistocervical *Axiodistogingival.

axiodistogingival Relating to the axial, distal and gingival walls of a buccal or lingual cavity in a molar or premolar.
a. angle The angle formed at the junction of these walls; a *point* angle.

axiodisto-incisal Relating to the axial, distal and incisal walls of a labial or lingual cavity in an incisor or canine.
a. angle The angle formed at the junction of these walls; a *point* angle.

axiodisto-occlusal Relating to the axial, distal and occlusal walls of a buccal or lingual cavity in a molar or premolar.
a. angle The angle formed at the junction of these walls; a *point* angle.

axiogingival Relating to the axial and gingival walls of a mesial, distal or proximo-occlusal cavity in an incisor or canine, or of a buccal or lingual cavity in a molar or premolar.
a. angle The angle formed at the junction of these walls; a *line* angle.

axio-incisal Relating to the axial and incisal walls of a mesial or distal cavity in an incisor or canine.
a. angle The angle formed at the junction of these walls; both a *line* angle and a *point* angle.

axiolabial Relating to the axial and labial walls of a mesial, distal or proximo-incisal cavity in an incisor or canine.
a. angle The angle formed at the junction of these walls; a *line* angle.

axiolabiocervical *Axiolabiogingival.

axiolabiogingival Relating to the axial, labial and gingival walls of a mesial, distal or proximo-incisal cavity in an incisor or canine.
a. angle The angle formed at the junction of these walls; a *point* angle.

axiolabiolingual Incisal edge of a tooth.

axiolingual Relating to the axial and lingual walls of a mesial, distal or proximo-incisal cavity in an incisor or canine.
a. angle The angle formed at the junction of these walls; a *line* angle.

axiolinguocclusal *Axiolinguo-occlusal.

axiolinguocervical *Axiolinguogingival.

axiolinguogingival Relating to the axial, lingual and gingival walls of a mesial, distal or proximo-incisal cavity in an incisor or canine.
a. angle The angle formed at the junction of these walls; a *point* angle.

axiolinguo-occlusal Relating to the axial, lingual and occlusal walls of a tooth cavity.

axiomesial Relating to the axial and mesial walls of a buccal or lingual cavity in a molar or premolar.
a. angle The angle formed at the junction of these walls; a *line* angle.

axiomesiocclusal *Axiomesio-occlusal.

axiomesiocervical *Axiomesiogingival.

axiomesiogingival Relating to the axial, mesial and gingival walls of a buccal or lingual cavity in a molar or premolar.

a. angle The angle formed at the junction of these walls; a *point* angle.

axiomesioincisal Relating to the axial, mesial and incisal walls of a labial or lingual cavity in an incisor or canine.

a. angle The angle formed at the junction of these walls; a *point* angle.

axiomesio-occlusal Relating to the axial, mesial and occlusal walls of a buccal or lingual cavity in a molar or premolar.

a. angle The angle formed at the junction of these walls; a *point* angle.

axio-occlusal Relating to the axial and occlusal walls of a buccal or lingual cavity in a molar or premolar.

a. angle The angle formed at the junction of these walls; a *line* angle.

axiopulpal Relating to the axial and pulpal walls in the step portion of a proximo-occlusal cavity in a molar or premolar.

a. angle The angle formed at the junction of these walls; a *line* angle.

axis 1. The line about which a body revolves. 2. *In anatomy*, the second cervical vertebra.

azzle tooth An old term for a molar tooth.

B

B Buccal.

BA Buccoaxial.

BAC Buccoaxiocervical.

Bact. Abbreviation for *Bacterium.*

BAG Buccoaxiogingival.

BBT Basal body temperature.

BC Buccocervical.

BD Buccodistal.

b.d. Abbreviation for *bis die*—twice a day; used in prescription writing.

BG Buccogingival.

b.i.d. Abbreviation for *bis in die*—twice a day; used in prescription writing.

bib. Abbreviation for *bibe*—drink; used in prescription writing.

BIPP Bismuth Iodoform Paraffin Paste; used in root canal treatment.

BL Buccolingual.

BM Buccomesial.

BO Bucco-occlusal.

BP 1. Buccopulpal. 2. Blood pressure. 3. British Pharmacopoeia; used in descriptions of drugs, to indicate the source of the formula in a prescription.

BPC British Pharmaceutical Codex. *Now called* Pharmaceutical Codex.

BTU, BThU British thermal unit; a measurement of heat. May also be written *Btu*.

'B' point *Supramentale.

Babbitt metal (I. Babbitt, 1799-1862. American inventor). An alloy sometimes used in dentistry; it contains copper, tin and antimony.

baccate Resembling a berry.

bacciform Shaped like a berry.

Bacillaceae A family of rod-shaped or spherical endospore-forming microorganisms, generally motile, aerobic or facultatively anaerobic, mostly occurring in soil.

bacillary Relating to or affected by a bacillus.

bacillicide Any agent used to destroy bacilli.

bacilliform In the shape of a bacillus.

Bacillus A genus of Gram-positive and aerobic or facultatively anaerobic bacteria, seen as rod-shaped or spherical organisms.
B. fusiformis **Fusobacterium nucleatum.*

bacillus (*pl.* bacilli) A term used, loosely, to denote any rod-shaped micro-organism of the genus *Bacillus*; many have now been reclassified under other genera.

bacillus, Vignal's **Leptotrichia buccalis.*

backing *In dentistry,* the metal plate in a denture or an artificial crown which protects or supports a tooth or tooth-facing.

bacteraemia A condition characterized by the transient presence of bacteria in the bloodstream.

bacteria (*sing.* bacterium) Microscopic unicellular vegetable organisms, having a single chromosome, no nuclear envelope and a rigid cell wall; they may be seen as rods, cocci or filaments and divide by binary fission.

bacterial Relating to or characterized by bacteria.

bactericide Any agent used for the destruction of bacteria.

bacteriology The study of bacteria.

bacteriolysis The destruction or disintegration of bacteria.

bacteriolytic Relating to bacteriolysis.

bacteriophage A micro-organism that attacks bacteria, sometimes resulting in their destruction.

bacteriosis Any disease caused by bacteria.

bacteriostasis The process of prevention or hindrance of growth of bacteria.

bacteriostat Any agent that inhibits the growth and multiplication of bacteria, such as any of the sulphonamide group of drugs.

bacteriostatic Relating to bacterio-stasis.

bacteritic Characterized or caused by bacteria.

Bacterium Former name for a genus of micro-organisms, all Gram-negative, and seen as rod-shaped or ellipsoid, and now reassigned to various different genera.

bacterium Singular form of *bacteria.

bacteroid Resembling bacteria.

Bacteroidaceae A family of anaerobic bacteria, Gram-negative and seen as either motile or non-motile, non-sporing rods.

Bacteroides The type genus of the family Bacteroidaceae, Gram-negative, non-motile, anaerobic micro-organisms commonly associ-ated with oral infections; species include *B. melaninogenicus, B. fragilis, B. oralis*.

Baelz's disease (E. von Baelz, 1845-1913. German physician). A disease characterized by the presence of painless papules on the labial mucous membrane.

Bailey's flask A type of investing box used in dentistry in the fabrication of dies and counterdies.

bake To harden by means of heat, e.g. as in the production of dental porcelain.

balance 1. An apparatus used for weighing. 2. Equilibrium.
occlusal b. Balanced *occlusion.

balancing contacts The contacts of the upper and lower teeth on the non-working side of a denture.

balancing side The side away from which the mandible has moved, during mastication.

balloon
sinus b. A plastic or rubber device, like a balloon, which can be expanded either with air or with liquid, and which is used to support depressed fractures of the zygomaxillary process.

band 1. Any structure or appliance that binds. 2. *In dentistry*, a thin metal strip formed to encircle the crown or root of a natural tooth.
adjustable b. A band that has some form of screw or mechanism whereby its size can be altered.
all-closing b. A band encircling the whole of a tooth.
anchor b. A band placed on one tooth to serve as anchorage for the movement of another in ortho-dontic treatment.
apron b. An orthodontic anchor band with a labial, gingival or incisal extension to aid in positioning the bracket and in retention.
clamp b. A band that is held in place by means of a screw and nut.
contoured b. A band shaped to the tooth.
lip furrow b. Vestibular *lamina.
matrix b. In dentistry, a thin band of metal used to provide a temporary tooth wall to support a filling.
orthodontic b. Anchor *band.
pier b. Any band constructed to fit an abutment tooth.
seamless b. A band stamped out from a metal tube, having no joins.

band adapter An orthodontic tool used to fit an orthodontic band on to a tooth.

band-driver An instrument used in orthodontics to seat a band over a tooth crown.

bandage A strip of gauze, muslin or other soft material, which may be in the form of a roll, triangular or tailed, bound round a part to hold dressings in place, to support or immobilize a part, or to apply pressure.
For eponymous bandages *see* under the personal name by which the bandage is known.

bands, Hunter-Schreger *Schreger's lines *in enamel.*

bar 1. A band or strip. 2. *In dentistry*, a metal rod or wire used either in prosthetics or orthodontics as part of an appliance. 3. That portion of the gums in the upper jaw of a horse which bears no teeth.
arch b. An orthodontic appliance consisting of a wire extending round the dental arch, to which the intervening teeth may be attached.
articulomachelian b. Embryonic cartilage from which the mandible develops.
labial b. A metal connector conforming to the labial mandibular arch and joining two parts of a lower partial denture.
lingual b. A metal bar fitted to the lingual arch of the lower jaw, and connecting two parts of a partial denture.
palatal b. A metal bar extending across the hard palate, connecting and strengthening two parts of an upper partial denture.
sublingual b. A metal connector on a mandibular partial denture which runs under the tongue, on the floor of the mouth.
For eponymous bars *see* under the personal name by which the bar is known.

bar, Passavant's *Passavant's ridge.

bar attachment A bar linking two or more teeth or tooth roots to support and retain a denture.

bar clasp A type of clasp in which the arms are a direct extension of the connector bars of the denture.

bar connector A bar or strip that connects the parts of a partial denture.

barb A fine backward-projecting point on a dental instrument, preventing its withdrawal.

barbiturate Any one of a group of hypnotic and sedative drugs: these are classified as *long-acting* (over 8 hours), used as sedatives and in epilepsy; *medium-* (6-8 hours) and *short-acting* (2-3 hours), used as hypnotics and in pre- or postoperative medication; and *ultra-short-acting*, used as intravenous anaesthetics and for induction prior to gaseous general anaesthesia.

barodontalgia Pain in the teeth experienced as a result of high-altitude flying; aerodontalgia.

barrel 1. The band of a metal tooth crown. 2. The reservoir of a hypodermic or other syringe.

bartholinitis Inflammation affecting Bartholin's duct.

Bartholin's duct (C. Bartholin, 1655-1738. Danish anatomist). The larger of the sublingual ducts.

Barton's bandage (J.R. Barton, 1794-1871. American surgeon). A figure-of-eight bandage used in fracture of the mandible.

basal Relating to a base.

basal vein Formed by the union of the anterior cerebral and deep middle cerebral veins. *See* Table of Veins—basalis.

base 1. The foundation on which a structure rests or is built. 2. *In dentistry*, denture *base.
cavity b. A material, usually a type of cement, used to line a prepared cavity before the insertion of a permanent restoration, to protect the pulp.
cement b. Cavity *base.
cranial b. The bony support for the brain, which divides the cranium from the facial skeleton and forms the floor of the cranial cavity.
denture b. That part of a denture which rests on the alveolar ridges, and which may extend over the palate, and to which the artificial teeth are attached.
record b. *Bite plate[1].
temporary b. *Bite plate[1].
trial b. *Bite plate[1].

base plane An imaginary plane used to estimate the retention in the construction of artificial dentures.

base plate 1. Denture *base. 2. *In orthodontics*, an acrylic plate, part of an orthodontic appliance, which is fitted to the mucosa and the necks of the teeth, and holds the springs or clasps.

basicranial Relating to the base of the skull.

basifacial Relating to the lower part of the face.

basilar Relating to the base.

basilar artery Supplies cerebellum and cerebrum. *See* Table of Arteries—basilaris.

basilar plexus A venous plexus into which drain the inferior petrosal sinuses. *See* Table of Veins—plexus basilaris.

basilomental Relating to the base of the skull and the chin.

basilosubnasal *Basinasial.

basinasial Relating to the basion and the nasion.

basioccipital Relating to the basilar part of the occipital bone.

basion The central point on the anterior edge of the foramen magnum.

basisphenoid Relating to the basilar part of the sphenoid bone.

basitemporal Relating to the lower part of the temporal bone.

batrachoplasty Plastic surgery in the cure of ranula.

Bauhin's glands (G. Bauhin, 1560-1624. Swiss anatomist). Lingual *glands.

beak The projecting jaws of pliers or forceps.

Bean crown Split-dowel *crown.

Bechterew *See* Bekhterev.

Béclard's triangle (P.A. Béclard, 1785-1825. French anatomist). The area comprised within the posterior border of the hyoglossus muscle, the greater cornu of the hyoid bone and the posterior belly of the digastric muscle.

Bednar's aphthae (A. Bednar, 1816-1888. Austrian physician). Two ulcers appearing symmetrically one on either side of the midline of the hard palate in infants, thought to be caused by the nipple or by thumb sucking or sucking hard objects. *Also known as* Valleix's aphthae.

Beers' crown (J.B. Beers, fl. 1873). *Morrison crown.

Begg appliance (P.R. Begg, 1898-1983. Australian orthodontist). An orthodontic light wire appliance used to tip tooth crowns.

Behçet's syndrome (H. Behçet, 1889-1948. Turkish dermatologist). The association of aphthous ulceration of the lips, tongue, buccal mucosa or palate with eye lesions and genital ulcerous lesions.

Bekhterev's reflex (V.M. Bekhterev, 1857-1927. Russian neurologist). Irritation of the mucosa on one side of the nasal cavity producing facial contraction on the same side; *also called* nasal reflex.

bell crown A crown of a tooth in which the diameter, mesiodistally, is much greater at the occlusal surface than at the cervix.

Bell's palsy (Sir C. Bell, 1774-1842. Scottish physiologist). Paralysis of the facial nerve, usually transient, the cause of which is unknown, and which results in facial hemiplegia.

belly *of a muscle* The bulging, fleshy part of a muscle.

benign Not malignant or recurrent; not endangering life or health. Describing a locally controlled growth or lesion, generally encapsulated, which does not produce metastases.

Bennett angle (Sir N.G. Bennett, 1870-1947. English dentist). The angle, during lateral movement of the mandible, between the sagittal plane and the path of the condyle.

Bennett movement (Sir N.G. Bennett, 1870-1947. English dentist). *Laterotrusion.

Berry-Franceschetti syndrome (Sir G.A. Berry, 1853-1940. English ophthalmologist; A. Franceschetti, b. 1896). Mandibulofacial *dysostosis.

bevel 1. An outward inclination cut or ground on any surface. 2. The outward inclination of the enamel edges of a prepared tooth cavity. 3. The act of making such an inclination.

bi- Prefix signifying *two*, or *twice*.

bibe Latin for *drink*; used in prescription writing, and abbreviated *bib*.

bibeveled, bibevelled Being bevelled on two sides.

Bichat's fossa (M.F.X. Bichat, 1771-1802. French anatomist). Pterygopalatine *fossa.

Bickel's ring (G. Bickel, 19th century German physician). The area of lymphoid tissue comprised by the pharyngeal and lingual tonsils and the lymphoid tissue of the soft palate.

biconcave Having two concave surfaces.

biconvex Having two convex surfaces.

bicuspid 1. Having two cusps. 2. A premolar *tooth.

bicuspidal, bicuspidate Having two cusps.

bidental, bidentate Having, or affecting, two teeth.

bifid Split into two branches, or parts.

biforate Having two openings or foramina.

bifurcate Forked, as the roots of molar or other teeth.

bifurcation 1. Division into two branches, as of tooth roots. 2. The place at which such a division occurs.

bihora Latin for *two hours*; used in prescription writing.

bilateral Occurring on, or relating to, two sides.

biligulate Resembling two tongues; having two tongue-like processes.

bilocular, biloculate Having two chambers or cavities.

bilophodont Having teeth with two transverse ridges forming the crown.

bimaxillary Relating to both jaws.

Bimler appliance (H.P. Bimler, 20th century German orthodontist). A type of removable myofunctional orthodontic appliance designed to produce tooth movement by reflex muscle activity. *Also called* Bimler stimulator.

binangle *Of an instrument:* having two angles in the shank.

binary 1. *In chemistry,* composed of two elements. 2. *In anatomy,* divided into two branches or parts. 3. *In mathematics,* to the base 2; i.e. a number system based on 0 and 1. This is used especially with digital computers.

Bing bridge (B.J. Bing, fl. 1865. American dentist). A bridge for a single tooth, attached to the adjoining teeth.

bio- Prefix signifying *life*.

biochemistry The chemistry of living organisms.

biointegration The formation of a biochemical union between the surface of an implant and the host tissue or bone.

biomaterial Any material, natural or man-made, which is relatively inert and can be used in implant surgery without adverse reactions from the tissues.

biomechanics The application of the laws of mechanics to the structures of the human body.
dental b. The study of the relationship between the function of oral structures and the effects of the introduction of a restoration or appliance within the mouth.

biometrics, biometry The application of statistical methods to biological sciences.

bionator A type of functional appliance; it is a tooth-borne passive appliance, much less bulky than an activator and is used to modify tooth eruption and reposition the mandible.

bio-occlusion Normal occlusion.

bioplasis *Anabolism.

biopsy Microscopic examination of tissue from a living body, generally for purposes of diagnosis.

biostatistics *Biometrics.

bis in die Latin for *twice a day*; used in prescription writing, and abbreviated *b.i.d.*; *also* written as *bis die*, abbreviated *b.d.*

biscuit Porcelain after it has been baked once, but before it has been glazed.

bisect To divide into two parts by cutting.

bistoury A long, narrow surgical knife, which may be either straight or curved.

bite 1. To grasp or to cut anything with the teeth. 2. An impression, in some plastic material, of the teeth or the gums in occlusion, to show their relationship; used for making artificial dentures. 3. A skin wound made by the teeth or by the mouth-parts of insects.
check b. Check *record.
close-b. A form of malocclusion in which there is abnormally deep overlap of the incisors when the jaws are closed.
counter-b. A bite[2] opposing that taken of the teeth in one jaw.
cross b. *See* crossbite.
edge-to-edge b. A form of malocclusion in which the anterior teeth occlude along the incisal edges and do not overlap.
end to end b. Edge-to-edge *bite.
jumping the b. The forcible movement forward of a retruded mandible to obtain normal occlusion.

locked b. Interlocking of the teeth in occlusion so that lateral movement of the mandible is restricted or prevented.
mush b. Squash *bite.
open b. 1. A form of malocclusion in which a group of teeth fail to come into contact when the dental arches are brought into occlusion. When the anterior teeth do not come into contact the condition is known as *anterior* open bite; when the posterior teeth do not contact on one side the condition is called *unilateral posterior* open bite, and when they do not contact on either side it is called *bilateral posterior* open bite. 2. *Apertognathia.
over b. See overbite.
rest b. See restbite.
squash b. A bite taken to register the relationship of the cusps of the upper and lower teeth, but not to give any clear reproduction of the teeth.
underhung b. A form of malocclusion in which the mandibular anterior teeth occlude with the labial surfaces of their maxillary antagonists.

bite block Occlusal *rim.

bite gauge An instrument designed to aid in the establishment of a correct occlusion in prosthetic dentistry.

bite lock A device that can be attached to the occlusal rims of a denture to retain them in the same position out of the mouth as they occupied in it.

bite plane 1. Occlusal *plane. 2. A form of *bite plate[2] on which the ledge against which the incisors strike is sloped and not flat.

bite plate 1. A temporary base plate of rigid material, carrying a rim of wax or plastic (occlusal rim) on which the bite is recorded. 2. An orthodontic appliance designed to correct an abnormal incisor relationship by providing a ledge of metal, vulcanite or acrylic in one arch, against which the opposing incisors strike. Where the ledge is sloped and not flat this appliance is known as a *bite plane*.

bite rim Occlusal *rim.

bitewing A form of individual x-ray film, held in place in the mouth by a central wing or *tab* on which the teeth can close. It shows the crowns of both the upper and lower teeth on one film.

bizygomatic Relating to the most prominent points on the zygomatic arches.

black copper cement A zinc phosphate cement containing cupric oxide, resulting in its characteristic black colour, which is used in restorations in primary teeth, for splint fixation and for orthodontic banding.

Black's amalgam (G.V. Black, 1836-1915. American dentist). A quaternary *amalgam.

Black's classification of cavities (G.V. Black, 1836-1915. American dentist). A classification of cavities in teeth based on tooth type, and sites or surfaces involved.
Class I: Cavities beginning in structural defects in the teeth; pits and fissures. These are located in the occlusal surfaces of the bicuspids and molars, in the occlusal two-thirds of the buccal surfaces of the molars, in the lingual surfaces of the upper incisors, and occasionally in the lingual surfaces of the upper molars.
Class II: Cavities in the approximal surfaces of bicuspids and molars.
Class III: Cavities in the approximal surfaces of the incisors and cuspids which do not

involve the removal and restoration of the incisal angle.

Class IV: Cavities in the approximal surfaces of the incisors and cuspids which do require the removal and restoration of the incisal angle.

Class V: Cavities in the gingival third - not pit cavities - of the labial, buccal or lingual surfaces of the teeth.

Black's crown (G.V. Black, 1836-1915. American dentist). A porcelain-faced crown for an anterior tooth, attached by a threaded post screwing into a gold-lined root canal.

blade The cutting portion of a knife or a pair of scissors.

bland 1. Mild. 2. Soothing.

Blandin's ganglion (P.F. Blandin, 1798-1849. French surgeon). Submandibular *ganglion.

Blandin's gland (P.F. Blandin, 1798-1849. French surgeon). Anterior lingual *gland.

Blandin's operation (P.F. Blandin, 1798-1849. French surgeon). An operation for the correction of double hare-lip by the excision of a triangular wedge from the vomer, with reduction of the projecting maxillary process.

blank *In orthodontics*, a short, slightly curved strip of metal used in banding.

Blasius' duct (G. Blasius, *or* Blaes, 1626(?)-82. Dutch anatomist). Parotid *duct.

blastoma A true tumour, exhibiting independent localized growth.

bleach 1. To whiten by means of chemicals; discoloured teeth may be so treated. 2. Any agent used for this purpose.

bleb A bulla or other skin blister filled with blood or serous fluid.

bleeding *Haemorrhage.

blenn-, blenno- Prefix signifying *mucus*.

blennoid Mucus-like.

blennostasis Suppression of excessive mucous discharge.

blepharal Relating to the eyelid.

blepharon The eyelid.

blister A vesicle caused by a localized accumulation of fluid beneath the skin.

block 1. A stoppage or obstruction. 2. A solid mass of material.

anaesthetic b. 1. Regional *anaesthesia. 2. The interruption of the nerve supply to an area because of trauma or a pathological lesion.

block anaesthesia Regional *anaesthesia.

blood The red fluid in the vessels of the circulatory system, which conveys oxygen and nutritive material to the tissues and removes carbon dioxide and waste matter.

blood poisoning *Septicaemia.

blood pressure The pressure exerted by the blood on the artery walls, dependent on the force of the heart action, the elasticity of the vessel walls, capillary resistance, and the volume and viscosity of the blood.

blood vessel Any of the tubes carrying blood through the body.

Bochdalek's ganglion (V.A. Bochdalek, 1801-1883. Austrian anatomist). The ganglion situated in the maxilla, and formed by the junction of the middle and superior alveolar nerves.

Bock's pharyngeal nerve (A.C. Bock, 1782-1833. German anatomist). The pterygopalatine *ganglion.

Bodecker's index The ratio between the number of tooth surfaces affected by caries, and the total number of surfaces that could be so affected.

Bohn's epithelial pearls, Bohn's nodules *Epstein's pearls.

boil A localized skin abscess, usually at the site of a hair follicle.

Boley gauge A finely-calibrated instrument used for intraoral measurements.

Bolton plane, Bolton-Broadbent plane (C.B. Bolton, sponsor; B.H. Broadbent, contemporary American orthodontist). The imaginary plane marking the division between the face and the skull, lying about a line from the Bolton point to the nasion.

Bolton point (C.B. Bolton, who, with Mrs C.C. Bolton, his mother, sponsored the research work of B.H. Broadbent which resulted in the designation of this point). The deepest point on the postcondylar notch of the occipital bone, seen on a lateral radiograph and marking the height of the curvature.

bolus 1. A rounded mass of food ready to be swallowed. 2. A large, rounded pill.

bonding Attaching securely to another object or surface either by the use of chemical reactions or with an adhesive.
direct b. A method of attaching an orthodontic appliance directly to the surfaces of teeth by techniques such as acid etch, without the use of a clasp or band.

bone 1. The material of the skeleton of most vertebrates, consisting of connective tissue containing ossein and impregnated with calcium salts. 2. Any separate part of the skeleton; *see* under the names of the individual bones for those of the skull.
articular b. The lower jaw in non-mammalian vertebrates.
basal b. The bone tissue of the mandible and maxillae, with the exception of their alveolar processes.
bundle b. That part of the bony wall of a tooth socket into which Sharpey's fibres are embedded.
cancellated, cancellous b. Spongy *bone.
compact b. The dense outer layers of fully developed bone.
cortical b. The thin outer layer of compact bone, made up of lamellated rings of collagen fibres.
lamellar, lamellated b. 1. Fully developed cortical bone with the collagen fibres in parallel rows. 2. Bundle *bone.
marginal b. Alveolar *margin.
non-lamellated b. Woven *bone.
primitive b. Woven *bone.
quadrate b. The upper jaw in non-mammalian vertebrates.
reticulated b. Woven *bone.
spongy b. The inner, spongy material found within the compact bone, made up of a latticework of bone trabeculae with intercommunicating spaces filled by bone marrow and linked to the central marrow of the bone.
woven b. A prenatal immature form of spongy bone, having connected vascular spaces with osteo-collagenous fibres forming a non-lamellated network round them. It is soon replaced by fully developed bone, but may be found in the lining of tooth sockets even in adults, in the process of normal bone repair, and in fast-growing bone tumours.

bone fibres *Sharpey's fibres.

bone marrow *See* marrow.

bone plate One or more perforated metal plates, either flat or L-shaped in cross-section, used in the

treatment of fractures, and which can be secured to bone fragments to immobilize them.
mandibular staple b. p. A form of transosseus *implant.

bonelet *Ossicle.

Bonwill crown (W.G.A. Bonwill, 1833-99. American dentist). A porcelain crown attached to the tooth root by a threaded post, and held in position by amalgam.

Bonwill triangle (W.G.A. Bonwill, 1833-99. American dentist). The adaptation and measurement of the mandible and mandibular arch as an equilateral triangle, with angles at the centre of each condyle and at the mesial contact area of the mandibular central incisors.

bony Relating to or resembling bone.

border An edge or boundary round an organ or tissue mass.
vermilion b. The red margin of the lips.

border moulding The shaping of impression material, either by hand or by tissue action, to the outline adjacent to the edges of the impression.

border seal The fit of the border of a denture with the adjacent tissues, rendering it airtight.

Borrelia (A. Borrel, 1867-1936. French bacteriologist). A genus of the Spirochaetaceae family, spiral bacteria, Gram-negative and anaerobic, which are parasitic on the mucous membranes of mammals, including man.

boss A rounded, knob-like prominence on the surface of a bone or a tumour.

bosselated Having knob-like protrusions or bosses.

bow Any curved, bow-shaped apparatus or instrument.
face b. See facebow.
hinge b. Adjustable axis *facebow.

Bowen's disease of the mouth (J.T. Bowen, 1857-1941. American dermatologist). A skin disease affecting the oral mucosa and characterized by reddish papules covered by a thick keratinized layer.

box *In dentistry,* that portion of a compound cavity, excluding the occlusal surface, which has four surfaces.

boxing *of an impression* The process of building up walls round an impression to produce a cast of the desired size and form, and to preserve the principal landmarks of the impression.

brace Any orthodontic appliance, especially one with bands or wires across the anterior teeth; a lay term.

brachiocephalic trunk The blood supply for the right upper limb and the right side of the head and neck; *also called* the innominate artery. *See* Table of Arteries—truncus brachiocephalicus.

brachiocephalic vein The vein found in the median portion of the root of the neck, deep to the sternocleidomastoid muscle, and draining into the superior vena cava. *See* Table of Veins—brachiocephalica.

brachiofaciolingual Relating to or affecting the arm, the face and the tongue.

brachy- Prefix signifying *short.*

brachycephalic Having an abnormally short head.

brachycheilia Shortness of the lip or lips; *also called* microcheilia.

brachydont *See* brachyodont.

brachyfacial Having an abnormally short and broad face.

brachyglossal Having an abnormally short tongue.

brachygnathia Abnormal shortness of the mandible.

brachygnathous Having an abnormally small lower jaw.

brachyodont Having teeth with short crowns and long roots.

brachyprosopic Having an abnormally short face.

brachypyrosopic *Brachyfacial.

brachyrhinia Abnormal shortness of the nose.

brachyrhyncus Abnormal shortness of both the nose and the maxilla.

brachystaphyline Having an abnormally wide palate.

brachyuranic Having an abnormally short and wide palate, with a palatal index above 115.

bracing Anything providing resistance to the horizontal components of force.

bracing arm That part of a partial denture which is designed to resist lateral movement or displacement.

bracket *In dentistry,* a type of downward-facing hook or clip on an orthodontic tooth band, used to attach ribbon archwire to banded teeth. *See also* attachment[2].

Brackett's probes (C.A. Brackett, 1850-1927. American dentist). Delicate, flexible probes, made of silver wire, used to explore fistulae of alveolar abscesses.

brady- Prefix signifying *slow.*

bradycardia Abnormal slowness of the heart and pulse rate.

bradyglossia Abnormal slowness of speech, due to difficulty in tongue movement.

bradylalia Slowness of speech, due to a central lesion.

bradylogia *Bradylalia.

bradypnoea Abnormal slowness of respiration, at a rate of less than 17 breaths a minute.

brain That part of the central nervous system within the cranium of vertebrates.

branch An offshoot from the main trunk or stem, as of blood vessels and nerves.

Branhamella (Named in honour of Sara Branham, who contributed to the knowledge of the Neisseriaceae family). A subgenus, from the genus *Moraxella,* of the Neisseriaceae family of bacteria, non-motile and non-spore-bearing cocci, Gram-negative and aerobic. *Moraxella (Branhamella) catarrhalis* is found in the oral cavity.

brass An alloy of copper and zinc.

breathing *Respiration.

bregma The junction of the coronal and sagittal sutures; the site of the anterior fontanelle.

bridge 1. A structure joining two distant or distinct points or parts. 2. *In dentistry,* an appliance, attached to remaining natural teeth, designed to restore aesthetics and function where teeth have been removed or failed to erupt.
arch b. Fixed *bridge.
cantilever b. A bridge of which one end only is attached to an abutment and the other is seated on the alveolar ridge.
dentine b. A layer of dentine which reseals an exposed pulp or forms over the excised surface after pulpotomy.
extension b. A dental bridge having a free pontic attached at one end beyond the point of anchorage.
fixed b. A dental bridge which is fixed in place permanently to its abutments.
Maryland b. A bridge in which the abutments are bonded to the acid-etched surfaces of the supporting teeth. Although the teeth undergo little preparation, the fitting

surfaces of the metal abutments are etched to improve the mechanical retention of the bonding agent.
removable b. A dental bridge which can be removed by the wearer for cleaning or other purposes.
Rochette b. A bridge in which the abutments are bonded to the acid-etched surfaces of the supporting teeth. Although the teeth undergo little preparation, the metal abutments are perforated to improve the mechanical retention of the bonding agent.
span b. Fixed *bridge.

bridge *of the nose* The bridge formed at the junction of the two nasal bones; the upper part of the nose.

broach A fine tapered hand instrument, either smooth or barbed, used to remove tooth pulp in the treatment of infected root canals, and as a reamer to enlarge root canals.
watchmaker's b. A tapered broach, sharp-angled and having four or five sides, used to enlarge root canals.

broch A developmental defect in tooth mineralization, seen as a projection on the surface at the cervical margin over which the surface enamel is absent.

bromopnoea Foetid breath.

bronch-, broncho- Prefix signifying relationship to the *bronchi.*

bronchial Relating to or affecting the bronchi.

bronchitis Inflammation of the bronchial tubes.

bronchodilator Any agent causing dilatation of the bronchi.

bronchospasm Spasmodic contraction of the bronchial tubes.

bronchus (*pl.* bronchi) One of a pair (*left* and *right*) of large air passages connecting the trachea with the lungs; in the lungs the passages branch repeatedly to form the 'bronchial tree'.

Brophy's operation (T.W. Brophy, 1848-1928. American surgeon). An operation for the closure of cleft palate by means of wire tension sutures held in place by lead plates, drawing the edges of the cleft together.

Brown crown (E.P. Brown, 1844-1916. American dentist). A porcelain crown with a convex base, into which is baked a platinum post for attachment to the tooth root.

bruise A superficial injury caused by a blow, with no laceration but with discoloration of the skin and subcutaneous tissue produced by an accumulation of blood.

bruxism Grinding or gnashing of the teeth, usually during sleep.

bruxomania A nervous disorder characterized by grinding of the teeth.

brycomania Insane tooth-grinding.

brygmus Grinding of the teeth.

bucca The cheek, especially the inner side in the mouth.

buccal Relating to the cheek.

buccal artery Supplies buccinator muscle, buccal mucous membrane and skin of cheek; *also called* buccinator artery. *See* Table of Arteries—buccalis.

buccal nerve The nerve supplying the skin and mucous membrane of the cheek and the buccinator muscle; *also called* N. buccinator. *See* Table of Nerves—buccalis.

buccal segment classification *See under* malocclusion.

buccellation The arrest of bleeding by means of a lint pad.

buccilingual Relating to the cheek and the tongue.

buccinator 1. The cheek muscle. *See* Table of Muscles. 2. A. buccalis, the artery supplying the buccal mucosa, the skin of the cheek, and the buccinator muscle. *See* Table of Arteries. 3. N. buccalis, the nerve supplying the buccinator muscle and the skin and mucous membrane of the cheek. *See* Table of Nerves.

bucco- Prefix signifying *cheek*.

buccoaxial Relating to the buccal and axial walls in the mesial or distal portion of a proximo-occlusal cavity in a molar or premolar.
b. angle. The angle formed at the junction of these walls; a *line* angle.

buccoaxiocervical *Gingivobucco-axial.

buccoaxiogingival *Gingivobucco-axial.

buccobranchial *Buccopharyngeal.

buccocervical 1. Relating to the cheek and the neck. 2. *Buccogingival[2].

buccoclusal *Bucco-occlusal.

buccoclusion A form of malocclusion in which the maxillary posterior teeth occlude buccally to their normal position.

buccodistal 1. Relating to the buccal and distal surfaces of a tooth. 2. Relating to the buccal and distal walls in the step portion of a proximo-occlusal cavity in a molar or premolar.
b. angle. The angle formed at the junction of these walls; a *line* angle.

buccofacial Relating to the cheek and the face.

buccogingival 1. Relating to the cheek and the gums. 2. Relating to the buccal and gingival walls in the mesial or distal portion of a proximo-occlusal cavity in a molar or premolar.
b. angle. The angle formed at the junction of these walls; a *line* angle.

buccoglossopharyngitis sicca Inflammation and dryness of the buccal and pharyngeal mucous membranes and of the tongue. Part of the complex known as *Sjögren's syndrome*.

buccolabial Relating to the cheek and the lip.

buccolingual Relating to the buccal and lingual surfaces of a tooth.

buccomaxillary 1. Relating to the cheek and the maxilla. 2. Relating to the buccal cavity and the maxillary sinus.

buccomesial Relating to the buccal and mesial surfaces of a molar or premolar, or to the buccal and mesial walls in the step portion of a proximo-occlusal cavity.
b. angle. The angle formed at the junction of these walls; a *line* angle.

bucconasal Relating to the cheek and the nose.

bucconasopharyngeal Relating to the cheek, the nose and the pharynx.

bucco-occlusal Relating to the buccal and occlusal surfaces of a molar or premolar tooth, or to the corresponding walls of a cavity.

buccopharyngeal Relating to the cheek and the pharynx.

buccopharyngeal muscle Part of constrictor pharyngis superior. *See* Table of Muscles—buccopharyngeus.

buccoplacement Displacement of a tooth buccally.

buccopulpal Relating to the buccal and pulpal walls in an occlusal cavity, or in the step portion of a proximo-occlusal cavity in a molar or premolar.
b. angle The angle formed at the junction of these walls; a *line* angle.

buccoversion The position of a tooth which is inclined outwards towards the cheek.

buccula The fleshy fold which forms a double 'chin'.

bud 1. A knob-like structure, the early stage in the growth of any plant, leaf or branch. 2. Any small anatomic structure resembling a bud.

taste b. One of the highly specialized sensory receptor cells within the surface epithelium and the epithelium of the fungiform and vallate papillae of the tongue, the terminal cells of the gustatory nerve and responsible for the ability to taste.

tooth b. A knob-like structure from the dental lamina in the primary development of a tooth, which later becomes the enamel organ within the dental sac.

bulboid Shaped like a bulb.

bulbous Resembling a bulb in either shape or nature; arising from or producing a bulb.

bulimia An eating disorder, occurring predominantly in adolescent or young adult females, and characterized by bouts of excessive eating, followed by vomiting, often self-induced; unlike *anorexia nervosa it does not lead to weight loss.

b. nervosa. *Bulimia.

bulla (*pl.* bullae) 1. A large vesicle. 2. *In anatomy,* a projecting, rounded structure.

bullous Relating to or characterized by bullae.

bunodont Having rounded cusps or cones on the molar teeth; a palaeontological term.

bunolophodont A palaeontological term for teeth having rounded crests.

bunoselenodont A palaeontological term for teeth having longitudinal rounded crests.

bur A rotary cutting instrument used in a dental handpiece for the preparation of cavities and the trimming of restorations. Burs are named according to the shape and pattern of the heads, or the purpose for which they are used.

cross-cut b. Dentate *bur.

dentate b. A bur having the cutting edges set with teeth for very rapid cutting.

finishing b. A bur having a more finely cut head, used in finishing and burnishing restorations.

fissure b. A cylindrical dental bur used for preparing a cavity involving the occlusal fissures of a molar or premolar tooth.

trephine b. A type of dental bur having either a hollow cylindrical or truncated cone head; it is primarily an end-cutting bur.

Burkitt's lymphoma (D.P. Burkitt, b. 1911. English surgeon). A malignant and rapidly growing lymphoma originally described in young children in East Africa, but now occurring in many other countries; it affects the jaws and the viscera, and is associated with the Epstein-Barr virus.

burn The injury resulting from the application of excessive heat, electric current, friction, or caustics to the skin or mucous membrane.

burnish To smooth or polish by friction either to obtain a high gloss or to secure the adaptation of two corresponding substances at a join.

burnisher An instrument used to finish and to polish fillings, crowns or dentures. Burnishers are named either by the material on which they are used or by the shape of the heads.

burn-out A term used in radiology to denote an area of excessive darkening on an otherwise normal radiograph, due to some non-penetration of the x-ray beam. *cervical b.* An area of excessive darkening on a dental radiograph seen at the cervical margin of a tooth; it may be mistakenly diagnosed as caries.

Burton's line (H. Burton, 1799-1849. English physician). Lead *line.

Buttner crown A porcelain-faced shell crown attached to the root by a post and a metal band.

button 1. A knob-like structure or device. 2. The excess metal which may be found on the end of the sprue after casting.

C

C 1. Abbreviation for *canine*, in the permanent dentition. 2. Chemical symbol for carbon. 3. One of the cervical vertebrae, numbered C1 to C7.

c. Abbreviation for *cum*—with; used in prescription writing.

CA 1. Cervicoaxial. 2. Chronological age. 3. Cardiac arrest.

Ca Chemical symbol for calcium.

cap. Abbreviation for *capsula*—a capsule; used in prescription writing.

cc Abbreviation for *cubic centimetre*.

cib. Abbreviation for *cibus*—food; used in prescription writing.

CLA Cervicolinguoaxial.

cm Abbreviation for *centimetre*.

Cr Chemical symbol for chromium.

Cu Chemical symbol for copper.

cable The flexible arm of a dental engine, which transmits power to the instrument to be used.

cachectic Relating to cachexia.

cachet A hollow capsule of rice paper enclosing a dose of some unpleasant medicine.

cachexia Generalized state of ill health due to some constitutional disorder.

cachou A tablet or pill for deodorizing or scenting the breath.

caco- Prefix signifying *bad, diseased*.

cacodontia An old term for any condition characterized by diseased teeth.

cacogeusia A bad taste.

cacoglossia The condition of having a diseased or gangrenous tongue.

cacostomia Any diseased condition of the mouth.

caecal 1. Relating to a blind tube or passage. 2. Relating to the caecum.

caecum 1. Any blind pouch, tube or passage. 2. The blind dilated pouch which is the beginning of the large intestine.

Caffey's disease (J. Caffey, 1895-1978. American paediatrician). An overgrowth of cortical bone, seen in infants and young children, and affecting in particular the clavicle and the mandible; it may be associated with swellings caused by trauma.

calcareous Relating to or containing calcium or calcium salts; chalky.

calci-, calco- Prefix signifying *calcium* or *calcium salts*.

calcific Lime-forming.

calcification The deposition in organic tissue of calcium salts, causing hardening.
diffuse pulp c. Calcification of the tooth pulp with deposits in columns or strands throughout the tissue.
pulp c. Deposition of calcium salts in the tissues of the tooth pulp, leading to hardening, mineralization and progressive narrowing of the pulp chamber; it may be caused by old age, caries or trauma.

calcification lines Incremental *lines.

calcified Hardened by the deposition of calcium salts.

calcigerous Calcium-producing or calcium-carrying.

calcination The reduction of a substance to powder, or the removal of volatile constituents from a compound by heat.

calcine To reduce to powder, to roast or to dry, by heat.

calcinosis A condition characterized by either localized or general depositions of calcium salts in nodules in the soft tissues.

calcium A bivalent metal, chemical symbol Ca, the basic component of lime, and occurring in almost all organic tissue.

calcium hydroxide Used in cavity base materials to provide a protective layer over freshly cut dentine. Used in root canal therapy to protect vital pulp and to stimulate dentine bridge formation following pulpotomy and in an attempt to promote continued root formation following pulpectomy in teeth with open apices.

calcium pyrophosphate A calcium salt, used as a polishing agent in toothpaste.

calcular Relating to calculus.

calculogenesis The production or formation of calcium deposits.

calculous Relating to or resembling a calculus.

calculus (*pl.* calculi) An abnormal concretion, occurring in the body, generally in the urinary system, bile duct, gall bladder, or salivary glands; it usually contains calcium salts.

dental c. A deposit of calcium salts in an organic matrix attached to the teeth.

salivary c. 1. An abnormal concretion occurring in a salivary gland or duct. 2. Supragingival *calculus.

serumal, seruminal c. Subgingival *calculus.

subgingival c. Dental calculus attached to the tooth within the gingival pocket.

supragingival c. Dental calculus attached to the tooth above the gingival margin.

Caldwell-Luc operation (G.W. Caldwell, 1834-1918. American surgeon; H. Luc, 1855-1925. French laryngologist). An operation for the relief of severe infection of the maxillary sinus by creating an opening into the supradental fossa. Adapted for other procedures such as the removal of a tooth root displaced into the antrum.

calibration 1. The measurement of the diameter of a canal or tube. 2. The marking of gradations on a measuring instrument from a given standard.

caliculus Taste *bud.

calipers An instrument, similar to a pair of compasses, having curved legs, and used to measure diameters of cylindrical bodies.

Callahan's method (J.R. Callahan, 1853-1918. American dentist). A method of root canal cleansing in which the application of sulphuric acid is used to aid in opening the canal and in the destruction of putrescent pulp.

callosity *Callus[2].

callus 1. The mesh of fibrous bony tissue surrounding and uniting the bone ends after a fracture; it is later replaced by hard bone. 2. An area of hard skin, usually caused by constant friction, pressure or irritation.

calvaria, calvarium The bony skull cap or cranium.

camera A box or chamber, especially the equipment used to take photographs.

Camper's angle (P. Camper, 1722-89. Dutch anatomist). Maxillary *angle.

Camper's line (P. Camper, 1722-89. Dutch anatomist). A line extending from the external auditory meatus to a point below the nasal spine; *also called* facial line.

Camper's plane (P. Camper, 1722-89. Dutch anatomist). A horizontal plane passing through the tragale of each ear and through the subnasale, and usually parallel with the occlusal plane; *also called* auriculonasal plane.

Campylobacter A genus of micro-organisms seen as slender spiral rods, motile and Gram-negative; found in the oral cavity and intestinal tract in man.

campylognathia Malformation of the jaw or lip in a rabbit-like appearance.

canal Any channel or duct which affords a passage, usually through bone.

alveolar c. Dental *canal.

alveolodental c. An old term for a dental *canal.

anterior condylar c., anterior condyloid c. The hypoglossal *canal.

anterior palatine c. 1. Incisive *canal. 2. Incisive *foramen.

auditory c. The auditory *meatus.

blunderbuss c. Term used to describe an incompletely formed root having the apical third of the root canal wider in diameter than the upper part.

carotid c. A passage in the petrous portion of the temporal bone, through which passes the internal carotid artery.

circulatory c. Nutrient *canal.

condylar c., condyloid c. An occasional canal in the floor of the condylar fossa, through which passes a vein from the transverse sinus.

dental c. Any one of the canals in the maxilla or in the mandible which afford passage to the vessels or nerves supplying the teeth. The *superior* dental canals are those in the maxilla, and the *inferior* dental canals are those in the mandible.

dentinal c. Dentinal *tubule.

ethmoid c. Any one of the canals between the ethmoid and frontal bones, through which pass the posterior ethmoid and the nasociliary nerves and the ethmoid vessels.

facial c. A canal extending from the petrous portion of the temporal bone to the stylomastoid foramen, through which passes the facial nerve; *also called* the aqueduct of Fallopius.

greater palatine c. The canal running from the pterygopalatine fossa to the greater palatine foramen, in the side wall of the nasal cavity, between the maxilla and the palatine bone, through which pass the greater palatine artery and nerve.

gubernacular c. The channel through the alveolar bone in which lies the gubernaculum dentis.

hypoglossal c. A passage for the hypoglossal nerve through the occipital bone; *also called* the anterior condylar canal.

incisive c. A canal leading from the incisive fossa to the floor of the nasal cavity.

infraorbital c. One of the passages from the infraorbital grooves to the infraorbital foramen in the maxilla, through which pass the infraorbital arteries and nerves.

interdental c. Nutrient *canal.

lesser palatine c. One of the branches of the greater palatine canal conveying branches of the greater palatine vessels to the tissues of the soft palate.

mandibular c. Inferior dental *canal.

maxillary c. Superior dental *canal.

nasolacrimal c. The canal in which runs the nasolacrimal duct.
nasopalatine c. Incisive *canal.
nutrient c. One of the tubular canals or grooves occurring in the alveolar bone structure of the maxilla and of the mandible, through which pass anastomosing blood vessels; *also called* Hirschfeld canal.
palatomaxillary c. Greater palatine *canal.
palatovaginal c. A narrow canal opening into the pterygopalatine fossa and the nasal cavity.
pharyngeal c. Palatovaginal *canal.
posterior condylar c., posterior condyloid c. Condylar *canal.
posterior palatine c. Lesser palatine *canal.
pterygoid c. A canal through the pterygoid plate of the sphenoid bone to the pterygopalatine fossa, conveying the pterygoid nerves and vessels; *also called* Guidi's canal.
pterygopalatine c. 1. Greater palatine *canal. 2. Palatovaginal *canal.
pulp c. Root *canal.
recurrent c. Pterygoid *canal.
root c. The canal, containing dental pulp, running through the root of the tooth to the pulp chamber.
sphenopalatine c. 1. Greater palatine *canal. 2. Palatovaginal *canal.
sphenopharyngeal c. Palatovaginal *canal.
superior maxillary c. *Foramen rotundum ossis sphenoidalis.
zygomaticofacial c. *Foramen zygomaticofaciale.
zygomatico-orbital c. *Foramen zygomatico-orbitale.
zygomaticotemporal c. *Foramen zygomaticotemporale.

canal, Hirschfeld Nutrient *canal.

canaliculus A minute canal.

canaliculus dentalis One of the minute canals carrying the processes of the cementoblasts to developing cementum.

canalis pterygoidei, artery Supplies levator and tensor veli palatini muscles, pharyngotympanic tube and upper portion of pharynx. *See* Table of Arteries—canalis pterygoidei.

canalis pterygoidei, nerve The nerve supply for the lacrimal gland and the glands of the nose and palate, via the pterygopalatine ganglion. *See* Table of Nerves.

cancellous Having a lattice-like, spongy structure; applied to bone tissue.

cancer Any of various malignant neoplasms that arise from the abnormal and uncontrolled division of cells, that then manifest invasiveness and a tendency to metastasize to new sites (WHO definition).

cancroid Cancer-like.

cancrum A gangrenous ulcer.

cancrum nasi Gangrene of the nasal mucous membrane.

cancrum oris Gangrene of the mouth; occurring in children, and starting on the mucous membrane of the cheek or the gum; *also called* noma.

Candida A genus of yeast-like fungi, commonly found in the normal flora of the skin, mouth and intestinal tract. It may become pathogenic where the balance of the flora is disturbed. A*lso called Monilia*.
C. albicans A pathogenic species that produces candidiasis.

candidiasis A condition resulting from infection by a pathogenic species of *Candida* fungus, usually *C. albicans*, and affecting various parts of the body.

atrophic c. Oral *candidiasis.
oral c. Infection of the mouth with *Candida albicans*; may be associated with precancerous conditions when chronic.
oral acute pseudomembranous c. *Thrush.

candidosis *Candidiasis.

canine muscle M. levator anguli oris. *See* Table of Muscles.

canine tooth A single-cusped tooth, resembling a dog's, found between the lateral incisor and the first molar or premolar. There is one in each quadrant in both the primary and the permanent dentition in man.

caniniform In the shape of or resembling a canine tooth.

canker Ulceration, especially of the mouth and lips; aphthous stomatitis.

cannula, canula A rigid or semirigid tube inserted into a duct, cavity or blood vessel.

cap 1. A protective covering over the head or the top of a structure. 2. *In dentistry,* any substance or structure covering an exposed pulp. 3. Lay term for an artificial *crown.
enamel c. The enamel covering the top of a developing tooth papilla.
skull c. *Calvaria.

cap crown Shell *crown.

cap splint A cast metal dental splint fitting accurately over the crowns and occlusal surfaces of the teeth and cemented into place; used to assist in immobilizing jaw fractures.

Capdepont syndrome (C. Capdepont, 1867-1917. French dentist). *Dentinogenesis imperfecta.

capillary 1. One of the very fine, thread-like blood vessels, connecting the veins and arteries. 2. Any very fine tube.

capitulum A small head; a bony articulating eminence.

capitulum mandibulae The articulating head of the lower jaw; the mandibular condyle.

capsula Latin for *capsule*; used in prescription writing, and abbreviated *cap.*

capsular Relating to a capsule.

capsule 1. The fibrous or membranous sheath or covering of an organ or part. 2. A soluble casing for enclosure of a drug.
enamel c. Enamel *cuticle[1].
nasal c. The cartilaginous structure around the embryonic nasal cavity.

capsulorrhaphy Surgical repair of a joint capsule.

capsulotomy The surgical opening of a joint capsule.

Carabelli's tubercle (G.C. Carabelli, 1787-1842. Austrian dentist). A small tubercle sometimes found on the lingual surface of a maxillary molar; usually hereditary.

carat The measure of purity of gold; pure gold is 24 carat.

carbohydrate An organic substance containing carbon, hydrogen and oxygen; included in this class of compounds are sugars, starches, dextrins and celluloses.

carboxymethylcellulose gelatin paste A paste capable of adhering to the oral mucosa; used to provide mechanical protection and as a vehicle for topical drugs.

carbuncle A staphylococcal infection of the sweat glands or hair follicles, causing inflammation of the surrounding subcutaneous tissues and discharging pus through several openings, finally sloughing away.

carcino- Prefix signifying *carcinoma.*

carcinogen 1. Any substance or agent producing a carcinoma. 2. Used more loosely for any agent producing a malignant tumour of any kind.

carcinogenesis The production of cancer.

carcinoma A malignant epithelial tumour, usually giving rise to metastases.
actinic c. Basal-cell type of carcinoma affecting the face and other uncovered body surfaces, caused by prolonged exposure to direct sunlight.
adenoid cystic c. A malignant epithelial tumour of the salivary glands containing both myoepithelial and duct-lining cells.
basal-cell c. Locally malignant carcinoma developing from the basal-cell layer of the epithelium and retaining its characteristics.
epidermoid c. A form of carcinoma derived from the stratified squamous epithelium; it can be differentiated into various types.
intraepithelial c. *Carcinoma-in-situ.
mucoepidermoid c. A malignant tumour, containing squamous cells and mucus-secreting cells, occurring in the salivary glands.
spindle-cell c. A variant of squamous-cell carcinoma, frequently mistaken for sarcoma or carcinosarcoma because of its spindle-shaped tumour cells.
squamous-cell c. Carcinoma developing from the squamous epithelium; a type of epidermoid carcinoma; said to be the most common malignant neoplasm of the oral cavity in its various forms, such as *fissured* or *ulcerative*.
verrucous c. A variant of squamous-cell carcinoma, with a low degree of malignancy, which erodes rather than invades the surrounding tissues; it is most often seen in the elderly.

carcinoma-in-situ That stage in the development of a tumour when it still remains within the tissue in which growth began.

carcinomatoid Resembling a carcinoma.

carcinomatous Relating to or affected by carcinoma.

carcinosarcoma A mixed tumour containing characteristics of both carcinoma and sarcoma.

cardi-, cardio- Prefix signifying *heart.*

caries Inflammatory decay of bone tissue.
dental c. Localized decay and disintegration of tooth enamel, dentine and/or cementum.

cariogenic Caries-producing.

cariology The scientific study of dental caries, its causes, prevention and treatment.

carious Relating to, or characterized by, caries.

Carmichael crown (J.P. Carmichael, 1856-1946. American dentist). A three-quarter *crown.

carnassial Relating to flesh eating; applied to those teeth designed to tear flesh.

carnivore Any animal that eats meat.

carnivorous Meat-eating.

caroticotympanic artery Branch of internal carotid supplying the tympanic cavity. *See* Table of Arteries—caroticotympanica.

caroticotympanic nerve Supplies the tympanic region and parotid gland. *See* Table of Nerves—caroticotympanicus.

carotid artery Common carotid, from the brachiocephalic trunk and the aortic arch, divides into the external and internal carotid arteries, supplying the brain and meninges, face, neck, side of head, and tongue. *See* Table of Arteries—carotis communis, carotis externa, carotis interna.

carotid nerves Supply filaments to the glands and smooth muscles of the head. *See* Table of Nerves—caroticus.

carpule A patent type of glass cartridge containing one dose of a drug solution, which can be loaded directly into a special hypodermic syringe for injection.

cartilage A form of elastic non-vascular connective tissue attached to articular bone surfaces and also forming some parts of the skeleton.
alar c. The U-shaped cartilage forming the tip of the nose.
gingival c. The tissue covering the cavity containing an unerupted tooth.
lateral nasal c. One of the two wing-like expansions of the septal cartilage, attached to the nasal bones and to the maxillae.
septal c. The cartilage lying within the nasal septum dividing the right and left nasal cavities.

cartilaginous Consisting of or relating to cartilage.

cartridge syringe A syringe in which the solution to be injected is delivered from a pre-packed cartridge in the form of a glass phial.

caruncle, caruncula A small fleshy elevation.
sublingual c. *Caruncula sublingualis.

caruncula salivaris *Caruncula sublingualis.

caruncula sublingualis A small elevation on either side of the lingual frenum, at the apex of the sublingual gland.

carver Any hand instrument used for carving and modelling, especially in the making of inlays, crowns and dentures.
amalgam c. A specially designed type of carver with a sharp blade, used for contouring amalgam restorations.
wax c. A type of carver with a blunt blade, specially designed for use in fashioning wax, and capable of being heated for this purpose.

caseous Cheese-like.

cassette *In radiography,* a holder for an x-ray plate or film.

cast *In dentistry,* a positive likeness of an object produced by the introduction of a plastic substance into a mould or impression of that object; e.g. a cast of the mouth made during the construction of dentures.
boxed c. An impression cast in a box or cup which has been built up round it of strips of soft metal or of wax, thus providing a cast which needs little trimming and which can be well vibrated.

cast core *Core.

casting 1. The forcing of molten metal into a mould. 2. The solid metal shape this produces. 3. The process of making a cast.

catabasis The abatement of a disease.

catabolism The process of breakdown of complex compounds by the body; destructive metabolism, as opposed to *anabolism.*

catalepsy An unconscious state, often associated with hypnosis, which is characterized by rigidity and loss of voluntary motion, the limbs of the patient remaining in any position in which they may be placed.

cataleptic Relating to or affected by catalepsy.

catamnesis Follow-up history of a discharged patient.

cataphasia A speech disorder in which the sufferer constantly repeats the same word or phrase.

cataplexy A state of muscular rigidity which may be caused by shock, by loss of muscle tone, or as a result of hypnosis.

catarrh Inflammation of the mucous membranes, especially those of the nose and throat, with a discharge of mucus.

catarrhal Relating to or affected by catarrh.

catenoid Chain-like; having a chain-like arrangement.

catgut Suture thread prepared from the lining of a sheep's intestine, cleansed, treated and rendered aseptic.

catheter A surgical tube used to evacuate fluid from body cavities, or to distend a canal or vessel.

cationic Relating to positively charged particles or molecules, which are attracted to a negative electrode.

catodont One who has mandibular teeth only.

cauda A tail or tail-like appendage.

caudal 1. Relating to a cauda. 2. Relating to the tail end of a body, as opposed to *rostral*.

caudate Having a tail.

causalgia A burning sensation arising after trauma to a sensory nerve.

caustic 1. Burning; destructive of tissue substance. 2. Any agent used to burn or to destroy tissue.

cauterization 1. The application of a cautery or caustic. 2. The result of such an application.

cautery 1. The destruction of tissue by burning with a caustic substance or a hot iron. 2. The substance or iron used for cauterization.

actual c. A white-hot iron used for cauterization.

chemical c. A chemical caustic used for cauterization.

cold c. The use of extreme cold, such as carbon dioxide snow, for cauterization.

caval Relating to a cavity.

cavernoma Cavernous *haemangioma.

cavernous Containing hollow spaces.

cavernous sinus A venous sinus at the side of the pituitary fossa, into which the ophthalmic and cerebral veins drain. *See* Table of Veins—sinus cavernosus.

cavilla The sphenoid bone.

cavitas pulpae The pulp *cavity.

cavity A hollow or space; in a tooth, the space either caused by caries or cut out to remove caries.

approximal c. A cavity affecting either a mesial or a distal surface; a Class III cavity.

complex c. 1. A carious lesion in a tooth, affecting three or more surfaces. 2. A prepared tooth cavity affecting two or more surfaces either because of caries or by extension.

compound c. 1. A carious lesion in a tooth, affecting two surfaces. 2. A complex *cavity.

labial c. A cavity in the labial surface of a tooth; a Class V cavity.

oral c. The area of the mouth within the lips, containing the teeth and their supporting structures, the tongue and the inside of the cheeks, back to the throat and tonsils; in ISO nomenclature the whole of the oral cavity is designated 00, the maxillary area 01 and the mandibular area 02.

proximal c. Approximal *cavity.

proximo-incisal c. A cavity affecting either a mesial or distal surface and

also the incisal edge of an incisor or canine; a Class IV cavity.
proximo-occlusal c. A cavity affecting either a mesial or distal surface and also the occlusal surface of a posterior tooth; a Class II cavity.
pulp c. The cavity at the core of a tooth, comprising the pulp chamber and the root canal.
simple c. One that involves only one tooth surface.

cavity angle The angle formed by the walls of a tooth cavity, named according to the walls which form it.

cavity classification *See* Black's cavity classification.

cavity floor That surface of a prepared cavity towards which the restoration is inserted.

cavity liner Material used in dentistry to protect and insulate the tooth tissues after the excavation of caries before the placing of a restoration in a prepared cavity.

cavity preparation Those operative procedures in restorative dentistry which are necessary to remove carious matter from a tooth and to shape the resultant cavity for filling.

cavity primer *Cavity liner.

cavity walls The walls that form the outline of a tooth cavity; they are named after the tooth surface towards which they face: *i.e.* mesial, distal, buccal, lingual, pulpal, axial, gingival, occlusal, incisal, labial.

cavum dentis The pulp *cavity.

CE marking Under the EC Medical Devices Directive all materials, instruments and equipment should carry the CE marking by June 13, 1998, to comply with the Medical Devices Regulations (S1 1994 no.3017). This marking indicates that the device satisfies the requirements of the Directive that it is of sufficient quality and fit for its intended use.

cebocephaly A congenital malformation of the head, marked by the absence of a nose, and with the orbital cavities close together, giving a general monkey-like appearance.

-cele Suffix signifying 1. *tumour* or *swelling*; 2. *cavity*.

cell One of the minute masses of protoplasm, containing a nucleus, which form the basis of all animal and plant structure.
embryonal c. One of the developmental cells.
enamel c. *Ameloblast.
epithelial c. One of the cells that make up the epithelium.
epithelial attachment c's. Reduced enamel *epithelium.
giant c. A large, multinuclear cell, such as an osteoclast.
plasma c. A bone-marrow cell of the lymphocytic series, which makes and secretes antibody.
prickle c. One having delicate processes connecting it to neighbouring cells.

cellular Composed of cells.

cellulitis Diffuse inflammation, often purulent, of the intercellular tissue and especially of subcutaneous tissue.

Celsius scale (A. Celsius, 1701-44. Swedish astronomer). A thermometric scale on which freezing point is 0° and boiling point 100°; *also called* centigrade.

cement 1. A non-metallic substance that will unite two opposed surfaces. 2. A non-metallic material that sets hard, used in dentistry to secure an inlay in a cavity, or as a filling material. 3. *Cementum.

black copper c. A zinc phosphate cement containing cupric oxide, resulting in its characteristic black colour, which is used in restorations in primary teeth, for splint fixation and for orthodontic banding.
glass-ionomer c. A translucent polyelectrolyte cement, composed of an aluminosilicate glass powder, which contains fluoride; it is used in restorations on anterior teeth, and to fill pits and fissures.
glass polyalkenoate c. Glass-ionomer *cement.

cementation The process of attaching restorations or fillings with cement.

cementicle A small calcareous body developing in the periodontal membrane.

cementification *Cementogenesis.

cementitis Inflammation of the cementum.

cementoblast A germ cell from which cementum is eventually formed.

cementoblastoma Benign *cementoma.

cementoclasia Resorption of the cementum.

cementocyte One of the cells incorporated in cementum.

cementodentinal Relating to both the cementum and the dentine of a tooth.

cemento-enamel Relating to both the cementum and the enamel of a tooth.

cemento-exostosis *Hypercementosis.

cementogenesis The process of cementum formation.

cementoid The unmineralized surface layer of developing cementum, thought to be resistant to resorption.

cementoma A benign tumour composed of cementum or cementum-like tissue.
benign c. A distinctive benign tumour containing sheets of cementum-like tissue, generally found about the root of a mandibular molar or premolar, the hard tissue of the lesion being fused to the root. It is most frequently seen in males under 25 years of age.
familial multiple c's. Gigantiform *cementoma.
gigantiform c. A type of cementoma characterized by a mass of dense, highly mineralized cementum, occurring in several parts of the jaw, often symmetrically; it is seen most frequently in middle-aged black women. *Also called* familial multiple cementomas.
true c. Benign *cementoma.

cementopathia *Periodontosis.

cementoperiostitis *Pyorrhoea alveolaris.

cementosis *Hypercementosis.

cementum Bony tissue, a layer of which surrounds the dentine of the root of a tooth in man, and provides attachment for the fibres of the periodontal ligament.
acellular c. The layer of cementum at the dentinocemental junction, which contains no cementocytes.
afibrillar c. A very thin layer of cementum, containing no banded collagen, found round the tooth cervix and thought to be produced by cementoblasts.

cementum exostosis *Hypercementosis.

cementum hyperplasia *Hypercementosis.

cementum inostosis A pathological thickening of cementum developing inwards into the dentine.

centi- Prefix signifying *one-hundredth*.

centigrade 1. Denoting a thermometric scale on which freezing point is 0 and boiling point is 100 ; now more usually called Celsius. 2. A term used by G.V. Black in his instrument formula; 1 centigrade = 3.6°.

central artery of the retina Branch of the ophthalmic artery supplying the retina. *Also called* Zinn's artery. *See* Table of Arteries—centralis retinae.

central bearing device A mechanical device used intraorally to record movements and positions of the mandible at selected jaw openings.

centrifugal Moving away from the centre.

centripetal Moving towards the centre.

cephal-, cephalo- Prefix signifying *head.*

cephalgia, cephalalgia Headache.

cephalic Relating to, or in the direction of, the head.

cephalodynia Headache.

cephalograph Cephalometric *radiograph.

cephalometric Relating to cephalometry.

cephalometry The science of measurement of the head, either directly or with tracings from radiographs, used in growth studies, orthodontics and facial plastic surgery.

cephalopharyngeal muscle M. constrictor pharyngis superior. *See* Table of Muscles.

cephalostat An apparatus designed to ensure the location of the head in a constant plane so that a series of x-ray photographs, taken over a long period, may be accurately superimposed for purposes of comparison.

cera Wax.

ceramics The art of making porcelain objects, and of processing porcelain.

dental c. The art of making porcelain teeth, crowns and inlays.

ceramodontics Dental *ceramics.

cerateous Wax-like.

ceratopharyngeal muscle Part of constrictor pharyngis medius. *See* Table of Muscles—ceratopharyngeus.

cerebellar Relating to the cerebellum.

cerebellar artery Supplies the cerebellum, the medulla and vermiform process; three branches: anterior inferior, posterior inferior, and superior. *See* Table of Arteries—cerebelli.

cerebellum That part of the brain which controls and co-ordinates movement; situated behind the cerebrum.

cerebral Relating to the cerebrum.

cerebral artery Supplies blood to the brain; three branches: anterior, middle, and posterior. *See* Table of Arteries—cerebri.

cerebral vein One of the veins draining the cerebrum. *See* Table of Veins—cerebri.

cerebralgia Headache.

cerebrum The main part of the brain, occupying the upper part of the cranium.

cereous Composed of wax.

cervical Relating to the cervix, or neck; especially, *in dentistry,* to the neck of a tooth, the narrow area at the junction of the tooth root with the crown.

cervical artery Supplies neck muscles, spinal cord and vertebrae; three branches: ascending, deep, and superficial (variable). *See* Table of Arteries—cervicalis.

cervical nerves Supply the muscles and skin of the neck, back and arms. *See* Table of Nerves—cervicales.

cervical third *of a tooth* That portion of the crown or root adjacent to the cervical line.

cervicoaxial *Axiogingival.

cervicobuccal 1. Relating to the buccal surface of the cervix of a posterior tooth. 2. *Buccogingival[2].

cervicobuccoaxial *Gingivobucco-axial.

cervicofacial Relating to the neck and the face.

cervicolabial 1. Relating to the labial surface of the cervix of an anterior tooth. 2. *Labiogingival.

cervicolingual 1. Relating to the lingual surface of a tooth cervix. 2. *Linguogingival.

cervix *In dentistry:* 1. The neck of a tooth; the narrowed part where the tooth enters the gum, at the cemento-enamel junction. 2. That part of a dental implant connecting the implanted appliance to the abutment through the mucosa.

chalinoplasty Plastic surgery operation at the angles of the mouth.

chamber 1. Any enclosed space. 2. *In anatomy*, a small or clearly defined cavity.

air c. A depression in the palatal portion of an upper denture, and once thought to assist in its retention; a vacuum chamber.

pulp c. The cavity at the core of a tooth crown, surrounded by dentine and containing dental pulp.

relief c. A recess in the surface of a denture base to reduce pressure on a specific area in the mouth.

suction c. Air *chamber.

vacuum c. Air *chamber.

chamecephalic Having a flattened skull.

chameprosopic Having a broad, low face.

chamestaphyline Having an abnormally low and flattened palatal arch.

chamfer To bevel.

chancre The primary syphilitic lesion, starting as a small papule and rapidly developing into an erosive ulcer.

chart 1. A visible record of data relating to a patient's illness, progress or treatment. 2. To record such data on a visible record.

dental c. A diagrammatic representation of the tooth surfaces of the upper and lower jaws, on which may be recorded details of cavities, fillings, extractions, or other relevant information.

check bite *Check record.

check record An impression taken in hard wax or in modelling compound to record the various occlusal positions of the teeth in the mouth, and used to check these positions in artificial dentures in an articulator.

cheek The side of the face below the eye.

cleft c. A developmental anomaly caused by the failure of some of the facial processes to unite.

cheekbone The *zygomatic bone.

cheil-, cheilo- Prefix signifying *lip*, or *edge*.

cheilalgia Neuralgic pain affecting the lip or lips.

cheilectomy The surgical removal of part of a lip.

cheilectropion Eversion of the lip.

cheilion The angle of the mouth.

cheilitis Inflammation of the lip.

angular c. Cheilitis affecting the angles of the mouth.

apostematous c. *Cheilitis glandularis.

impetiginous c. Impetigo affecting the lip.
migrating c. *Cheilosis.
solar c. *Cheilitis actinica.

cheilitis actinica Cheilitis caused by exposure to sunlight.

cheilitis exfoliativa Recurrent crust formation which affects the vermilion border of the lip, and peels off.

cheilitis glandularis Inflammation of the labial glands, causing swelling and hardening of the lips.

cheilitis venenata Contact dermatitis caused by cosmetic or chemical irritants.

cheilocarcinoma Cancer of the lip.

cheilognathopalatoschisis Congenital malformation marked by fissure of the upper lip, the maxillary alveolar process and the palate; hare-lip and cleft palate.

cheilognathoprosoposchisis A fissure involving the upper lip and the maxilla, associated with an oblique facial cleft.

cheilognathoschisis Congenital fissure of the upper lip and the maxillary alveolar process.

cheilognathouranoschisis Hare-lip and cleft palate; cheilognathopalatoschisis.

cheilognathus *Hare-lip.

cheiloncus A tumour of the lip.

cheilopalatognathus Congenital fissure of the maxillary alveolar process combined with cleft palate.

cheilophagia Biting the lips.

cheiloplasty The repair of a lip defect by plastic surgery.

cheilorrhaphy Suture of the lips.

cheiloschisis *Hare-lip.

cheilosis A non-inflammatory condition of the lips, frequently associated with riboflavin deficiency, and characterized by chapping and fissures.
angular c. A form of cheilosis affecting the angles of the mouth; perlèche.

cheilostomatoplasty The repair of lip and mouth damage by plastic surgery.

cheilotomy Excision of part of a lip.

cheloid *See* keloid.

chemical 1. Any specific substance whose composition, properties and reactions are known. 2. Relating to chemistry.

chemical cautery A chemical caustic used for cauterization.

chemico-parasitic theory of caries A theory of the cause of dental decay advanced in 1889; it postulated that caries was the result of demineralization of the tooth enamel due to the action of acids produced by bacteria.

chemistry The science and study of the composition of matter, and the analysis and transformation of substances.
biological c. *Biochemistry.
histological c. *Histochemistry.
pharmaceutical c. The chemistry of drugs.

chemoprophylaxis The use of chemical drugs in the prevention of disease.

chemotherapy 1. The treatment of disease by chemicals which affect the pathogenic organism without harming the patient. 2. The treatment of malignant neoplasia by chemical means.

chemotherapy mucositis Oral lesions producing a burning sensation, areas of redness and possibly ulceration, the ulcers becoming numerous and large; relatively infrequent side-effect of chemotherapy.

cheoplastic Relating to cheoplasty.

cheoplasty The moulding of artificial teeth by means of a low-fusing alloy; now obsolete.

cherubism The round, chubby features and upturned eyes characteristic of facial fibrous dysplasia.

chiasm *See* chiasma.

chiasma (*pl.* chiasmata) 1. Any crossing over; a decussation. 2. The crossing of the fibres of the optic nerve; the optic chiasm.

chiasmal, chiasmatic, chiasmic Relating to a chiasma.

Chievitz's organ (J.H. Chievitz, 1850-1901. Danish anatomist). The mandibular branch of the parotid duct.

child Human young, up to the age of puberty.

chilitis *See* cheilitis.

chill A cold sensation with shivering, often characteristic of the onset of fever.

chin The central prominence of the lower jaw.

chin reflex Closure of the mouth produced by stroking the chin.

chincap A cap-like pad fitted over the chin and used to supply attachment for extra-oral traction during orthodontic treatment.

chip syringe A type of air syringe consisting of a metal nozzle and a rubber bulb, used to remove loose debris during operative procedures, or for drying the area.

chirurgical Relating to surgery.

chisel A hand instrument used in surgery for chipping away bone, and in dentistry for cutting tooth enamel; it is bevelled on one side of the blade only.

chloroma A condition characterized by multiple myeloid tumours, of a greenish colour, affecting particularly the face and skull, and associated with a blood picture of leukaemia.

chloropercha A mixture of chloroform and gutta-percha, in the form of a paste, used with a solid core to seal root canals.

chlorosarcoma *Chloroma.

choana (*pl.* choanae) 1. Any funnel-shaped opening. 2. One of the posterior nasal orifices; a nostril.

chondr-, chondro- Prefix signifying *cartilage*.

chondral Relating to cartilage.

chondrocranium The cartilaginous cranium of the embryo.

chondrofibrosarcoma *Chondrosarcoma.

chondroglossal muscle Draws back and depresses the tongue. *See* Table of Muscles—chondroglossus.

chondroliposarcoma *Chondrosarcoma.

chondroma A benign tumour composed of cartilaginous tissue.

chondromalacia A condition characterized by abnormal softness of cartilage.

chondropharyngeal muscle Part of constrictor pharyngis medius. *See* Table of Muscles—chondropharyngeus.

chondrosarcoma A malignant, cartilaginous sarcoma.

chondrosis Cartilage formation.

chorda tympani nerve Supplies the submandibular and sublingual glands and the taste buds on the front of the tongue. *See* Table of Nerves.

choroid artery Supplies the choroid plexus of the lateral ventricle. *See* Table of Arteries—choroidea anterior.

Christensen's phenomenon *In prosthetic dentistry*, the development of a gap between the opposing ends of flat occlusal rims when the mandible is protruded. *Also called* Christensen's cleft.

chrom-, chromo- Prefix signifying *colour.*

chrome *Chromium.

-chrome Suffix signifying *colour.*

chrome-cobalt *See* cobalt-chromium casting alloy.

chromium A hard, brittle, silvery metal, chemical symbol Cr, used mainly as protective plating.

chronic Long continued; as opposed to *acute.*

cibus Latin for *food*; used in prescription writing and abbreviated *cib.*

cicatricial Relating to a cicatrix or scar.

cicatrix (*pl.* cicatrices) A scar.

cicatrization The process of wound healing which leaves a scar.

ciliary Relating to or resembling the eyelash.

ciliary artery Supplies blood to the eyeball; three branches: anterior, long posterior, short posterior (*also called* uveal). *See* Table of Arteries—ciliaris.

ciliary muscle Muscle of accommodation of vision. *See* Table of Muscles—ciliaris.

ciliary nerve Supplies the eyeball and ciliary muscles. *See* Table of Nerves—ciliaris.

ciliated Having hair-like processes, or a fringe of hair.

ciliiform Hair-like.

cingulum (*pl.* cingula) 1. *In anatomy,* any encircling part or structure. 2. Basal ridge in the cervical third on the lingual surface of the anterior teeth.

cionectomy *Uvulectomy.

cionitis *Uvulitis.

cionoptopsis *Uvuloptosis.

cionorraphy *Staphylorraphy.

cionotomy *Uvulotomy.

circa Latin for *about*; abbreviated *c.*

circle of Willis (T. Willis, 1621-75. English anatomist and physician). *Circulus arteriosus cerebri.

circular In the shape of or resembling a circle.

circulation Movement or flow in a circle, retracing its course repeatedly; applied especially to the flow of blood through the body.

circulatory Relating to circulation; applied especially to the circulation of the blood.

circulus arteriosus cerebri The circular arterial system at the base of the brain, formed by the anterior and posterior cerebral, the anterior and posterior communicating, and the internal carotid arteries; *also called* the circle of Willis.

circulus arteriosus halleri *Circulus vasculosus nervi optici.

circulus vasculosus nervi optici A circle of arteries round the entrance of the optic nerve to the sclera; *also called* Zinn's circle or circulus arteriosus halleri.

circum- Prefix signifying *around, surrounding.*

circumcoronitis *Pericoronitis.

circumoral Around the mouth.

circumtonsillar About a tonsil.

circumvallate Surrounded by a wall, as the circumvallate, or vallate, papillae of the tongue.

clamp 1. A screw or spring type of device for holding anything in position. 2. A surgical device used to apply compression.
rubber-dam c. A form of spring clip which holds the rubber dam round the neck of an exposed tooth.

clamp band A band which is held in place by means of a screw and a nut.

clams *Actinomycosis.

Clapton's line (E. Clapton, 1830-1909. English physician). A greenish line on the gums, seen in copper poisoning.

Clarke's tongue (Sir Charles M. Clarke, 1782-1857. English physician). The fissured tongue of syphilitic glossitis sclerosa.

-clasia Suffix signifying *destruction* or *degeneration.*

clasp *In dentistry,* any hook or band attached to a natural tooth and used to anchor a partial denture or any orthodontic appliance.
arrowhead c. A form of orthodontic attachment consisting of a wire clasp round a molar tooth, fitting under the mesial and distal bulges, to which removable appliances may be fastened. The Adams clasp is a modified form of arrowhead clasp.
bar c. A type of clasp in which the arms are a direct extension of the connector bars of the denture.
circumferential c. A clasp that surrounds more than half of the abutment tooth.
continuous c. Continuous bar *retainer.
flyover c. A clasp used to attach a removable orthodontic appliance to a band, usually on an upper first permanent molar.
molar c. A form of orthodontic clasp for a partially erupted molar tooth, designed to pass over the occlusal surface and to give positive inward pressure; it is anchored at both ends by embedding in the base of the appliance.

clasp, Adams *See* Adams clasp.

class The primary division in biological classification, subdivided into orders.

claudication Lameness, limping.
jaw c. Pain caused when chewing; seen in giant cell arteritis.

clearance
interocclusal c. The slight gap between the upper and lower teeth when the mandible is at rest.

cleat 1. *In orthodontics,* a metal loop or spur on an appliance to which elastic bands or other means of traction may be anchored. 2. *In prosthetic dentistry,* occlusal *rest.

cleft A fissure.
alveolar c. A cleft in the alveolar process, sometimes seen in association with cleft lip and palate.
facial c. A developmental anomaly caused by the failure of any of the facial processes to unite.
gingival c. A narrow, V-shaped split in the marginal gingiva, sometimes seen in pocket formation, and most commonly found in the labial gingiva of the mandibular incisors and the buccal gingiva of the maxillary molars.

cleft cheek A developmental anomaly caused by the failure of some of the facial processes to unite.

cleft palate Congenital fissure of the palate, due to defective development in embryo; it may be associated with hare-lip. There is a wide range of deformity, from a bifid uvula to complete bilateral cleft of both palate and lip.

cleidocranial Relating to the clavicle and the cranium.

cleoid A claw-like instrument used in cavity excavation, or in carving amalgam restorations.

cliche metal A fusible alloy of tin, lead, antimony and bismuth, used in dentistry.

clinical 1. Relating to the observation and treatment of disease in the patient, as opposed to theoretical and experimental investigation. 2. Relating to a clinic.

clinocephalic Saddle-headed; having a congenital defect of the skull, in which there is a concavity in the vertex.

clonic Relating to or characteristic of a clonus.

clonus Convulsive spasm, with alternating contraction and relaxation of muscles.

close-bite, closed bite A form of malocclusion in which there is abnormally deep overlap of the incisors when the jaws are closed.

Clostridium A genus of anaerobic, Gram-positive, spore-bearing bacteria, seen as spindle- or rod-shaped organisms.

clutch

dental c. A metal casting of the dental arch with space for the tooth crowns, which can be fitted over the teeth, leaving the occlusal surfaces free, and following the indentations of the teeth on both the lingual and buccal surfaces; it is used as attachment for a facebow or other measuring instrument.

clyers *Actinomycosis.

coagulation The process of clotting.

coalesce To fuse or unite separate parts.

coalescence The fusion or union of parts previously separate.

coarctation Narrowing or constriction, applied to blood vessels.

coarticulation Fibrous *joint.

cobalt-chromium casting alloy A hard and corrosion-resistant alloy of cobalt and chromium, used in the construction of partial dentures.

coccal Relating to or resembling a coccus.

coccus (*pl.* cocci) A spherical bacterium, whose genera are differentiated by the grouping of their cells: completely separate cocci are called *micrococci*; those that are paired, *diplococci*; those arranged in chains, *streptococci*; and those arranged in clusters, *staphylococci*.

cochlea A spiral tube forming part of the inner ear.

cochlear Relating to the cochlea.

cochlear nerve Supplies the spiral organ of the cochlea. *See* Table of Nerves—cochlearis.

coffer dam *Rubber dam.

Coffin split plate (C.R. Coffin, 1826-91. American dentist). An orthodontic appliance used formerly for expanding the dental arch by means of a divided plate, constructed to exert controlled lateral pressure on the lingual edges of the arch.

Coffin spring (C.R. Coffin, 1826-91. American dentist). A heavy-gauge wire spring used to expand or contract posterior sections of an orthodontic appliance.

cohesion The force uniting the molecules of a substance.

cohesive Relating to cohesion; sticking together.

cohesiveness The quality of being cohesive.

col

gingival c. A depression in an interdental papilla between the two peaks, one on each side of the contact area.

cold sore *Herpes labialis.

collagen An albuminoid, one of the main constituents of bone, cartilage, and connective tissue.

collagen fibres Soft, flexible fibres, made up of bundles of fibrils and often themselves formed into larger bundles; they are the main constituent of fibrous tissue and the principal component of the periodontal ligament.

collagen fibrils Very fine, delicate fibrils which are made up into bundles to form collagen fibres.

collagenous Relating to collagen.

collar 1. A band encircling the neck of any structure. 2. *In dentistry*, a narrow metal band round a tooth cervix.

collar crown An artifical crown attached to the tooth root by a metal band.

collet A *collar.

collimation *In radiography*, the use of a cone, diaphragm or slit apparatus to restrict the size of an x-ray beam.

collimator *In radiography*, any piece of apparatus used to reduce the size of an x-ray beam.

colloid 1. A state of matter in which individual particles of one substance, either as large single molecules or collections of smaller molecules (the disperse phase), are uniformly distributed in a dispersion medium of another substance. 2. Glue-like. 3. The colourless, gelatinous secretion of the thyroid gland.

colloidal Relating to or having the properties of a colloid.

collutory A gargle or mouthwash.

coma A state of complete unconsciousness from which a patient cannot be roused even by determined external stimulation.

comatose The condition of being in a coma.

commensal An organism that lives on or within another organism to its own advantage and without detriment to the host.

comminuted Broken into small pieces.

commissure The point of union between similar parts or bodies.
labial c. The corners of the mouth where the upper and lower lips join.

communicating artery Forms part of the circulus arteriosus cerebri. *See* Table of Arteries—communicans.

community dentistry That branch of dentistry providing for the treatment and prevention of dental disease within the community, and the promotion of good oral health.

Community Periodontal Index of Treatment Needs An index (CPITN) designed for the WHO, to assess treatment needs rather than periodontal status; it may be used for epidemiological surveys or oral health screening of individuals. Examination, using the WHO ball-pointed periodontal probe, is based on three maxillary and three mandibular sextants within the mouth, excluding the third molars. For surveys certain index teeth in each sextant are scored, and for individual screening the worst finding for all teeth in a sextant, recording 0 for no sign of disease, 1 for gingival bleeding, 2 for supragingival or subgingival calculus, 3 for pathological pocketing from 4mm to 6mm, and 4 for pocketing of 6mm or over. Treatment needs are recorded as 0 = no treatment; I = improvement in personal oral hygiene (Code 1); II = I + scaling (Codes 2 & 3); III = I + II + complex treatment (Code 4).

complex muscle M. semispinalis capitis. *See* Table of Muscles.

component Any one of the parts of an appliance.
transmucosal c. Implant *abutment.

composite Composite *resin.

compound 1. Made up of two or more substances. 2. Any material so composed. 3. *Impression compound.

compression moulding The process of shaping under pressure in a mould.

compressor naris muscle *See* Table of Muscles—nasalis, pars transversa.

concave Having an inward curve or a hollowed surface.

concha (*pl.* conchae) Any anatomic structure resembling a shell, as the centre of the external ear, or the turbinate bone.
nasoturbinal c. *Agger nasi.

concrement *Concretion.

concrescence *In dentistry*, the joining of the roots of two adjacent teeth by a deposit of cementum.

concretion Any hardened or solidified mass in the tissues; a calculus.

concussion 1. A violent blow or shock; generally used of a blow on the head. 2. The condition resulting from such a blow.

condensation 1. The act of making more compact or denser. 2. *In dentistry*, the act of packing a filling into a tooth cavity, used particularly of a gold-foil filling.

condenser *In dentistry,* an instrument with a blunt, serrated edge, used for packing and compressing gold-foil or amalgam fillings.
amalgam c. An instrument used to condense amalgam in a tooth cavity.
foil c. Gold *condenser.
gold c. An instrument used to condense and compact direct filling gold into a prepared cavity.
mechanical c. An instrument used to condense gold or amalgam in restorations; the blow is produced either by hand operation, with a dental engine, or with compressed air.

conduction anaesthesia, conduction analgesia Regional *anaesthesia.

condylar Relating to a condyle.

condyle A rounded articulating prominence on a bone, especially one of the rounded articulating prominences of the mandible.

condylectomy Surgical removal of a condyle.

condylion A point on the lateral tip of the mandibular condyle.

condyloid Relating to or resembling a condyle.

condyloma acuminatum A papillomatous growth resulting from venereal disease; oral manifestations do occur but are very rare.

condylotomy Surgical division of or incision into a condyle.

cone, silver Silver *point.

cone-socket instrument One in which the shank and blade or nib are separate from the handle, and screw into it.

congenital Present at birth.

conical Cone-shaped.

conjunctiva The mucous membrane covering the front of the eyeball and lining the eyelid.

conjunctival Relating to the conjunctiva.

conjunctival arteries Supply the conjunctiva. *See* Table of Arteries— conjunctivalis.

conjunctivitis Inflammation of the conjunctiva.

connector *In prosthetic dentistry,* any part of a partial denture whose function is to link two of the major components of the denture.
bar c. A bar or strip that connects the parts of a partial denture.
major c. The rigid framework of a partial denture to which all the various components are attached;

it may be *labial, lingual,* or *palatal.*
minor c. Bar *connector.
saddle c. Major *connector.

conoides Canine teeth, so named from their cone-like shape.

conservation Restoration and preservation of health, or of injured parts, such as teeth.

constitution *In medicine,* the functional habit of the body, taking into account inherited qualities and the effects of environment on the physical and mental development.

constitutional Relating to or affecting the constitution as a whole.

constriction A contraction or drawing together in one part; tightness.

constrictor pharyngis muscles Constrict pharynx. *See* Table of Muscles.

contact area Any one of the areas of contact on the approximal surfaces of adjacent teeth.

contact point *Contact area.

contact surface Approximal *surface.

contaminate To soil or make impure by the addition of foreign material or organisms.

contamination The condition of being soiled or impure as a result of the addition of foreign material or organisms.

contiguous In close proximity to, or in contact with.

contour 1. The external shape of any object. 2. To carve or otherwise create the external form, as of artificial teeth or fillings.

contour alloy One suitable for fillings which can be anatomically contoured.

contra- Prefix signifying *against* or *opposed to.*

contra-angle A double angle or a series of angles in the shank of an instrument bringing its point or edge into line with the axis of the handle.

contraction 1. A decrease in size, either of length, area or volume. 2. The shortening and tensing of a muscle.

contraindication Any symptom or additional condition which makes a particular form of treatment unsuitable.

contralateral 1. Relating to the side opposite a structure or lesion. 2. Referring to the non-working side of a denture.

contrast *In radiology,* the difference in density seen in a radiograph as a result of the difference in radio-pacity of the object x-rayed.

contusion A *bruise.

convex Having an outward curve or a domed surface.

cope A metal plate used to cover the root of a tooth before attaching an artificial crown; a diaphragm.

coping 1. A thin metal cap. 2. A *cope. 3. *In implant dentistry,* *cover screw.
healing c. *Cover screw.
impression c. *Cover screw.

copper A reddish metallic element, chemical symbol Cu, soft and malleable, with poisonous salts; it is much used in alloys.

copper amalgam An amalgam alloy containing mainly copper and mercury.

copper line A line, which may be greenish or purple, on the edge of the gums; seen in copper poisoning; *also called* Corrigan's line.

copula linguae Hypobranchial *eminence.

cord Any long, flexible structure, circular in cross-section.
enamel c. A temporary structure in the developing tooth linking the enamel knot to the outer dental lamina.

gubernacular c. *Gubernaculum dentis.

cordate Heart-shaped.

core *In restorative dentistry,* a metal casting, suitably shaped, and generally held in place by a post, over which an artificial crown can be fitted; *also called* a cast core.

corium The layer of connective tissue between the epidermis and the subcutaneous tissue; the dermis or true skin.
gingival c. The connective tissue or lamina propria of the gingiva.

cornu (*pl.* cornua) A horn or horn-shaped process.

cornual Relating to a cornu.

coronal 1. Relating to a crown. 2. In the direction of the coronal suture.

corone The coronoid *process of the mandible.

coronion *In craniometry,* the point or tip of the coronoid process of the mandible.

coronofacial Relating to the crown of the head and the face.

coronoid 1. Crown-shaped. 2. Curved, like a beak.

coronoid process A thin and flattened projection of bone from the anterior upper border of the ascending ramus of the mandible into which the temporal muscle is inserted.

coronoidectomy The surgical removal of the coronoid process of the mandible.

coronoidotomy The surgical division of the coronoid process of the mandible.

coronoplasty Alteration to the crown of a natural tooth by abrasion.

Corrigan's line (Sir D.J. Corrigan, 1802-80. Irish physician). *Copper line.

corrugator supercilii muscle Draws eyebrow down and wrinkles forehead. *See* Table of Muscles.

cortex 1. The external layer of an organ, within the capsule. 2. The outer layer of grey matter of the brain.

cortical 1. Relating to a cortex. 2. Relating to the bark of a tree; applied to the outer bone tissue.

corticalosteotomy *Corticotomy.

corticotomy Surgical section through the alveolar bone cortex at the base of the dento-alveolar segment, serving to weaken the resistance of the bone to the application of orthodontic forces.

Corynebacterium A genus of slender rod-shaped micro-organisms, often with club-shaped swellings, Gram-positive, facultatively anaerobic, although some organisms are aerobic, and generally non-motile.
C. fusiforme **Fusobacterium nucleatum.*

coryza The common cold; a catarrhal inflammation of the nasal mucous membrane.

Costen's syndrome (J.B. Costen, 1895-1962. American otolaryngologist). Referred pain associated with temporomandibular joint destruction through faulty occlusion, occurring in the head, the eye, the tongue, and nasal sinuses; there may also be painful muscle spasm during mastication.

costocervical trunk The blood supply for the deep muscles of the neck and back, 1st and 2nd intercostal spaces and the vertebral column. *See* Table of Arteries—truncus costocervicalis.

cotton-wool roll A small and tightly packed roll of cotton wool used in the mouth to absorb saliva and assist in keeping the operative field dry.

Cotunnius' nerve (D. Cotugno (Cotunnius), 1736-1822. Italian anatomist). The *nasopalatine nerve.

counter-bite A bite[2] opposing that taken of the teeth in one jaw.

counter-irritant 1. Producing or causing counter-irritation. 2. Any agent used to produce counter-irritation.

counter-irritation The deliberate production of superficial irritation in order to mask or relieve an existing irritation or pain.

counterdie The reverse image of a die.

countersink 1. A bevelled depression in a surface to accommodate the head of a screw or rivet. 2. The instrument used to make this depression.

cover screw A thin covering designed to fit the implant abutment and connect it to the prosthesis or superstructure; *also called* impression coping *or* healing coping.

cranial Relating to the cranium.

cranial nerve Any one of twelve pairs of peripheral nerves arising directly from the brain stem. *See* Table of Nerves—craniales.

cranio- Prefix signifying *cranium.*

craniobuccal Relating to the cranium and the oral cavity.

craniocleidodysostosis Cleidocranial *dysostosis.

craniofacial Relating to the cranium and the face.

craniomalacia A condition characterized by softness of the bones of the skull; usually seen in infants.

craniomandibular Relating to the skull and the mandible.

craniometry The science of measuring the skull for the comparative study of racial types in humans and of variations with other primates.

craniostat *Cephalostat.

craniostosis Ossification of the cranial sutures, occurring prematurely.

cranium The skull.

cranter A third molar; an obsolete term.

crater A localized depression, usually circular and having a raised edge or rim.
gingival c. A depression in the interproximal gingiva caused by necrotic destruction of the papilla.

crazing A pattern of minute cracks which may appear on the surface of plastic or porcelain teeth.

crepitation A crackling noise; occurring in joints, in the lungs when affected by certain diseases, and in other parts.

crepitus *Crepitation.

crescent 1. In the shape of a new moon. 2. Any structure so shaped.
lingual c. The area between the lingual wall of the mandible and the floor of the mouth beneath the tongue.

crest A prominent raised edge or border.
alveolar c. One of the highest points on the alveolar process, between the tooth sockets.
buccinator c. A ridge from the base of the anterior border of the coronoid process of the mandible to the molar teeth, providing attachment for the buccinator muscle.
conchal c. of the maxilla An oblique ridge on the nasal surface of the maxilla, anterior to the lacrimal sulcus and articulating with the inferior nasal concha.

conchal c. of the palatine bone A sharp horizontal ridge near the posterior end of the nasal surface of the palatine bone, articulating with the inferior nasal concha.
dental c That portion of the maxillary ridge on which the incisor teeth develop; *also called* Kölliker's dental crest.
ethmoidal c. of the maxilla A small oblique ridge on the medial surface of the frontal process of the maxilla, supporting the middle nasal concha.
ethmoidal c. of the palatine bone A narrow ridge near the upper end of the medial surface of the palatine bone, articulating with the middle nasal concha.
gingival c. Gingival *margin.
inferior turbinal c. of the maxilla Conchal *crest of the maxilla.
inferior turbinal c. of the palatine bone Conchal *crest of the palatine bone.
nasal c. of the maxilla A ridge on the medial border of the maxillary palatal process, articulating with the vomer.
nasal c. of the palatine bone A ridge on the medial border of the palatal bone, articulating with the vomer.
palatine c. A thin, transverse ridge of bone across the back of the hard palate.
superior turbinal c. of the maxilla Ethmoidal *crest of the maxilla.
superior turbinal c. of the palatine bone Ethmoidal *crest of the palatine bone.

crevice A narrow split or fissure in a tooth.
gingival c. Gingival *sulcus.

crevicular Relating to a crevice, particularly applied to the gingival crevice.

crib 1. A removable form of anchorage used with orthodontic appliances. 2. An orthodontic appliance designed to be habit-breaking.

cribriform Perforated like a sieve.

crico- Prefix signifying *ring*.

cricoarytenoid muscles Open or narrow rima glottidis. *See* Table of Muscles—cricoarytenoideus.

cricopharyngeal muscle Part of constrictor pharyngis inferior. *See* Table of Muscles—cricopharyngeus.

cricothyroid artery Supplies the cricothyroid muscle. *See* Table of Arteries—cricothyroidea.

cricothyroid muscle Tenses the vocal folds. *See* Table of Muscles—cricothyroideus.

crossbite A form of malocclusion caused by an abnormality of the lateral relationship of the jaws to each other, thus preventing normal occlusion because the buccolingual relationships of opposing teeth are the reverse of normal.

Crouzon's disease (O. Crouzon, 1874-1938. French neurologist). Craniofacial *dysostosis.

crowding *In dentistry*, displacement or malposition of teeth in the dental arch caused by disproportionately large teeth or a disproportionately small dental arch.

crown 1. That part of a tooth, covered by enamel, which is exposed above the gum. 2. An artificial cap to fit over the stump of a carious or of a fractured tooth.
abutment c. An artificial crown used to support or retain a dental prosthesis or orthodontic appliance.
acrylic veneer c. A metal crown covered by a thin veneer of acrylic.
anatomical c. That part of the tooth which is covered by enamel, not all of which may be visible above the gum.

basket c. A form of three-quarter crown, with an acrylic facing, used as a semi-permanent restoration for a fractured or malformed incisor in a school-child.

bell c. A crown of a tooth in which the diameter, mesiodistally, is much greater at the occlusal surface than at the cervix.

cap c. Shell *crown.

clinical c. That part of the tooth crown which projects above the gum surface.

collar c. An artifical crown attached to the tooth root by a metal band.

dowel c. Post *crown.

half-cap c. A form of crown covering all but the labial or buccal surface of a tooth, and attached by a metal band.

hood c. A half-cap crown covering the lingual, approximal and occlusal surfaces of a tooth.

jacket c. A porcelain or acrylic veneer crown which is placed over the prepared remains of a vital natural tooth.

open-face c. Half-cap *crown.

partial c. Three-quarter *crown.

pivot c. An artificial crown attached by means of a metal post into the root canal of the natural tooth.

platinum bonded c. A porcelain jacket crown fused on to a platinum matrix.

porcelain cusp c. A crown having porcelain and not metal on the occlusal surface.

porcelain veneer c. A metal crown covered by a thin veneer of porcelain.

post c. Any artificial crown attached to the tooth root by means of a post or dowel; *also called* a pivot crown.

seamless c. A shell crown contoured from a metal cap, without soldering.

shell c. A crown consisting of a metal shell, contoured to fit over the crown of an existing natural tooth; *also called* a cap crown.

shoulder c. An artificial crown shaped at the base to sit on a prepared root without a metal collar.

split-dowel c. A removable crown attached to the tooth by means of a split-pin, which is fitted into a gold-lined root canal.

telescope c. A double metal crown, composed of two tubular or conical crowns, placed one over the other.

three-quarter c. A form of shell crown, retained by cement and slotted into the tooth, covering all but the labial or buccal surface; *also called* a Carmichael crown.

two-piece c. A crown made from a contoured metal band joined to a swaged cap.

verrucous c. A wart-like overgrowth of enamel on a tooth crown.

visible c. That part of the anatomical crown visible for examination above the gum.

window c. A type of artificial crown which has a thin veneer of porcelain or acrylic resin on the outer surface only.

crownwork 1. The construction or fitting of artificial crowns to the teeth. 2. The actual prosthesis, when in place in the mouth.

Crozat appliance (G.B. Crozat, b. 1876. American orthodontist). A removable orthodontic appliance consisting of a palatal archwire joining retention clasps on the first molars which have a claw-like grip; used as a base for various types of attachment to provide tooth movement; *also called* a Walker appliance.

crucial 1. In the form of a cross. 2. Decisive.

crude Raw, unrefined.

Cruveilhier's nerve (J. Cruveilhier, 1791-1874. French anatomist and pathologist). An occasional branch of the facial nerve.

Cryer's elevator (M.H. Cryer, 1840-1921. American oral surgeon). One of a pair of elevators for removing molar roots, one for the distal and one for the mesial, being reversible for opposite sides of the jaw.

cry- , cryo- Prefix signifying *cold.*

cryocautery Cold *cautery.

cryoprobe An instrument used for cryosurgery.

cryosurgery The use of extreme cold for surgical destruction of tissue.

cryotherapy The treatment of disease with the use of extreme cold.

crypt A pit or follicle.
dental c. The bony space within the jaw containing the developing tooth.

cryptococcosis A chronic fungal infection caused by *Torula histolytica (Cryptococcus neoformans)*; violet-coloured verrucous lesions may be found on the oral mucous membranes and may become ulcerated.

cuff
epithelial c. Epithelial *attachment.

culture 1. The growth of micro-organisms in an artificial medium. 2. A group of micro-organisms so grown.
direct c. Any culture produced by direct transfer of the micro-organisms from a natural source to the culture medium.
mixed c. A culture containing several different species of micro-organisms.
needle c. Stab *culture.
plate c. A bacterial culture grown on a glass plate, or in a Petri dish.
pure c. A culture containing only one species of micro-organism.
slant c. One grown on a slanting surface to obtain a greater area for growth.
stab c. A culture made by inoculating the medium by means of a needle thrust deeply into it.

culture medium (*pl.* media) Any substance used to cultivate bacteria; the principal media are broth, milk, blood serum, agar and potato.

cum Latin for *with*; used in prescription writing and abbreviated *c.*

cuneate Wedge-shaped.

cupreous Relating to copper.

cure 1. To treat a disease or injury successfully. 2. Any method or drug used in treatment. 3. To harden materials such as those used for denture bases.

curet *See* curette.

curettage 1. The removal of foreign matter from the walls of a bony cavity. 2. *In dentistry*, the removal of material from root surfaces and periodontal pockets.
apical c. Periapical *curettage.
gingival c. The removal of inflamed or diseased epithelial tissue from the wall of a periodontal pocket.
periapical c. Surgical removal of chronic diseased tissue from the bony socket surrounding the apex of a tooth root.
subgingival c. Removal of the epithelium at the bottom of the gingival sulcus and the lining of a periodontal pocket.
ultrasonic c. Removal of diseased tissue from the surface of a tooth root and from the periodontal pocket with an ultrasonic instrument.

curette An instrument used in curettage.

curve of Monson (G.S. Monson, 1869-1933. American dentist). The curved plane on which lie the occlusal surfaces of the posterior teeth; it conforms to the segment of the surface of a sphere of 102mm radius.

curve of Spee (F. von Spee, 1855-1937. German embryologist). An imaginary line joining the buccal cusps of the upper or the lower posterior teeth, viewed from the side, which curves upwards.

curve of Wilson A cross-arch, cross-tooth curve indicating the height difference between supporting and non-supporting cusps in occlusion.

Cushing's syndrome (H.W. Cushing, 1869-1939, American neurosurgeon). A syndrome resulting from hyperfunction of the adrenal cortex and producing obesity, 'moon face', and a characteristic hump at the base of the neck. It may also produce osteoporosis in the facial bones.

cushion of Passavant *Passavant's ridge.

cusp 1. A pointed, conical or rounded projection on the crown of a tooth, on or near the occlusal surface. 2. One of the triangular sections of a cardiac valve.
supplemental c. Any abnormal or extra cusp on a tooth surface.

cusp angle The angle of incline of the sides of a cusp made with a perpendicular line bisecting the cusp, measured mesiodistally or buccolingually.

cuspal Relating to a cusp.

cuspid 1. Having a cusp. 2. A canine *tooth.

cuspidate Pointed; having one or more sharp points or cusps.

cuspidor A form of spittoon with running water to keep it constantly flushed out.

cutaneous Relating to the skin.

cutaneous colli nerve N. transversus colli. *See* Table of Nerves.

cuticle 1. The outer layer of the skin. 2. A layer covering the free surface of an epithelial cell.
acquired c., acquired enamel c. Acquired *pellicle.
dental c. 1. Reduced enamel *epithelium. 2. Acquired *pellicle. 3. Secondary *cuticle.
enamel c. 1. An acellular layer of organic material secreted onto the surface of the enamel; it is thought to be the final product of ameloblasts. As it cannot be seen with an electron microscope, it is thought by some to be an artefact; *also called* primary enamel cuticle. 2. Acquired *pellicle.
post-eruption c. Acquired *pellicle.
primary enamel c. See enamel cuticle.
secondary c. An occasional layer below reduced enamel epithelium, thought to be either the product of epithelial cells or the result of a blood leak following slight trauma.

cuticula dentis Reduced enamel *epithelium.

cutis The dermis, or skin.

cyanosis Bluish discoloration of the skin and mucous membranes, often due to deficient oxygenation of the blood.

cylinder Any solid or hollow body having parallel sides and a circular cross-section in one direction.

cylindrical Shaped like a cylinder.

cylindroma Adenoid cystic *carcinoma.

cymbocephalic Having a hollowed or boat-shaped skull.

cynodont A canine *tooth.

cynodontism Having teeth with long roots and a small pulp chamber entirely confined to the crown.

cyst A membranous sac containing fluid, gas, or soft matter.
adventitious c. A cyst that forms about a foreign body.
aneurysmal bone c. A benign, expansile cyst comprising many blood-filled spaces, which may affect the jaw bones.
antral c. A benign mucosal cyst of the maxillary antrum.
apical c. Periapical *cyst.
branchial c., branchial cleft c. A superficial and symptomless cyst, thought to arise from the remnants of the branchial arches, and found on the side of the neck near the angle of the jaw; it is seen as a smooth, rounded and mobile swelling.
calcifying odontogenic c. A cystic lesion occurring in bone or in the soft tissues of the tooth-bearing area, showing well-defined layers of cells within the epithelial lining, and masses of 'ghost' epithelial cells, which may become calcified.
dental c. Any cyst affecting a tooth, or tooth-bearing structure.
dentigerous c. A cyst of odontogenic origin, arising from the enamel organ of an unerupted tooth; it is most often associated with maxillary canines, mandibular second premolars and with third molars in both arches.
dermoid c. A developmental cyst containing hair follicles, teeth, and sweat or sebaceous glands.
developmental c. 1. A form of cyst arising from developmental anomalies in the surrounding tissue. 2. Inclusion *cyst.
epidermoid c. A cyst lined with stratified squamous epithelium and containing keratin but lacking other structures of epithelial origin.
eruption c. A cyst of odontogenic origin occurring about the crown of an erupting tooth, and presenting as a bluish swelling in the eruption area; a form of dentigerous cyst.
extravasation c. A cyst formed following haemorrhage into the tissues.
fissural c. 1. A cyst which develops at the lines of union of the embryonic processes which form the jaws. 2. Inclusion *cyst.
follicular c. A dentigerous *cyst.
gingival c. A small, circumscribed and painless cyst on the gingiva, arising from epithelial debris.
globulomaxillary c. A cyst arising in the region of the maxillary lateral incisors and canines.
incisive canal c. Nasopalatine duct *cyst.
inclusion c. Any cyst arising from epithelial residues within connective tissue; in bone such cysts occur along lines of fusion.
lateral periodontal c. A cyst found at the side of a tooth; it may be of inflammatory or developmental origin.
median anterior maxillary c. Nasopalatine duct *cyst.
multilocular c. Any cyst having many interconnected compartments.
nasolabial c. A developmental cyst of soft tissue in the nasolabial fold.
nasopalatine duct c. The most common type of inclusion cyst, seen in the midline of the maxilla, in or near the incisive canal.
odontogenic c. Any cyst arising from the epithelium of odontogenic tissue.
paradental c. Lateral periodontal *cyst.
periapical c. A cyst occurring about the root of a tooth, arising from a granuloma in that area.
periodontal c. Periapical *cyst.
primordial c. An uncommon cyst of odontogenic origin, arising where a tooth has failed to develop; it is

characterized by a thin fibrous capsule lined with keratinized squamous epithelium.
radicular c. Periapical *cyst.
residual c. A periapical cyst which remains or develops after the extraction of the affected tooth.
retention c. One caused by the retention of glandular secretion, and lined with epithelium; a mucocele.
sebaceous c. A cyst caused by the blocking of the duct of a sebaceous gland and the retention of its secretion.
solitary (simple) bone c. A cyst of the skeleton, which in the jaws forms an empty or fluid-filled cavity beneath the teeth, lined with thin fibrous tissue.
sublingual c. *Ranula.
thyroglossal c. A cyst occurring in or arising from the thyroglossal duct.
traumatic c. One caused by some traumatic injury.
unilocular c. A cyst having only one cavity.

cystadenofibroma *Adenofibroma.

cystadenoma A cystic tumour composed of adenomatous tissue.

cystadenoma lymphomatosum, papillary *Adenolymphoma[1].

cystic Relating to a cyst; cyst-like.

-cyte Suffix signifying *cell.*

cyto- Prefix signifying *cell* or *cells.*

cytology The study of cells in health and disease.
exfoliative c. The examination of cells shed or deliberately removed from a body surface.

Czermak's lines (J.N. Czermak, 1828-73. Austrian physiologist). Rows of interglobular spaces, following the outline of the dentine of a tooth, visible in histological sections.

D

D Distal.

DB Distobuccal.

DBO Distobucco-occlusal.

DBP Distobuccopulpal.

DC Distocervical.

def The expression used to indicate the number of **d**ecayed, **e**xtracted or **f**illed teeth in the primary dentition; it gives an index of the caries experience of both individuals and of groups. Sometimes used to describe the state of primary teeth present in the mouth; indicating the numbers of teeth **d**ecayed but restorable, carious and in need of **e**xtraction, and filled.

DG Distogingival.

DI Disto-incisal.

DL Distolingual.

DLa Distolabial.

DLaI Distolabio-incisal.

DLaP Distolabiopulpal.

DLI Distolinguo-incisal.

DLO Distolinguo-occlusal.

DLP Distolinguopulpal.

dmf The expression used to indicate the number of **d**ecayed, **m**issing or **f**illed teeth in the primary dentition.

DMF The expression used to indicate the number of **D**ecayed, **M**issing or **F**illed teeth in the permanent dentition; it gives an index of the caries experience of both individuals and of groups.

DMFS The expression used to indicate the number of **D**ecayed, **M**issing or **F**illed **S**urfaces on permanent teeth; it gives an index of the caries experience of both individuals and of groups.

DO Disto-occlusal.

DP Distopulpal.

DPL Distopulpolingual.

DPLa Distopulpolabial.

dacryon The point of juncture of the frontal, lacrimal and maxillary bones; one of a pair of craniometric landmarks.

dakryon *See* dacryon.

dam *See* rubber dam.

dappen dish A small decagonal glass stand, cupped at both ends, used to hold small quantities of medicaments during operative procedures on the teeth.

d'Arcet's metal (J. d'Arcet, 1727-1801. French chemist and physician). An alloy of tin, lead and bismuth, formerly used in dentistry, particularly for dies.

Darling's disease (S.T. Darling, 1872-1925. American physician). *Histoplasmosis.

dartrous Herpetic.

Daubenton's angle (L.J.M. Daubenton, 1716-1800. French physician). Occipital *angle.

Davis crown A ready-made porcelain detachable post crown, having the post cemented into the artificial crown and into the tooth root.

de- Prefix signifying *from, loss of, taken from*; it also indicates the reversal of a process, or a negative effect.

de Salle's line (E.F. de Salle, 1796-1873. French physician). Nasal *line.

dead 1. Without life. 2. Without sensation.

dead tracts Areas of dentine tubules beneath a carious lesion in which the odontoblast processes have died and the pulpal ends have been blocked by calcific matter.

débridement The removal of dead tissue and foreign matter from a wound.

debris 1. Any foreign matter attached to the surface of a tooth. 2. Any pieces of tooth substance removed by operation.
food d. Food remnants and bacteria loosely attached to the tooth, which can be removed by rinsing.
organic d. Remains after the degeneration of micro-organisms or of necrotic tissue; may be found, for example, in a root canal.

deca- Prefix signifying *ten*.

decalcification Loss or removal of the calcium salts in bone or calcified tissue.

decalcify To remove calcium salts in bone or calcified tissue.

decay 1. The progressive decomposition of organic matter. 2. The gradual decline in health, especially in old age. 3. Dental *caries.

deci- Prefix signifying *one-tenth*.

deciduous Regularly or naturally shed; not permanent.

decongestant 1. Producing or aiding in the reduction of swelling or congestion. 2. Any agent used for this purpose.

decuspation Removal of a tooth cusp, or cusps.

decussate To intersect or form an X-shaped crossing; used of nerve and muscle fibres.

decussation An intersection or X-shaped crossing of symmetrical parts; a chiasma.

dedentition Loss of teeth, more especially due to atrophy of the sockets in old age.

deep Some distance below the surface; as opposed to *superficial*.

deep temporal nerve Motor nerve to the temporal muscles. *See* Table of Nerves—temporalis profundi.

deficiency disease Any disease caused by absence or shortage of some element vital to bodily health.

deflect To alter the course or direction of anything.

deflection A turning to one side; altering the course or direction.

deformity Malformation of an organ or part.

degeneration Gradual deterioration of tissue, with loss of function and chemical change within the tissue.
calcareous d. Degeneration accompanied by deposit of calcareous material in the degenerative tissue.
calcific d. Diffuse pulp *calcification.

degloving A surgical procedure to turn back a mucoperiosteal flap and so expose a large area of bone.

deglutition Swallowing.

deglutitive, deglutitory Relating to deglutition.

degradation The reduction of an organic chemical compound to one containing a smaller number of carbon atoms.

degustation The function of tasting.

dehiscence The development of an opening or split.
implant d. A split in the covering epithelium leaving one area of an implant exposed.
mandibular d. Extreme resorption of the mandible, resulting in the exposure of the inferior alveolar nerve.
root d. A pathological condition in which the vestibular surface of a tooth root is exposed to the oral cavity over some or all of the apical two-thirds of its length.

dehydration 1. Loss or removal of water from the body, or from any tissues. 2. The condition resulting from this removal or loss.

deleterious Harmful, injurious.

demi- Prefix signifying *one half.*

demineralization Loss or removal of minerals from the body.

demulcent 1. Bland, soothing, allaying irritation of inflamed surfaces, particularly of the mucous membrane. 2. Any soothing substance.

denervation Removal or resection of a nerve or nerves.

dens (*pl.* dentes) Latin for *tooth*; used in anatomical nomenclature.
d. acutus An incisor tooth.
d. adversus An incisor tooth.
d. angularis A canine tooth.
d. bicuspidatus A premolar tooth.
d. caninus A canine tooth.
d. cariosus A carious tooth.
d columellari A molar tooth.
d. deciduus A deciduous tooth.
d. evaginatus A condition in which the pulp horn extends into a core of dentine on the occlusal surface of a first or second premolar; it is most often found in individuals of Oriental origin.
d. excertus A tooth projecting in front of the dental arch.
d. incisivus An incisor tooth.
d. invaginatus 1. A form of tooth anomaly where there is a deep fold on the lingual surface of an incisor, either partially or totally lined with enamel. 2. *Dens in dente.
d. lacteus A primary tooth.
d. permanens A permanent tooth; a tooth of the second dentition.
d. premolaris A premolar tooth.
d. primoris An incisor tooth.
d. sapientiae A third molar, or wisdom tooth.
d. serotinus A third molar tooth.
d. tomici An incisor tooth.

dens in dente A condition in which a tooth-like structure is present within the pulp chamber of a tooth.

dent-, denta-, dento- Prefix signifying *tooth or teeth.*

dentagra 1. Toothache. 2. A key or forceps for tooth extraction.

dental Relating to the teeth and gums.

dental artery 1. British terminology for *alveolar* artery. *See* Table of Arteries—alveolaris. 2. One of the branches of the alveolar artery supplying the teeth in the maxilla or the mandible. *See* Table of Arteries—dentalis[2].

dental nerve In new terminology, branches of the alveolar nerve supplying the teeth. *See* Table of Nerves—dentalis. *Also* British terminology for *alveolar* nerve. *See* Table of Nerves—alveolaris.

dentalgia Toothache.

dentaphone A type of deaf-aid which transmits vibrations from the teeth to the auditory nerve.

dentarpaga An old instrument used in tooth extraction.

dentary One of the several lower jaw bones which may be present in non-mammalian vertebrates.

dentate Having teeth, or projections like teeth on a serrated edge.

dentation The condition of having tooth-like projections or processes.

dentelation *Dentation.

dentia praecox Premature eruption of the primary teeth.

dentia tarda Delayed eruption of the primary teeth.

dentiaskiascope A dental x-ray apparatus.

dentibuccal Relating to the teeth and the cheek.

denticle 1. A small tooth or tooth-like process. 2. A pulp stone.

denticulate Having tooth-like projections.

dentification The process of tooth formation.

dentiform In the shape of a tooth.

dentifrice Paste, powder or liquid used in cleaning the teeth.

dentigerous Containing or bearing teeth.

dentilabial Relating to the teeth and the lips.

dentilave A mouthwash.

dentilingual Relating to the teeth and the tongue.

dentilinimentum National Formulary name for drops prescribed for toothache.

dentimeter An instrument used to measure teeth.

dentin *See* dentine.

dentinal Relating to dentine.

dentinalgia Pain or sensitiveness of the dentine.

dentine, dentin The mineralized organic tissue forming the body of the tooth, surrounding the pulp and covered by enamel or cementum.
adventitious d. Irregular secondary *dentine.
calcified d. Transparent *dentine.
circumpulpal d. The inner layer of dentine surrounding the pulp chamber; it contains fine collagen fibres which run at right angles to the tubules.
cover d. Mantle *dentine.
functional d. Regular secondary *dentine.
hereditary opalescent d. *Dentinogenesis imperfecta.
interglobular d. Poorly mineralized patches of dentine, where the globules have not fused together.
intratubular d. The mineralized matrix found in the tubules of *orthodentine.
mantle d. The thin, superficial outer layer of dentine.
peritubular d. The layer of highly mineralized dentine lining the walls of dentinal tubules.
primary d. The dentine that is present in the tooth when it is fully formed.
reparative d. Irregular secondary *dentine.
sclerotic d. Transparent *dentine.
secondary d. A new deposit of dentine laid down as a result of normal or traumatic stimuli after the completed formation of the tooth. It may be *regular* - associated with normal stimuli; or *irregular* - formed as a result of trauma or disease.
tertiary d. Irregular secondary *dentine.
transparent d. Dentine having some tubules which have been calcified, giving a translucent appearance. It may be caused by injury, abrasion or ageing.
vitreous d. A very hard type of dentine, having few dentinal tubules.

dentine bridge A layer of dentine that reseals an exposed pulp or forms over the excised surface after pulpotomy.

dentinification The formation of dentine; dentinogenesis.

dentinitis Inflammation of the dentinal tubules.

dentinoblast One of the cells from which dentine is formed; an odontoblast.

dentinoblastoma A benign tumour composed of dentine-forming cells.

dentinocemental Relating to both the dentine and the cementum of a tooth.

dentinogenesis The process of dentine formation.

dentinogenesis imperfecta Defective mineralization of dentine, characterized by an opalescent appearance of the teeth; it is an hereditary condition.

dentinoid 1. Resembling dentine. 2. A tumour composed of dentine. 3. *Predentine.

dentinoma A very rare benign tumour containing odontogenic epithelium and immature connective tissue, characterized by the formation of abnormal, poorly mineralized dentine; it is most commonly found in bone.

dentinosteoid A mixed tumour composed of dentine and bone tissue.

dentiparous Relating to the formation of teeth.

dentiphone *Dentaphone.

dentist Any person who practises dentistry, and is qualified and licensed to do so.

dentistry That branch of medicine concerned with oral and dental diseases and their prevention and treatment, and with oral prostheses.
community d. That branch of dentistry providing for the treatment and prevention of dental disease within the community, and the promotion of good oral health.
conservative d. That branch of restorative dentistry concerned with the treatment and restoration of individual diseased or injured teeth.
cosmetic d. That branch of dentistry concerned with restoration or improvement of appearance.
forensic d. That branch of dentistry concerned with the examination, interpretation and presentation of evidence relating to dental or oral matters in a legal context.
implant d. That branch of dentistry concerned with the design and use of prostheses involving some form of oral implant surgically inserted into hard or soft tissue within the mouth.
paediatric d. The care and treatment of teeth and oral conditions in children.
preventive d. Prevention and preventive treatment for diseases of the mouth and teeth, and for malformation and the promotion of good oral health.
prosthetic d. Restoration of function and appearance by replacement of missing teeth with full or partial dentures, bridges, etc.
public health d. That branch of dentistry concerned with dental health in the community, its promotion through health education, the provision of preventive and other forms of treatment for dental disease, and associated research.
restorative d. A comprehensive term, which may include conservative dentistry, prosthetics and periodontal therapy, and also orthodontics, for that branch of dentistry concerned with the provision of a healthy and functional dentition for the dentate or the edentulous.

dentitia praecox *Dentia praecox.

dentitia tarda *Dentia tarda.

dentitio difficilis Teething troubles.

dentition 1. The teeth in the jaws. 2. Also used occasionally to mean the eruption of the teeth.
deciduous d. Primary *dentition.
mixed d. That stage of development during which both primary and permanent teeth may be found together in the mouth.
permanent d. The second teeth, normally thirty-two in man: four incisors, two canines, four

premolars, and six molars in each jaw.

primary d. The first teeth to erupt, which are gradually shed; usually twenty in number in man: four incisors, two canines and four molars in each jaw.

dentoalveolar Relating to the teeth and the alveolar process.

dentoalveolitis *Pyorrhoea alveolaris.

dentocemental *Dentinocemental.

dentofacial Relating to that area of the face that contains and is supported by the teeth and the gums.

dentography A description of the teeth.

dentoid In the form of a tooth; tooth-like.

dentoidin The basic organic substance of a tooth.

dentolegal Relating to dental juris-prudence.

dentology *Dentistry.

dentoma A dentinal tumour; an odontoma.

dentomechanical Relating to dental mechanics.

dentomental Relating to the teeth and the chin.

dentonasal Relating to the teeth and the nose.

dentonomy The classification of the teeth.

dentosurgical Relating to dental surgery.

dentotropic Attracted to those tissues which compose the teeth.

dentulous Having natural teeth present in the mouth; as opposed to *edentulous*.

dentural Relating to a denture.

denture 1. A full set of natural teeth. 2. A set of artificial teeth.

complete d. A denture that replaces all the teeth in either the upper or the lower jaw, or both.

continuous gum d. An obsolete form of denture constructed by fusing a porcelain base and teeth on to a platinum matrix.

full d. Complete *denture.

immediate d., immediate replacement d. A denture constructed for insertion immediately after the removal of the natural teeth.

implant d. An artificial denture supported by a framework fastened to the alveolar process beneath the periosteum, and having protruding abutments; it may be *complete* or *partial*.

partial d. A denture that replaces some of the natural teeth in one jaw.

skeleton d. A form of partial denture which is mainly tooth-borne, and which has connectors of the smallest size consistent with adequate strength, leaving the mucous membrane and the gingival margins exposed.

spoon d. A form of upper partial denture for the restoration of one or more anterior teeth, the teeth being attached to a plastic base plate which extends over the whole of the hard palate, but does not cover the gingival margins of the natural teeth.

trial d. A trial plate, complete with artificial teeth, for fitting in the mouth and for adjustments before the final completion of a denture.

denture base *In dentistry,* that part of a denture which rests on the alveolar ridges, and which may extend over the palate, and to which the artificial teeth are attached.

denture flange The buccal, labial or lingual vertical extension from the denture base into the oral cavity.

denturist A dental technician who has been further trained, qualified and licensed to make and supply dentures to the general public.

deossification The loss or removal of those materials that give bone its characteristics; the absorption of bony material.

depigmentation The loss or removal of pigment.

depolymerization The process whereby a polymer is broken down into its constituent molecules.

deposit 1. Sediment. 2. *In dentistry,* soft or hard material adhering to the tooth surface.

depression 1. An indentation in a surface. 2. A general state of emotional dejection or unhappiness.

depressor muscles Any of the muscles that depress or pull down. *See* Table of Muscles.

derma-, dermato-, dermo- Prefix signifying *skin.*

dermal Relating to the skin.

dermatostomatitis Erythema multiforme with involvement of the conjunctiva and the oral tissues; Stevens-Johnson syndrome.

dermoid 1. Skin-like. 2. A dermoid cyst.

dermolabial Relating to the skin and the lips.

descending cervical nerve, descending hypoglossal nerve *Ansa cervicalis.

desensitization *of dentine* The reduction of sensitivity in exposed dentine by the application of a prophylactic preparation.

desiccation The process of drying.

desmodont, desmodontium Periodontal *ligament.

desmodontal Relating to the periodontal *ligament.

desmoid 1. Resembling a ligament; fibrous. 2. A hard form of fibroma.

desmosome The structure forming the site of contact between adjacent cells, especially epithelial cells.

desquamation Peeling off of the outer epithelial layer.

desquamative Relating to desquamation.

detergent A surface-active cleansing agent in solution; it may be used to cleanse or purify a wound, ulcer, etc.

detrital Relating to or composed of detritus.

detrition Wearing away, as of teeth, by abrasion.

detritus 1. Any waste matter from disintegrated tissue. 2. *In dentistry,* waste matter adhering to a tooth surface or to disintegrated tooth substance.

deuterocone The mesiobuccal cusp of a maxillary premolar in a mammal.

deuteroconid The mesiobuccal cusp of a mandibular premolar in a mammal.

deuteromere The lingual half of the enamel organ of a tooth.

deviation A turning away from a regular, normal course, position or standard.

devitalization The destruction of vitality, especially, *in dentistry,* the vitality of the dental pulp.
pulp d. Any procedure that destroys the vitality of the dental pulp.

devitalize To destroy vitality; *in dentistry,* to destroy the vitality of the dental pulp.

dexiotropic Relating to a clockwise spiral—i.e. one turning from left to right.

diagnosis The recognition of a disease or the location of an injury from observation of symptoms and signs.

diagnostic Relating to diagnosis.

diaphanoscopy *Transillumination.

diaphragm 1. *In anatomy*, a thin musculomembranous partition or septum. 2. *In dentistry*, a thin metal plate adapted to form a cap over a tooth root and soldered to the collar of an artificial crown.
oral d. The partition dividing the submandibular region from the sublingual, and formed by the hyoglossus and the mylohyoid muscles.
root d. That part of the epithelial root sheath which angles beneath the dental papilla early in tooth development.

diaplasis The reduction of a fracture or dislocation.

diaplastic Relating to diaplasis.

diapyema An abscess.

diapyesis *Suppuration.

diarthrosis Synovial *joint.

diastema An abnormally wide space between two adjacent teeth, occurring naturally.

diastematocheilia Congenital longitudinal fissure of the lip.

diastematoglossia Congenital longitudinal fissure of the tongue.

diastole The dilatation period in each heart beat, following the systole.

diastolic Relating to the diastole.

diathesis An hereditary condition or combination of attributes predisposing a person to susceptibility to a certain disease or diseases.

diathetic Relating to diathesis.

diatoric Referring to pinless teeth—artificial teeth which have pierced bases to allow rubber to flow in and so, when vulcanized, attach them to the denture base.

dicheilia Double *lip.

dichotomy Division into two equal branches or parts.

die A metal impression or mould from which casts or models can be made.
amalgam d. A model cast in amalgam from an impression and from which inlays or crowns may be fabricated.

die plate A sheet of metal containing dies for forming cusps on a shell crown.

diet The nutritional intake of a person.

diffuse Widespread, scattered.

digastric muscle Raises and stabilizes the hyoid bone. *See* Table of Muscles —digastricus.

digestion The process whereby food is converted into materials for assimilation or absorption by the body.

diglossia Double or bifid tongue; a developmental anomaly.

dilaceration 1. Tearing apart. 2. *In dentistry*, a condition caused by damage or fracture of a tooth during development, resulting in distortion without interruption of the normal mineralization.

dilatation, dilation The condition of being stretched or enlarged beyond the normal size.

dilatator naris muscle, dilator naris muscle M. nasalis, pars alaris. *See* Table of Muscles.

diphtheria An acute infectious disease characterized by the formation of patches of false membrane on mucous surfaces, especially of the throat and upper respiratory tract.
labial d. A localized form of diphtheria in which membrane formation occurs on the outer edges of the lips; it has been noted as a complication of cheilosis.

diphyodont Having two successive sets of teeth, the first being deciduous, and giving place to the second, permanent dentition.

diplococcal Relating to a diplococcus.

diplococcus A form of coccus which occurs attached in pairs.

Diplococcus Former name for a genus of micro-organisms, parasitic and Gram-positive, seen as elongated cells, occurring in pairs or short chains, now reassigned to other genera.
D. pneumoniae **Streptococcus pneumoniae.*

diploë The bony tissue between the tables of the cranial bones.

diploic Relating to diploë.

diprotodont Having two incisors in the lower jaw.

disc 1. A flat, circular or rounded plate-like object or structure. 2. *In dentistry,* a round, solid ring of some material such as carborundum or emery, which can be revolved in the handpiece of a dental engine and is used for polishing, cutting, or grinding teeth.
articular d. A fibrous plate between articulating bone surfaces in a joint.
interarticular d. A fibrocartilaginous plate found in some synovial joints, such as the temporomandibular joint, filling the space between the articular cartilage surfaces and held in place by a ligament.
suction d. A flexible disc attached to the fitting surface of an upper denture in an attempt to improve its retention. This method is no longer used.

discharge 1. An emission or secretion. 2. To release or set free.

disclosing agent, solution, tablet A staining agent, which, when applied to the tooth surface either as a tablet to be chewed or in a mouthwash, attaches to the bacterial plaque and other surface deposits and shows them up in some distinct colour against the normal clean enamel.

discoid 1. In the shape of a disc. 2. *In dentistry,* a type of instrument having a disc-like blade, used for excavating caries or for carving amalgam restorations. 3. A disc-shaped tablet.

discrete Separate, composed of separate parts, not joined or blended; as, for example, some lesions.

disease Any illness or abnormal state of health either of the whole body or of specific parts or organs, having characteristic symptoms. *See also* syndrome.
contagious d. A disease communicated by direct contact with an affected person, with any object with which such a person has been in contact, or with his or her secretions.
deficiency d. Any disease caused by absence or shortage of some element vital to bodily health.
degenerative d. A process of general degeneration with no specific cause, commonly found in old age.
infectious d. A disease caused by pathogenic organisms.
marble bone d. *Osteopetrosis.
occupational d. One caused by the patient's occupation; it may be organic or functional.
periodontal d. Any disease affecting the gingiva or the supporting tissues of the teeth.
pink spot d. Internal tooth *resorption.

For eponymous diseases *see* under the personal name by which the disease is known.

disinfectant Any agent that destroys pathogenic organisms.

disinfection The destruction of pathogenic organisms and their products.

disintegration Decay or decomposition.

disjunction Non-union.
craniofacial d. *Le Fort fracture of the maxilla, Class III.

disk *See* disc.

dislocation Displacement of any part from its normal position; commonly used of bones and joints.

disocclude To grind the occlusal surface of a tooth so that it does not occlude with the opposing tooth in the other jaw during mastication.

displacement 1. Removal from the normal position. 2. *In dentistry,* the malposition of a tooth, or teeth, where the whole tooth has moved in the same direction, without tilting.

disseminated Dispersed or scattered over a wide area.

distal Away from the midline; *in dentistry*, those surfaces farthest from the midline of the dental arch.

disto- Prefix signifying *distal.*

disto-angular Relating to any distal angle.

distobuccal 1. Relating to the distal and buccal surfaces of a tooth. 2. Relating to the distal and buccal walls of an occlusal cavity in a molar or premolar.
d. angle The angle formed at the junction of these walls; a *line* angle.

distobucco-occlusal Relating to the distal, buccal and occlusal surfaces of a tooth.

distobuccopulpal Relating to the distal, buccal and pulpal walls in an occlusal cavity, or in the step portion of a proximo-occlusal cavity, in a molar or premolar.
d. angle The angle formed at the junction of these walls; a *point* angle.

distocclusal *Disto-occlusal.

distocervical 1. Relating to the distal surface of a tooth cervix. 2. *Distogingival.

distoclusion A form of malocclusion in which the teeth of the lower jaw are displaced distally in relation to those in the upper jaw.

distogingival Relating to the distal and gingival walls of a buccal or lingual cavity in a molar or premolar.
d. angle The angle formed at the junction of these walls; a *line* angle.

disto-incisal 1. Relating to the distal surface and the incisal edge of an anterior tooth. 2. Relating to the distal and incisal walls in a labial or lingual cavity.
d. angle The angle formed at the junction of these walls; a *line* angle.

distolabial 1. Relating to the distal and labial surfaces of a tooth. 2. Relating to the distal and labial walls in the step portion of a proximo-incisal cavity.
d. angle The angle formed at the junction of these walls; a *line* angle.

distolabio-incisal Relating to the distal and labial surfaces and the incisal edge of an anterior tooth.

distolingual 1. Relating to the distal and lingual surfaces of a tooth. 2. Relating to the distal and lingual walls of an occlusal cavity in a molar or premolar.
d. angle The angle formed at the junction of these walls; a *line* angle.

distolinguocclusal *Distolinguo-occlusal.

distolinguo-incisal Relating to the distal and lingual surfaces and the incisal edge of an anterior tooth.

distolinguo-occlusal Relating to the distal, lingual and occlusal surfaces of a tooth.

distolinguopulpal Relating to the distal, lingual and pulpal walls of an occlusal cavity, or in the step

portion of a proximo-occlusal cavity in a molar or premolar.
d. angle The angle formed at the junction of these walls; a *point* angle.

distomolar A small supernumerary tooth which may erupt behind the molar teeth.

distomus Accessory *jaws.

disto-occlusal 1. Relating to the distal and occlusal surfaces of a tooth. 2. Relating to the distal and occlusal walls in a buccal or lingual cavity.
d. angle The angle formed at the junction of these walls; a *line* angle.

distoplacement Distal displacement of a tooth or teeth.

distopulpal Relating to the distal and pulpal walls of an occlusal cavity, or in the step portion of a proximo-occlusal cavity in a molar or premolar.
d. angle The angle formed at the junction of these walls; a *line* angle.

distopulpolabial Relating to the distal, pulpal and labial walls of a cavity in an incisor or a canine.
d. angle The angle formed at the junction of these walls; a *point* angle.

distopulpolingual Relating to the distal, pulpal and lingual walls of a tooth cavity.
d. angle The angle formed at the junction of these walls; a *point* angle.

distortor oris muscle M. zygomaticus minor. *See* Table of Muscles.

distoversion The position of a tooth inclined away from the median line.

ditching *In dentistry,* a defect occurring at the junction of a restoration with the tooth substance, which produces a characteristic ditch-like appearance.

Dodge crown A porcelain crown baked to a hollow metal cone and attached to the tooth by a wooden post.

Dolder bar A metal bar attached to the jaw or to abutment teeth, used to provide retention for an overlay denture.

dolicho- Prefix signifying *long.*

dolichocephalic Having an abnormally long skull.

dolichocranial *Dolichocephalic.

dolichoeuromesocephalic Having an abnormally long skull which is also very broad in the temporal region.

dolichoeuro-opisthocephalic Having an abnormally long skull which is also very broad in the occipital region.

dolichoeuroprocephalic Having an abnormally long skull which is also very broad in the frontal region.

dolichofacial Having an abnormally long face.

dolicholeptocephalic Having an abnormally long and narrow skull.

dolichoplatycephalic Having an abnormally long and broad flat skull.

dolichoprosopic *Dolichofacial.

dolichouranic Having an abnormally long palate, with a palatomaxillary index of less than 110.

dolorimetry The measurement of pain.

dolorogenic Pain-producing.

Donaldson broach (R.B. Donaldson, contemporary American dentist). A fine, barbed broach used particularly for removing the contents of pulp canals.

dormant 1. Inactive, quiescent. 2. Potential, concealed.

dorsal Relating to the dorsum or back; as opposed to *ventral.*

dorsalis linguae artery Supplies the dorsum of the tongue, tonsils and fauces. *See* Table of Arteries.

dorsalis nasi artery Supplies the skin of the dorsum of the nose. *See* Table of Arteries.

dorsonasal Relating to the bridge of the nose.

dorsoventral From the back to the front.

dorsum The back of any organ.

dose One measured portion of any medicine which is to be taken at one time.

dovetail A flared cavity, like the spread of a dove's tail, serving as a lock in a metal or wooden joint; *in dentistry* it is applied to the flared cavity which serves to lock a filling or inlay in place in a tooth.

dowel *Post.

drainage The gradual removal of fluid from a cavity or wound.

dressing 1. A medicament used to promote wound healing. 2. A covering for a wound used for protection or to assist healing. 3. *In dentistry*, a temporary filling or restoration.

drift The horizontal movement or displacement of a tooth.

drifting *of the teeth* Movement of the teeth within the arch.

drill An instrument with spiral flukes used in a dental engine for boring or cutting holes in a tooth or in bone.

drop
enamel d. *Enameloma.

dropsy The abnormal accumulation of serous fluid in the tissues or in the body cavity.

drug Any medicinal substance.

Dubreuil-Chambardel syndrome (L. Dubreuil-Chambardel, 1879-1927. French dentist). A syndrome characterized by caries of the maxillary anterior teeth developing in teenagers aged between 14 and 17 years, and followed by caries in the other teeth later.

duct A tube or canal serving as an outlet for secretion; used especially of glandular outlets.
lingual d. Caecal *foramen of the tongue.
nasolacrimal d. The membranous canal through which tears pass from the lacrimal sac to the nasal cavity.
nasopalatine d. A small opening in the midline of the palate in the embryo, which persists for a time between the primitive palate and the palatal processes of the maxilla but is finally closed by epithelial fusion; its position in the hard palate is taken by the incisive canal.
parotid d. The duct through which saliva secreted by the parotid gland flows into the mouth; its opening lies opposite to the maxillary molars on the buccal surface. *Also called* Blasius' duct.
salivary d. Any one of the ducts from the salivary glands through which the saliva flows.
sublingual d. One of the ducts of the sublingual gland; Bartholin's duct.
submandibular d., submaxillary d. The duct through which saliva from the sublingual and submandibular glands flows into the mouth; its openings are on either side of the lingual frenum. *Also called* Wharton's duct.
thyroglossal d., thyrolingual d. A duct extending from the thyroid gland to the base of the tongue; found in the embryo and occasionally persisting into adult life.

For eponymous ducts *see* under the name of the person first describing the duct.

Dutch gold An alloy of zinc and copper.

dwarfism The condition of being a dwarf; underdevelopment of the body.

dys- Prefix signifying *difficult, painful.*

dysaesthesia An impairment of feeling or sensation; a condition in which normal stimuli produce disagreeable sensations.

dysallilognathia The condition of having dissimilar, not matching, jaws.

dyscephaly Any malformation of the facial bones or the skull.

dysfibrinogenaemia *Afibrinogenaemia or *hypofibrinogenaemia.

dysfunction Impairment or abnormality of function.

dysgnathic Relating to imperfectly developed and malrelated jaws.

dyskeratosis Abnormal or premature keratinization of the epithelial cells of the skin or mucous membrane; sometimes associated with premalignant lesions.

dyslalia Impairment of speech due to some abnormality of the speech organs.

dysodontiasis Painful, difficult or delayed eruption of the teeth.

dysosteogenesis *Dysostosis.

dysostosis Congenital defective bone formation.

cleidocranial d. A rare form of dysostosis characterized by defective formation of the cranial bones and partial or complete absence of the clavicles; eruption of the teeth is often affected, and there may be partial anodontia.

craniofacial d. An hereditary disease of bone characterized by maxillary hypoplasia, mandibular prognathism, short upper lip and protruding lower lip, protrusion of the frontal bones, hypertelorism and exophthalmos; *also called* Crouzon's disease.

mandibulofacial d. A rare congenital malformation of the face and jaws, characterized by hypoplasia of the facial bones, anti-mongoloid slanting of the lower eyelids, deformity of the pinna, macrostomia and a general fish-like facies; *also called* Berry-Franceschetti syndrome.

dysphagia The condition of being unable to swallow or of experiencing great difficulty in swallowing.

sideropenic d. *Plummer-Vinson syndrome.

dysplasia Abnormal formation or development.

chondro-ectodermal d. *Ellis-van Creveld syndrome.

cleidocranial d. Cleidocranial *dysostosis.

dentinal d. An hereditary disorder affecting both the primary and the permanent dentitions; it may be *radicular* or *coronal*, and is characterized by atypical dentinal tubule formation and either obliteration of the pulp chamber or the presence of multiple pulp stones.

dento-alveolar d. Any developmental anomaly of the dento-alveolar structures.

ectodermal d. An hereditary disease characterized by defective development of all dermal structures, including the teeth.

fibrous d. of the jaws. A benign lesion in which normal bone is replaced by cellular fibrous tissue, fusing directly to the surrounding bone with no line of demarcation; it is generally found in the young, the familial form producing cherubism.

odontogenic d. *Odontodysplasia.

periapical cemental d. A type of cementoma, similar in structure to a cementifying fibroma, occurring in the incisor region of the mandible and seen most commonly in post-menopausal women.
periapical fibrous d. Periapical cemental *dysplasia.

dyspnoea Laboured breathing; shortness of breath.

dyspnoeic Relating to or characterized by dyspnoea.

dystrophic Relating to or affected by dystrophy.

dystrophy Defective nutrition.

E

e- Prefix signifying *from, out of, without.*

EBV Epstein-Barr virus.

exhib. Abbreviation for *exhibeatur*—let it be given; used in prescription writing.

ext. Abbreviation for *extract.*

ear The organ of hearing.

Ebner's fibrils (V. von Ebner, 1842-1925. Austrian histologist). Connective tissue fibres pervading the dentinal matrix.

Ebner's glands (V. von Ebner, 1842-1925. Austrian histologist). Serous lingual glands.

Ebner's lines (V. von Ebner, 1842-1925. Austrian histologist). Fine incremental lines in dentine, representing daily growth during tooth development.

ebur dentis *Dentine.

eburnation An increase in hardness or density of tooth or bone structure following a pathological change.

eburneous Like ivory.

eburnitis An increase in hardness or density of dentine structure, usually seen in exposed dentine; there may also be discoloration to brown or even black.

eccentric Situated away from a centre.

ecchymosis A diffuse extravasation of blood into the tissues; also discoloration of the skin which this causes.

ecderon The outer layer of the mucous membrane and the skin.

eclabium Eversion of a lip, or lips.

ecto- Prefix signifying *outside*, or *on.*

ectoconchion The point on the lateral border of the orbit which marks the greatest breadth measured from the dacryon or from the maxillofrontale; one of a pair of craniometric landmarks.

ectoderm The outermost of the three primary germ layers of the embryo, from which are developed the epidermis, the external sense organs, and the oral and anal mucous membrane.

ectoloph The outer ridge on an equine upper molar.

ectomesenchyme One of the tissues of the embryonic neural crest which migrates to the head to form the cartilages of the branchial arch and participates in the inductive interactions of odontogenesis.

ectopic In an abnormal place or position.

ectosteal Relating to, or situated on, the outside of a bone.

ectropion *Eversion, especially of the eyelid or eyelashes.

edema *See* oedema.

edentate *Edentulous.

edentia *Anodontia.

edentulism The condition of having no natural teeth in the mouth; it may be *partial* or *complete.*

edentulous Having no teeth.

efferent Carrying or conveying away from a centre or from a part; as opposed to *afferent.*

Ehrenritter's ganglion (J. Ehrenritter, d. 1790. Austrian anatomist). The superior ganglion of the glossopharyngeal nerve, in the jugular foramen.

eisanthema *Enanthema.

elastic *In orthodontics*, an elastic or rubber band used for the purposes of traction.

intermaxillary e's. Orthodontic elastic bands attached to wires or appliances and stretched between the jaws.
intramaxillary e's. Orthodontic elastic bands attached to wires or appliances within one jaw.
rubber dam e's. Orthodontic elastics made from rubber dam material.
vertical e's. Elastics applied with the traction vertical, perpendicular to the occlusal plane, to improve intercuspation.

elastomer A polymer having elastic, rubber-like properties; used in impression materials.

electro- Prefix signifying *electricity.*

electroanaesthesia, electroanalgesia Anaesthesia or analgesia induced by the use of an electric current.

electrocautery 1. Cauterization by low-voltage current producing burn-like tissue repair, but with no control over the extent or quality of tissue destruction. 2. The apparatus used for this purpose.

electrocision The cutting of tissues by electrocautery or electrotome.

electrocoagulation Biterminal application of damped high-frequency alternating current, dehydrating cells and coagulating their contents in a necrotic zone limited to the surface of the area to which it is applied; as, for example, in haemostasis.

electrodent The negative electrode on a vitalometer.

electrodesiccation Deeply penetrating tissue dehydration produced by the insertion of electrodes into the tissue.

electroexcision *Electrocision.

electromallet An electrically or electronically operated instrument used to pack and condense gold into a prepared cavity.

electromedication *Iontophoresis.

electroresection Excision by electrosurgery.

electrosection Biterminal application of undamped high-frequency alternating current used with a surgical electrode moved along the tissue surface to create precise surgical incisions.

electrosterilization The use of electrolysis to decontaminate a root canal; a rarely used procedure.

electrosurgery High-frequency alternating current used for dehydration, coagulation and sectioning of tissues; able to be controlled in use.

elephantiasis gingivae Gingival *fibromatosis.

elevator An instrument used as a lever to remove sunken or embedded parts or particles; *in dentistry*, an instrument used to remove tooth roots, or those teeth that cannot be extracted with forceps.
angular e. One in which the blade is set at an angle to the shaft.
apical e. One designed to remove from the socket a fractured and retained tooth apex.
root e. One designed to remove a fractured and retained root; root elevators may come in pairs, left and right.
screw e. An instrument that can be screwed into a retained root in order to draw it out.
straight e. One in which the blade, shaft and handle are all in one straight line.
wedge e. One designed for use in tooth extraction; it fits into a hole drilled in the tooth root, and is used to work the tooth loose.

For eponymous elevators *see* under the name of the designer.

elinguation Removal of the tongue.

Ellis-van Creveld syndrome (R.W.B. Ellis, b. 1902. English paediatrician; S. van Creveld, b. 1894. Dutch paediatrician). A disease characterized by defective development of the nails, teeth and hair; in the mouth there may be tooth defects and delayed eruption or absence of teeth.

elongation 1. The process of becoming longer. 2. The condition of being lengthened. 3. *In dentistry*, pathological tooth movement out of the socket; extrusion.

emaciation A wasted condition; the result of extreme loss of flesh.

emaculation The removal of skin lesions and freckles, and more particularly of skin tumours.

emailloblast *Ameloblast.

emailloid A tumour arising from the tooth enamel.

embed *In histology*, to fix tissue in some rigid material, such as wax, in order to cut thin sections for microscope study.

embolism The sudden blockage of a blood vessel by a clot or other obstruction within the blood stream, causing failure of the circulation.

embolus An obstruction or clot in the blood stream blocking a vessel and so restricting or stopping the circulation.

embrasure The space on each side of the contact point, created by the rounding of the approximal surfaces away from each other.
buccal e. The space between molars or premolars, opening towards the cheek.
labial e. The space between incisors or canines, opening towards the lip.
lingual e. The space between any two teeth, opening towards the tongue.

embryo The fertilized ovum during the early stage of development; in man it is the foetus in the first three months of growth.

embryology The science and study of the embryo and of its development.

embryonic Relating to an embryo; in an early stage of development.

eminence Any prominent or projecting part, especially one on a bone surface.
canine e. The ridge on the anterior surface of the maxilla, occurring over the canine tooth socket.
hypobranchial e. A median swelling between the tongue and the laryngotracheal groove in the embryo, from which is developed the epiglottis and the aryepiglottic folds, and the posterior third of the tongue.

emollient 1. Soothing or softening. 2. Any agent used to soften or soothe the skin, or to soothe an irritated or inflamed internal surface.

emphragma salivare *Ranula.

emphysema A distention caused by air in the interstices of the connective tissues, or of the alveolar tissue of the lungs.
cervicofacial e. Accumulation of air in the tissues of the face and neck, producing rapid and painful unilateral swelling; it may occur after mid-face fractures, tooth extraction, or the use of compressed air in treatment of a periodontal pocket or root canal.

empyema The accumulation of pus in a body cavity or hollow organ.

enamel *In dentistry*, vitreous calcific tissue covering the dentine of the tooth crown.
aprismatic e. A form of enamel consisting of a solid layer without prisms, found on the outer surface

of dental enamel and in the initial layers.

curled e. Enamel in which the prismatic rods are curled round.

dwarfed e. Nanoid *enamel.

gnarled e. Enamel in which the prismatic rods are twisted in various directions.

mottled e. Hypoplasia and discoloration of the tooth enamel due to ingestion of excessive amounts of fluorine during the developmental period; chronic endemic (dental) fluorosis.

nanoid e. Enamel that is thinner than normal.

straight e. Enamel in which the prismatic rods run straight.

enamel agenesis *Hypoplasia of the enamel.

enamel cap The enamel covering the top of a developing tooth papilla.

enamel capsule *Enamel cuticle[1].

enamel cell *Ameloblast.

enamel cord A temporary structure in the developing tooth linking the enamel knot to the outer dental lamina.

enamel cuticle 1. An acellular layer of organic material secreted on to the surface of enamel; it is thought to be the final product of ameloblasts. As it cannot be seen with an electron microscope, it is thought by some to be an artefact; *also called* primary enamel cuticle. 2. Acquired *pellicle.

enamel drop *Enameloma.

enamel fibre *Enamel prism.

enamel fissure *Fissure[2].

enamel hatchet A type of chisel with a contra-angled shaft giving it a hatchet form.

enamel hypoplasia *Amelogenesis imperfecta.

enamel knot An aggregation of epithelial cells at the base of the enamel organ, which have not yet differentiated into stellate reticulum.

enamel lamellae The flat, organic bands running transversely through the enamel of a tooth.

enamel matrix The organic secretion of the ameloblasts within which the inorganic enamel crystallites are laid down.

enamel niche One of a pair of funnel-shaped depressions in the dental lamina of a developing tooth.

enamel nodule *Enameloma.

enamel organ A proliferation of the dental lamina enclosing the dental papilla; it determines the shape of the tooth crown and forms the dental enamel.

enamel pearl *Enameloma.

enamel prism One of the prismatic rods of which tooth enamel is made up.

enamel proteins Those proteins synthesized by the ameloblasts during amelogenesis and forming part of the enamel matrix. Those that are newly secreted are termed *young* enamel proteins, and those remaining in the fully developed enamel are termed *mature* enamel proteins.

enamel pulp The stellate *reticulum.

enamel rod *Enamel prism.

enamel spindles Short extensions into the enamel, across the amelo-dentinal junction, of dentinal tubules.

enamel striae of Retzius (M.G. Retzius, 1842-1919. Swedish anatomist). Lines visible under a microscope which mark the successive layers of mineralization in tooth enamel.

enamel tufts Bundles of poorly mineralized enamel rods extending into the tooth enamel from the amelodentinal junction.

enamelins Mature *enamel proteins.

enameloblast *Ameloblast.

enameloblastoma *Ameloblastoma.

enameloma A benign tumour arising from embryonic enamel tissue.

enanthema, enanthem An eruption occurring on a mucous surface, or on any surface within the body; as opposed to *exanthema.*

enarthrosis Spheroidal *joint.

encapsulated Enclosed in a capsule.

encephalo- Prefix signifying *brain.*

Endamoeba See Entamoeba.

endemic Prevalent in a particular region.

endepidermis *Epithelium.

endermic, endermatic Absorbed through the skin.

endo- Prefix signifying *within.*

endocarditis Inflammation of the endocardium, the lining of the interior of the heart, generally affecting the valves.

endochondral Within a cartilage; developing in cartilage.

endocrine gland Any one of the ductless glands (adrenal, thyroid, etc.) supplying internal secretions to the body directly through the blood stream.

endocrinodontia The study of internal glandular secretion in relation to tooth development.

endodontics, endodontia That branch of restorative dentistry which is concerned with the diagnosis and treatment of injuries and diseases affecting the tooth root, tooth pulp and periapical tissues.

endodontitis Inflammation of the tooth pulp; *also called* pulpitis.

endodontium The tissues of the dentine and the dental pulp.

endodontology The scientific study of the tooth root, tooth pulp and periapical tissues in health and disease.

endodontoma Internal tooth *resorption.

endogenous Arising or developing within an organism.

endognathion The hypothetical inner portion of the premaxilla.

endolarynx The interior of the larynx, the laryngeal cavity.

endolymph The liquid in the membranous labyrinth of the ear.

endolymphatic Relating to, or derived from, the endolymph.

endomolare The point marking the most lingual margin of the alveolus in the region of the maxillary permanent second molars; one of a pair of craniometric landmarks.

endosteal Within the bone.

endothelial Relating to, or derived from, the endothelium.

endothelioma A tumour arising from the endothelial cells.

endothelium The membrane lining the heart and blood vessels.

endotoxin A heat stable, phospholipid-polysaccharide-protein complex contained as a structural part of the cell of many Gram-negative bacteria, released by the disintegration of the cell.

enervation Removal of a nerve or of part of a nerve.

engine

dental e. The apparatus used to drive instruments for cutting, drilling and polishing the teeth; the interchangeable parts are held in an angled handpiece, and the driving power is supplied by some form of motor, generally electric.

engomphosis *Gomphosis[1].

engorgement 1. Excess of blood in any part of the body. 2. Localized congestion or distention.

enostosis A localized morbid bone growth arising within the bone cavity.

Entamoeba A genus of amoeba, including species parasitic to humans.
E. buccalis **Entamoeba gingivalis.*
E. gingivalis A species found about the gums and in the plaque on teeth.

Enterobacteriaceae Former name for a large family of micro-organisms of the order Eubacteriales, Gram-negative, facultatively anaerobic and rod-shaped, now reassigned to other genera.

enthlasis A depressed and comminuted fracture of the skull.

ento- Prefix signifying *inside, within.*

entocone The lingual posterior cusp of a maxillary molar.

entoconid The lingual posterior cusp of a mandibular molar.

entoglossal Occurring within the tongue.

entomion The point at the tip of the mastoid angle of the parietal bone where it crosses the parietal notch of the temporal bone.

entopic Occurring in the normal position.

entostosis *Enostosis.

entropion *Inversion, especially of the eyelid or eyelashes.

enucleate To remove an organ or part, or a circumscribed, space-filling lesion entire from its outer sheath or covering.

enula The inner aspect of the gums.

envelope 1. Any outer covering. 2. A surrounding membrane or capsule.

epactal Supernumerary.

ephemeral Of short duration, temporary.

epi- Prefix signifying *upon* or *above*.

epiagnathus One having a deficient upper jaw.

epicranius muscle Muscular cover of the scalp. *See* Table of Muscles.

epidemic 1. Affecting a large number of people within an area or region. 2. A period during which some particular disease is so affecting many people.

epidemiology That branch of science concerned with the study of a disease or condition through its frequency and distribution.

epidermis Cuticle; the outer layer of the skin.

epidermoid 1. Resembling the epidermis. 2. An epidermoid *carcinoma.

epiglottis Fibrocartilage behind the base of the tongue covering the opening at the upper end of the larynx.

epimandibular Upon the mandible.

epipalatus Congenital *teratoma of the mouth.

epipharynx *Nasopharynx.

episphenoid Congenital *teratoma of the mouth.

epistaxis Nose-bleed.

epistropheus The second cervical vertebra, the axis.

epithelial Relating to the epithelium.

epithelioid Resembling epithelium.

epithelioma Any tumour derived from the epithelium, or composed of epithelial cells.

epithelium A thin cellular layer covering or lining the organs and tissues of the body.
columnar e. Epithelium composed of prismatic column cells; it may be *simple* or *stratified*.

crevicular e. Non-keratinized epithelium lining the gingival crevice.
cuboidal e. Epithelium composed of cube-shaped cells; it may be *simple* or *stratified*.
dental e. Enamel *epithelium.
enamel e. The inner ameloblastic layers of the enamel matrix and the enamel organ.
gingival e. The layer of stratified squamous epithelium which covers the gingival tissues.
inner zone e. Reduced enamel *epithelium.
junctional e. Epithelial *attachment.
keratinized e. A type of stratified epithelium in which the outer cells acquire deposits of keratin and become scale-like and hard on the surface.
laminated e. Stratified *epithelium.
oral e. The epithelium lining the oral cavity: that lining the hard palate, gingiva, and upper surface of the tongue is keratinized; that lining the tonsils, soft palate, cheeks, lips and sublingual region is non-keratinized.
pavement e. Simple squamous *epithelium.
pocket e. The epithelium lining a periodontal pocket.
reduced dental e. Reduced enamel *epithelium.
reduced enamel e. A cellular layer, the remnants of the enamel organ, attached to the enamel surface of a tooth on eruption.
simple e. Any form of epithelium composed of only a single layer of cells.
squamous e. Epithelium composed of flat, or flattened, cells; it may be *simple* or *stratified*.
stratified e. A type of epithelium made up of layers of cells.
sulcal e., sulcular e. Crevicular *epithelium.
tabular e. Squamous *epithelium.
united enamel e. Reduced enamel *epithelium.

epitympanic Above the tympanum.

eponym The name of an organ, syndrome, disease, etc., that contains or is derived from a proper name; *e.g.* Bartholin's duct.

eponymous Relating to an eponym.

epostoma *Exostosis.

epoxy resin A synthetic form of resin containing a hardening agent; it is used in dies and for coating, and for adhesive purposes, and is resistant to heat and chemicals.

Epstein-Barr virus (M.A. Epstein, b. 1921. English physician; Y.M. Barr, contemporary English virologist). A distinct type of herpes virus, the cause of glandular fever, and thought to have some causal relationship with Burkitt's lymphoma.

Epstein's pearls (A. Epstein, 1849-1918. Bohemian paediatrician). Small, slightly elevated, yellowish-white masses seen on either side of the median line of the hard palate at birth; gingival cysts.

epulis (*pl.* epulides) Any tumour of the gums; more especially either a fibrous or a giant-cell tumour.
congenital e. A benign granular-cell tumour of the mandible or the maxilla, usually in the region of the central incisors, which develops *in utero*.
fibrous e. An inflammatory pedunculated overgrowth of gum tissue.
giant-cell e. Peripheral giant-cell *granuloma.
malignant e. Old term for a sarcoma that affects the jaw and presents as an epulis.

myeloid e. Malignant *epulis.
e. of the newborn Congenital *epulis.
pregnancy e. A form of epulis developing during or as a result of pregnancy.

epulis fibromatosum Inflammatory fibrous hyperplasia of the gingiva, caused by chronic irritation.

epulis granulomatosum An inflammatory hyperplastic lesion developing from the socket of an newly extracted tooth, caused, for example, by a sharp spicule of bone.

epulofibroma A fibroma affecting the gums.

epuloid Resembling an epulis.

epulosis *Cicatrization.

epulotic Relating to epulosis.

equi- Prefix signifying *equal.*

equilibration The maintenance or restoration of equilibrium.
occlusal e. The restoration of normal occlusion within the mouth by mechanical means.

equilibrium A state of equal balance or counteraction.

erode To wear away, producing erosion.

erosion 1. A shallow ulcer. 2. *In dentistry*, the wearing away of a tooth surface due to chemical or abrasive action.

erosive 1. Relating to erosion. 2. Relating to a substance that tends to erode a surface.

eruption 1. The act of appearing, or pushing through, as of teeth coming through the gums. 2. A visible skin lesion, occurring in disease.

eruption cyst, eruption haematoma A cyst of odontogenic origin occurring about the crown of an erupting tooth, caused by an accumulation of blood or tissue fluid, and presenting as a bluish swelling in the eruption area; a form of dentigerous cyst.

eruptive Relating to or characterized by an eruption.

erythema Redness of the skin, either diffuse or patchy, caused by congestion of the subcutaneous capillaries.

erythema migrans linguae Geographic *tongue.

erythema multiforme An acute inflammatory disease affecting the skin and oral mucosa, and producing oral macules or papules.

erythro- Prefix signifying *red.*

erythrocyte One of the red cells found in blood which carry oxygen and are produced by the bone marrow.

erythrodontia The condition of having a reddish brown stain on the teeth.

erythroplakia A precancerous condition of the epithelial mucosa, characterized by circumscribed red velvety lesions which may be interspersed with fine white nodules of leukoplakia; often carcinoma-in-situ. *Also called* Queyrat's erythroplasia.

erythroplasia Painless erythematous eruptions, papular or macular in nature, affecting mucous membrane.

eschar A dry slough, the result of burning or contact with a corrosive agent.

escharotic 1. Caustic or corrosive; producing an eschar. 2. A caustic or corrosive substance.

Esmarch's operation (J.F.A. Esmarch, 1823-1908. German surgeon). Surgical treatment of temporomandibular ankylosis by mandibular osteotomy.

esophagus *See* oesophagus.

esosphenoiditis Osteomyelitis affecting the sphenoid bone.

esquillectomy The surgical removal of bone fragments after a fracture caused by a projectile.

etchant Any agent used for etching.

etching *See* acid etching.

ethanol *Alcohol.

ethmocranial Relating to the ethmoid bone and the skull.

ethmofrontal Relating to the ethmoid and frontal bones.

ethmoid 1. Sieve-like; cribriform. 2. Relating to the ethmoid bone.

ethmoid artery Supplies the dura mater, frontal and ethmoidal sinuses. *See* Table of Arteries—ethmoidalis.

ethmoid nerve Supplies the mucosa of the ethmoid sinuses and of the nasal cavity. *See* Table of Nerves—ethmoidalis.

ethmolacrimal Relating to the ethmoid and the lacrimal bones.

ethmomaxillary Relating to the ethmoid bone and the maxilla.

ethmonasal Relating to the ethmoid bone and the nasal bones.

ethmopalatal Relating to the ethmoid bone and the palate.

ethmosphenoidal Relating to the ethmoid and the sphenoid bones.

ethmovomerine Relating to the ethmoid bone and the vomer.

ethyl alcohol *See* alcohol.

etiology *See* aetiology.

eugenol The principal constituent of clove oil.

eugnathic Relating to well-developed, normal jaws.

eurodontia Old term for dental caries.

eury- Prefix signifying *broad* or *wide*.

eurycephalic, eurycranial Having an abnormally wide skull.

eurygnathic Having an unusually broad jaw.

euryon One of two points on the skull at either end of its greatest transverse diameter.

euryprosopic Having an abnormally low and wide face.

Eusol (*Edinburgh University solution of lime*). A solution of chlorinated lime with boric acid used as an antiseptic and disinfectant cleansing agent.

Eustachian tube (B. Eustachio, ?1513-74. Italian physician). Auditory *tube.

eutectic Easily melted, melting at a low temperature. *See also* eutectic *alloy.

evacuator

oral e. *Aspirator.

evagination Protrusion from a sheath or outer covering.

evanescent Disappearing quickly; unstable.

Evans gold crown (G. Evans, fl. 1888. American dentist). An all-gold seamless crown contoured to the anatomical form of the natural tooth.

evaporation The conversion of a solid or a liquid substance into vapour.

eversion A turning outwards, or a state of being turned outwards.

Every denture (R.G. Every, contemporary New Zealand dental surgeon). An upper partial denture designed in such a way that, apart from the occlusion, the only contact made with the natural teeth is at their contact points; the denture base is extended to make contact with the distal surface of the most posterior tooth in the arch.

Ewing's sarcoma (J. Ewing, 1866-1943. American pathologist). A rare, highly malignant tumour of bone which occasionally arises in or metastasizes to the jaws; found in children and young adults.

ex- Prefix signifying *without, beyond, from, out of*.

exacerbation An increase in the severity of a disease, or of any symptoms.

examination Investigation for diagnostic purposes.

exanthema, exanthem 1. Any skin eruption. 2. Any eruptive fever.

exanthematous Relating to an exanthema.

excavation 1. A hollow or cavity. 2. The process of cutting such a cavity. 3. *In dentistry*, the cavity prepared in a tooth, in which is placed a filling or inlay; also the process of preparing such a cavity.

excavator Any instrument used for hollowing or scooping out; the cutting blade is curved.
cleoid e. A type of dental excavator having a triangular blade with two cutting edges.
dental e. A hand instrument used in dentistry for excavation and removal of caries, especially of dentinal caries.
discoid e. A type of dental excavator with a semispherical blade having a circumferential cutting edge.
spoon e. A type of dental excavator having a spoon-shaped head, with the cutting edge on the concave side of the blade.

excementosis *Hypercementosis.

excise To cut out, or to remove by surgery.

excision Removal of any part by cutting.

excochleation The operation of curetting a cavity or scooping out foreign or diseased matter.

excoriation Superficial loss of surface skin; a graze.

excrete To expel waste material from the body.

excretion 1. The process by which waste matter is expelled from the body. 2. The matter thus expelled.

excursion Any movement of a movable part from a resting position during the performance of some function. *In dentistry*, used of the various movements of the mandible during mastication: these may be to the side (*lateral*), forward (*protrusive*) or slightly backwards (*retrusive*).

exelcymosis *Extraction.

exesion The gradual eating away of superficial tissue or of bone, as in an ulcerative condition.

exfoliatio areata linguae Geographic *tongue.

exfoliation 1. A peeling off in layers or in scales. 2. *In dentistry*, the natural shedding of the deciduous teeth.

exfoliative Relating to or causing exfoliation.

exhibeatur Latin for *let it be given*; used in prescription writing and abbreviated *exhib.*

exo- Prefix signifying *outside* or *towards the outside*.

exodontia, exodontics Tooth extraction.

exodontist One who specializes in the extraction of teeth.

exodontosis Exostosis affecting the root of a tooth.

exogenous Arising or developing outside an organism.

exognathia *Prognathism.

exognathion The maxillary alveolar process.

exolever A dental *elevator.

exophthalmos Abnormal protrusion of the eyeball.

exophytic Relating to something growing outwards, used of tumours projecting above the normal surface contours.

exorbitism *Exophthalmos.

exostosis A bony swelling developing on the bone surface, or on a tooth root.

exostotic Relating to exostosis.

exotoxin A toxic secretion of bacterial cells which causes damage in sites distant from the focus of infection.

expansion An increase in size, either of length, area or volume.
maxillary e. In orthodontics, a method of obtaining increased arch width by using appliances that expand the palatal bones and sutures; where considerable force is applied the technique is known as *rapid maxillary expansion (RME)*; where only slight force is used it is called *slow maxillary expansion.*

expansion arch An orthodontic appliance used to assist in the lateral movement of the teeth.

expansion plate An orthodontic appliance consisting of a divided base plate fitted with a screw which will separate the parts and so apply pressure to the teeth.

expansion wire An orthodontic appliance of wire, conforming to the dental arch, and used for anchorage in the movement of teeth.

explorer Any instrument used in diagnostic investigation; especially hand instruments with sharp flexible points used *in restorative dentistry* to examine tooth surfaces for breaks or early signs of dental caries, and *in periodontology* to examine root surfaces for subgingival deposits.

exposure 1. The laying open of a covered or protected area. 2. *In dentistry*, the removal of the protecting enamel and dentine from the pulp of a tooth by caries or trauma, thus laying it open to the mouth.

extension bridge A dental bridge having a free pontic attached at one end beyond the point of anchorage.

extension outline The outline on the surface of a cast, including the entire area of the denture base.

external Outside; as opposed to *internal.*

external nasal vein The vein draining the side of the nose. *See* Table of Veins—nasalis externa.

external palatine vein Drains the palatal region. *See* Table of Veins—palatina externa.

extirpation Complete eradication of a part.

extra- Prefix signifying *outside.*

extrabuccal Outside the oral cavity.

extracoronal Outside the tooth crown.

extraction The process of pulling out or removing.
progressive e. Serial *extraction.
rubber band e. A method of tooth extraction which may be used for haemophiliac or other patients with blood disorders. A rubber band is placed over the crown of the tooth and encouraged to work its way down to the root, thus detaching the tooth from the socket without causing any loss of blood.
selective e. Serial *extraction.
serial e. An orthodontic procedure to relieve crowding during the eruption of permanent teeth; it involves the selective extraction of primary teeth timed to coincide with the eruption of their permanent successors, and it may

also involve the extraction of permanent premolars.

extractor Any instrument used in dentistry for the extraction of teeth.

extradental Outside a tooth or teeth.

extragingival Outside the gums.

extraoral Outside the mouth.

extravasation 1. The escape of fluid from a vessel into the surrounding tissues. 2. The fluid that escapes in this way.

extravascular Outside a vessel or vessels.

extrinsic Having its origin outside and separate from a body, organ or part; as opposed to *intrinsic*.

extrudocclusion *Extrusion.

extrusion *In dentistry*, the condition of a tooth that has been pulled or pushed up slightly out of its socket; it may be due to a pathological condition or it may be part of orthodontic treatment.

exudate The matter that passes out into the adjacent tissue through vessel walls in inflammation.

exudation The passage of matter into the adjacent tissues through vessel walls in inflammatory conditions.

exuviation The shedding of any epidermal structure, such as the deciduous teeth.

eye The organ of sight.

eye tooth A maxillary canine *tooth.

eyelet wiring Interdental eyelet *wiring.

Eysson's bone (H. Eysson, 1620-90. Dutch physician). The ossa mentalia at the symphysis menti.

F

F 1. Chemical symbol for fluorine. 2. Abbreviation for *Fahrenheit*.

f. Abbreviation for *fiat*—make; used in prescription writing.

Fe Chemical symbol for iron.

f.h. Abbreviation for *fiat haustus*—make a draught; used in prescription writing.

fl. Abbreviation for *fluid*.

f.m. Abbreviation for *fiat mistura*—make a mixture; used in prescription writing.

f.p. Abbreviation for *fiat pilula*—make a pill; used in prescription writing.

ft Abbreviation for *foot*.

ft. Abbreviation for *fiat*—make; used in prescription writing.

face 1. The front of the head, from the forehead to the chin. 2. Any exterior surface or presenting aspect.

facebow 1. In *dental prosthetics*, an instrument, designed originally by G.B. Snow, used for determining the relationship of the teeth to the axis of movement of the mandible and transferring the bite-blocks to an articulator so that this movement may be reproduced in making the denture. 2. *In orthodontics,* any extraoral wire arch or bow used to attach an internal appliance to an external anchorage.
adjustable axis f. A form of facebow that can be adjusted to locate the axis of rotation of the mandible.

faceometer An instrument used for taking facial measurements.

facet A small abraded area on a bone or on a tooth surface.

facial Relating to the face.

facial artery Supplies the pharynx, soft palate, tonsil, submandibular gland, part of the orbit and lacrimal sac. *See* Table of Arteries—facialis.

facial nerve The seventh cranial nerve, supplying the muscles of facial expression, and also the posterior belly of the digastric muscle, the stapedius and the stylohyoid muscles. *See* Table of Nerves—facialis.

facial veins Those veins that drain the muscles and tissues of the face. *See* Table of Veins—facialis.

facies 1. A face, or the appearance of a face. 2. A specific surface.

facing A thin piece of porcelain trimmed to represent the outer surface of a tooth and to be reinforced with gold or other backing, used to restore the full form of a tooth.
reverse pin f. A porcelain facing in which the pins attaching it to the metal crown are fixed into the tooth.

facio- Prefix signifying *face*.

faciocervical Relating to the face and the neck.

faciolingual Relating to the face and the tongue.

facioplasty Plastic surgery operations on the face.

facioplegia Facial paralysis.

factitial *Factitious.

factitious Artificially or unintentionally produced.

Fahrenheit (G.D. Fahrenheit, 1686-1736. German physicist). Denoting a thermometric scale on which freezing point is 32° and boiling point 212°; this scale was until recently used for clinical thermometers. It has now been superseded by the Celsius scale.

Fallopius, aqueduct of (G. Fallopius, 1523-62. Italian anatomist). Facial *canal.

falx cerebelli A sickle-shaped process of the dura mater between the cerebellar hemispheres.

falx cerebri A sickle-shaped vertical partition between the cerebral hemispheres.

familial Relating to a family, or affecting several of its members.

family In biological classification, the principal division of an order, which itself divides into genera.

fang 1. A sharp-pointed tooth, such as a canine or the tooth of a wild animal. 2. An old term for a tooth root.

Farabeuf's triangle (L.H. Farabeuf, 1841-1910. French surgeon). A triangle of the neck, formed by the internal jugular vein, the facial vein and the hypoglossal nerve.

fascia 1. The layers of areolar tissue beneath the skin (*superficial* fascia). 2. The layers of areolar tissue investing the muscles, nerves and other organs (*deep* fascia).

fascial Relating to a fascia.

fauces The throat.
pillars of f. Curved muscular folds on either side of the pharyngeal opening, running from the palate to the base of the tongue and the pharynx; they enclose the tonsils. The *anterior* pillars are also known as the palatoglossal arch and the *posterior* as the palatopharyngeal arch.

Fauchard's disease (P. Fauchard, 1678-1761. French dental surgeon). *Pyorrhoea alveolaris.

faucial Relating to the fauces.

febrile Feverish.

Fede's disease (F. Fede, 1832-1913. Italian physician). Sublingual papillomatous ulceration, found especially in infants, and caused by trauma from the lower incisors during suckling; *also called* Riga-Fede's disease.

fenestrate To pierce with one or more holes, sometimes used on the walls of bony defects in an attempt to stimulate repair.

fenestration 1. The surgical procedure by which one or more holes are pierced in hard tissue. 2. An opening not normally present, such as the absence of bone over the root of a tooth.

Fergusson's operation (Sir W. Fergusson, 1808-77. Scottish surgeon). 1. Excision of the maxilla for a malignant tumour. 2. An operation for the repair of hare-lip.

ferric Relating to iron as a trivalent metal.

ferrous Relating to iron as a bivalent metal.

-ferrous Suffix signifying *producing* or *bearing*.

ferrule *In dentistry*, a metal band placed round the root or the crown of a tooth for strength.

festoon The natural curved outline of the gums about the necks of the teeth.

fetid *See* foetid.

fetus *See* foetus.

fever 1. Abnormal increase in body temperature. 2. Any disease characterized by a high temperature, accompanied by other symptoms such as restlessness, delirium, rapid pulse.
uveoparotid f. A form of sarcoidosis affecting the parotid gland and characterized by firm, painless swelling accompanied by xerostomia.

fiat Latin for *make* (imperative); used in prescription writing, and abbreviated *f.* or *ft.*

fiber *See* fibre.

fibre A thread-like structure found in organic tissue.
bone f's. *Sharpey's fibres.
collagen f's. Soft, flexible fibres, made up of bundles of fibrils and often themselves formed into larger bundles; they are the main constituent of fibrous tissue and the principal component of the periodontal ligament.
dentinal f's. Odontoblast *processes.
dentinogenic f's. *Korff's fibres.
enamel f. Enamel *prism.
odontogenic f's. Those fibres which make up the connective tissue layer of the tooth matrix, surrounding the pulp.
For eponymous fibres *see* under the name of the person first describing them.

fibril A small fibre.
collagen f's. Very fine, delicate fibrils which are made up into bundles to form collagen fibres.

fibrilloblast *Odontoblast[2].

fibrin An insoluble fibrous protein formed by the action of thrombin on fibrinogen; it provides the network that retains corpuscles in the mechanism of blood clotting.

fibrinogen A soluble blood protein, occurring in blood plasma, which is converted into the insoluble fibrin in the process of clotting.

fibrinogenopenia *Afibrinogenaemia.

fibrinous Relating to fibrin.

fibro- Prefix signifying *fibre*.

fibroadamantinoblastoma Ameloblastic *fibroma.

fibroadenoma *Adenofibroma. *Also called* f. xanthomatodes, foetal f., pleomorphic f.

fibroblast One of the germ cells from which connective tissue is formed.

fibrocartilage Cartilage that also contains dense fibrous tissue.

fibroma A benign tumour composed of fibrous tissue.
ameloblastic f. A benign tumour containing both odontogenic epithelium and connective tissue resembling that of the dental papilla, usually found in the mandible in individuals under 21 years of age.
cementifying f. A benign tumour of odontogenic origin, similar to ossifying fibroma, occurring in the mandible in older persons; it starts with the development of cellular fibrous tissue, which becomes progressively more cementum-like as it mineralizes.
odontogenic f. A type of fibroma containing odontogenic fibrous tissue.
ossifying f. A benign tumour containing fibrous tissue with some bone cells and mineralized masses, very similar in structure to fibrous dysplasia but separated within a capsule from the surrounding bone.

fibromatosis The development of multiple fibromas.
gingival f. Fibrous overgrowth of the gingiva, localized or general; it may be hereditary, idiopathic or drug-induced, and is especially associated with phenytoin anticonvulsive therapy. *Also called* elephantiasis gingivae.

fibro-odontoma
ameloblastic f. A benign tumour resembling an ameloblastic fibroma, but containing dental hard tissues.

fibro-osteoma Ossifying *fibroma.

fibropapilloma *Adenofibroma.

fibrosarcoma A malignant tumour derived from fibroblasts.

ameloblastic f. A tumour similar in structure to an ameloblastic fibroma, but with the mesenchymal component showing the malignant features of a sarcoma.

fibrosis Fibrous degeneration; the abnormal formation of fibrous tissue.

oral submucous f. A disease characterized by progressive fibrosis beneath the oral mucous membranes, especially in the cheek, with atrophy of the overlying epithelium; it may be a precancerous condition.

fibrous Relating to a fibre or fibres; composed of fibres.

Filatov's spots (N.F. Filatov, 1847-1902. Russian paediatrician). *Koplik's spots.

file A hard steel tool with a roughened surface, for abrading or polishing.

filiform Filamentous; thread-like.

filling 1. The material inserted into a prepared cavity in a tooth; *also called* a restoration. 2. The operation of inserting such material into a prepared cavity.

post-resection f. Retrograde root *filling.

retrograde root f. The placing of a root filling in the apex of a tooth, which is surgically exposed, to seal the end of the root canal after apicectomy; the material is inserted upwards through the apex, rather than through the pulp chamber.

reverse root f. Retrograde root *filling.

root f. 1. Any material used to fill up and seal a root canal. 2. The process of inserting the material into the root canal.

filtration The separating out of a solid from a liquid by passing it through a filter.

fimbria A border, edge or fringe.

fimbriated Having a fringed edge.

first arch syndrome A congenital abnormality syndrome, which includes cleft lip and palate, mandibulofacial dysostosis, hypertelorism and deformities of the ear, all stemming from developmental deficiency in the first branchial arch.

fissural Relating to a fissure.

fissure 1. A small groove, slit or trough. 2. *In dentistry,* used especially of the small grooves in the enamel surface of a tooth, caused by a fault in its structure.

auricular f. of the temporal bone Tympanomastoid *fissure.

basilar f. Spheno-occipital *fissure.

enamel f. *Fissure².

gingival f. Gingival *cleft.

inferior orbital f. A long cleft between the floor and lateral wall of the orbit, opening into the infratemporal fossa.

lip f. *Hare-lip.

mandibular f. One of the grooves on the lower part of the developing face in the embryo, occurring at the midline of the mandibular arches and where these arches contact the maxillary processes.

occipitosphenoidal f. Spheno-occipital *fissure.

oral f. The opening into the oral cavity between the lips.

palpebral f. The opening slit between the eyelids.

petrosquamous f. The narrow cleft between the petrous and squamous portions of the temporal bone.

petrotympanic f. The narrow opening posterior to the mandibular fossa, through which passes the chorda tympani nerve; *also called* Glaserian fissure.

pterygoid f. The angular cleft between the pterygoid processes of the sphenoid bone.

pterygomaxillary f. A narrow cleft between the lateral pterygoid plate and the maxilla, through which passes the maxillary artery.
pterygopalatine f. Greater palatine *sulcus of the palatine bone.
sphenoid f. Superior orbital *fissure.
sphenomaxillary f. 1. Inferior orbital *fissure. 2. Pterygopalatine *fossa.
spheno-occipital f. The line of junction lying between the sphenoid bone and the basilar portion of the occipital bone, filled with cartilage until it becomes ossified.
superior orbital f. An elongated cleft between the great and small wings of the sphenoid bone, giving passage to various blood vessels and nerves.
tympanic f. Petrotympanic *fissure.
tympanomastoid f. A cleft between the tympanic portion and the mastoid process of the temporal bone, through which passes the auricular branch of the vagus nerve.
zygomatic f. Infratemporal *fossa.
zygomaticosphenoid f. A fissure between the zygoma and the orbital surface of the great wing of the sphenoid bone.

fissure, Glaserian Petrotympanic *fissure.

fissure bur A cylindrical dental bur used for preparing a cavity involving the occlusal fissures of a premolar or molar tooth.

fissure sealing The filling up of developmental pits and fissures in posterior teeth to prevent the onset of occlusal caries.

fissure sealant An impermeable material, usually a form of resin, used for pit and fissure sealing.

fistula An abnormal tract between two organs or an organ and the outer surface, lined with epithelium; often leading from a suppurating cavity.
alveolar f. One leading from a cavity of an alveolar abscess; an alveolar sinus.
antral f. 1. A tract leading from an antral abscess or from a bone cavity. 2. A surgically created tract between the maxillary antrum and the nose, used for drainage in chronic sinusitis.
antro-oral f. Oroantral *fistula.
blind f. A fistula that has an opening at one end only; a **sinus*[4].
branchial f. A congenital opening in the face or neck resulting from the persistence of some part of one of the embryonic branchial arches, or its associated pouches or grooves.
cervical f. A type of branchial fistula which connects the pharynx with the outer surface on the side of the neck.
cervicoaural f. Branchial *fistula.
dental f. Alveolar *fistula.
external f. One opening from a body cavity or abscess to the surface of the skin.
internal f. A fistula between two internal organs or cavities, with no opening to the outer surface.
labial f., lip f. A minute tract or congenital depression on the edge of the lower lip; a labial sinus.
oroantral f. A fistula leading from the maxillary antrum into the oral cavity, most commonly found in the region of the molar teeth.
orofacial f. A fistula leading from the oral cavity, opening on to the surface of the face.
oronasal f. A fistula leading from the nose into the mouth, usually in the region of the hard palate.
salivary f. An abnormal tract leading from a salivary gland or salivary duct either on to the outer surface or into the mouth, through which saliva may drain.

submental f. A type of salivary fistula which opens in the skin below the chin.

fistulous Relating to or resembling a fistula.

fixation The act of fastening in a rigid position.
craniomandibular f. A method of fastening the mandible to the head by rods connected either to a head frame or to bone plates and to dental splints.
craniomaxillary f. A method of stabilizing a fractured maxilla by external rods connected to some form of headcap or frame and to a maxillary dental splint.
external skeletal f. A method of immobilizing the ends of a fractured bone by external metal pins or screw appliances, used especially for an edentulous mouth.
intermaxillary f. A method of immobilizing the mandible by fastening it to the maxilla.
internal skeletal f. The immobilization of a fractured bone by direct wiring, by the use of bone plates or by fixation by medullary pins.
intramedullary f. A method of uniting the ends of a fractured bone by means of a metal pin within the bone marrow cavity.

flagellar, flagellate Relating to or possessing flagella.

flagellum (*pl.* flagella) A thin, whip-like process, seen on certain micro-organisms.

flange An external or internal rim, either for strength or as an attachment or guide to some other part.
denture f. The buccal, labial or lingual vertical extension from the denture base into the oral cavity.

flange splint A metal splint used in fracture of the mandible; it is cemented to several of the posterior mandibular teeth and has a high flange which rests on the buccal surfaces of the opposing maxillary teeth.

flap A partially detached layer of skin or tissue, either surgically produced for access or repair, or accidentally formed.

flash Excess material squeezed out of a die during casting.

flask 1. Any glass or metal bottle with a narrow neck. 2. A metal box or frame containing plaster of Paris, in which dentures are enclosed and embedded for vulcanizing or curing.

flasking The process of packing a denture into a flask prior to vulcanizing or curing it.

flav-, flavo- Prefix signifying *yellow.*

Fleischmann's bursa (F.L. Fleischmann, fl. 1841. German anatomist). An occasional sublingual bursa.

Fleischmann's follicle (F.L. Fleischmann, fl. 1841. German anatomist). An inconstant follicle on the floor of the mouth, near the edge of the genioglossus muscle.

flexible Not rigid; readily bendable without breaking.

flexion reflex, flexor reflex Nociceptive *reflex.

floor
cavity f. That surface of a prepared cavity towards which the restoration is inserted.

flora
oral f. Those micro-organisms normally found in the mouth.

floss, dental; floss silk, dental Soft waxed thread or tape, used to clear and to clean interproximal spaces.

Flower's index (Sir W.H. Flower, 1831-99. English physician). Dental *index.

fluid 1. Any substance that flows; it may be a liquid or a gas. 2. Descriptive of any substance having this property.
body f's. Any of the liquids within the body and necessary for its normal functioning.
crevicular f. Gingival *fluid.
extracellular f. Any of the body fluids outside the cells and membranes and supplying nutrients, etc.
gingival f. A transudate of blood plasma collecting in the gingival sulcus, produced by leakage from the capillaries in the free gingiva.
interstitial f. Extracellular fluid within tissue spaces which is not lymph, plasma or transcellular fluid.
intracellular f. The fluid within the cells of the body.
lymphatic f. *Lymph.
oral f. *Saliva.
synovial f. A viscid, transparent alkaline and albumen-like fluid contained in joint cavities and tendon sheaths, secreted by synovial membranes; *also called* synovium.
transcellular f. Extracellular fluid that has been excreted or secreted through the cell membranes.

fluoridation *See* water fluoridation.

fluoride 1. A compound of fluorine with another element. 2. A salt of hydrofluoric acid.
topical f. Any agent containing fluoride that is applied to the surfaces of the teeth to improve their resistance to the onset of caries. It may take the form of a gel, paste, varnish, solution or mouthwash.

fluoridization The use of any fluoride, in any form, for the prevention of dental caries.

fluorine A non-metallic element of the halogen group, having the chemical symbol F.

fluoroapatite The compound formed when a fluoride reacts with the enamel of a tooth; it aids in resistance to the onset of caries.

fluorosis 1. Fluorine poisoning. 2. A chronic condition resulting from prolonged ingestion of excessive amounts of fluorides and characterized by increased density of the skeletal bones, and hypoplasia and discoloration of the teeth.
chronic endemic (dental) f. Hypoplasia and discoloration of the tooth enamel due to ingestion of excessive amounts of fluorine during the developmental period; mottled enamel.

flux 1. A material used in soldering to prevent oxidation and aid the flow of the solder. 2. A material used in ceramic and vitreous substances to aid in melting.

focal Relating to a focus.

focus (*pl.* foci) The chief centre of activity or the point of convergence.

focus *of infection* The chief centre of pathogenic activity from which the infection spreads to surrounding areas.

foetal Relating to a foetus.

foetal fibroadenoma *Adenofibroma.

foetid Having an unpleasant or foul smell.

foetor oris Foetid breath; halitosis.

foetus, fetus The developing embryo in the womb, especially, in humans, after the first three months of growth.

foil Metal in a very thin sheet or ribbon, especially gold, tin or platinum.

foil carrier An instrument used to transfer strips of gold foil to a prepared tooth cavity.

foil condenser Gold *condenser.

fold 1. To bend or be bent over so that one part lies back over the other. 2. The part or edge produced in this way. 3. *In anatomy*, a folding over of tissue or skin producing a rolled edge; plica.
fimbriated f. The fold of fringed mucosa extending from the lingual frenum to the base of the tongue; plica fimbriata.
glosso-epiglottal f. One of the mucosal folds or ridges that extend from the base of the tongue to the epiglottis; plica glossoepiglottica.
mucobuccal f. The folding back of the alveolar mucosa from the maxilla or the mandible to the cheek, creating the limits to the vestibule of the mouth.
mucolabial f. The fold of the alveolar mucosa from the maxilla or the mandible to the lip; in the midline this forms the frenulum.
mucosobuccal f. Mucobuccal *fold.
palatine f. One of the ridges on the anterior portion of the hard palate; plica palatina transversa.
pterygomandibular f. The fold of mucosa stretching from the region of the pterygoid hamulus to the retromolar pad on each side of the oral cavity.
salpingopharyngeal f. A vertical fold of mucous membrane within the nasopharynx, covering the salpingopharyngeus muscle and running from the edge of the auditory tube to the lateral wall of the pharynx; plica salpingopharyngea.
sublingual f. A horseshoe-shaped fold or ridge of mucosa covering the sublingual salivary glands; plica sublingualis.

follicle A minute sac or gland.
dental f. The fibrocellular sac containing the unerupted tooth within the alveolar process.

follicular Relating to or resembling a follicle.

fontanelle, fontanel The membranous and cartilaginous structure present between the ossifying skull bones of a new-born infant.

food debris Food remnants and bacteria loosely attached to the tooth, which can be removed by rinsing.

foramen (*pl.* foramina) A small hole in a bone, through which pass either blood vessels or nerves, or both.
alveolar f. One of the openings of the alveolar canals on the infratemporal surface of the maxilla, through which the posterior superior alveolar nerves and vessels pass to the molar and premolar teeth. *Also called* posterior superior alveolar foramen.
anterior ethmoid f. A canal between the ethmoid and frontal bones, through which pass the nasal branch of the ophthalmic nerve and the anterior ethmoid vessels.
anterior palatine f. Incisive *fossa[1].
apical f. The small opening at the apex of the tooth by which the nerve and blood supply of the pulp enter.
caecal f. of the tongue A depression above the root and dorsum of the tongue, the site of the former opening of the thyroglossal duct; *also called* Morand's foramen.
condylar f. Condylar *canal.
greater palatine f. The opening of the greater palatine canal into the hard palate, between the horizontal

portion of the palatine bone and the adjacent maxilla.
incisive f. One of two to four openings of the incisive canal on the floor of the incisive fossa; *lateral*: on the hard palate behind the incisors, transmitting branches of the greater palatine artery; *median*: in the midline of the hard palate, transmitting the nasopalatine nerves.
inferior dental f. Mandibular *foramen.
infraorbital f. The external opening of the infraorbital canal, through which pass the infraorbital artery and nerve.
jugular f. The opening formed by the jugular notches of the temporal and occipital bones, through which pass a jugular vein and the ninth, tenth and eleventh cranial nerves.
lesser palatine f. One of the openings of the lesser palatine canals, on the anterior surface of the hard palate.
malar f. *Foramen zygomatico-faciale.
mandibular f. An oblong opening in the internal surface of the ramus, through which pass the inferior dental nerve and artery; *also called* the inferior dental foramen.
mastoid f. A small opening behind the mastoid process, through which pass an artery and a vein.
maxillary f. Maxillary *hiatus.
mental f. A large foramen in the mandible, below the second premolar, through which pass the mental branches of the inferior dental nerve, and their accompanying blood vessels.
nutrient f. One of the foramina in the maxilla and the mandible through which the nutrient canals pass.
occipital f. *Foramen magnum.
orbitomalar f. *Foramen zygomatico-orbitale.
posterior superior alveolar f. Alveolar *foramen.
sphenopalatine f. The space between the orbital and sphenoid processes of the palatine bone, opening into the nasal cavity.
spinous f. *Foramen spinosum.
stylomastoid f. An opening between the styloid and the mastoid processes, through which pass the stylomastoid artery and the facial nerve.
superior maxillary f. *Foramen rotundum ossis sphenoidalis.
supraorbital f. The foramen formed by the bridging over of the supraorbital notch, on the supraorbital margin of the frontal bone; through it pass the supraorbital nerve and vessels.

foramen caecum linguae Caecal *foramen of the tongue.

foramen lacerum An interosseous foramen between the apex of the petrous bone and the attachment of the great wing of the sphenoid bone, through which the carotid artery passes.

foramen magnum A large opening in the lower portion of the occipital bone, through which passes the medulla oblongata.

foramen ovale An opening between the auricles of the heart in the foetus.

foramen ovale alae majoris An opening in the great wing of the sphenoid bone, through which pass the inferior dental nerve and the accessory meningeal artery.

foramen rotundum ossis sphenoidalis A round opening in the great wing of the sphenoid bone, through which passes the maxillary branch of the trigeminal nerve.

foramen spinosum An opening in the great wing of the sphenoid bone near to its posterior angle, through which passes the middle meningeal artery.

foramen zygomaticofaciale The external opening on the surface of the zygomatic bone, through which the zygomatic nerve and vessels pass.

foramen zygomatico-orbitale The canal through the zygomatic bone through which passes the zygomatic branch of the maxillary nerve.

foramen zygomaticotemporale The opening on the temporal surface of the zygomatic bone, through which passes the zygomaticotemporal nerve.

forceps An instrument having two blades and handles, used for holding, compressing, or removing.
dental f. Forceps used for the extraction of teeth.
haemostatic f. Scissor-like instruments with grooved blades, used to constrict and clamp blood vessels during surgery.
rubber-dam clamp f. Specially designed forceps for placing rubber-dam clamps on the teeth.

Fordyce's spots, Fordyce's granules (J.A. Fordyce, 1858-1925. American dermatologist). Small yellowish spots, of no pathological significance, occurring on the vermilion border and the inner surface of the lips and cheeks.

former An instrument used for shaping or forming.
angle f. One of a pair (*left* and *right*) of hand cutting instruments with blades sharpened on all edges; they are used in finishing a prepared cavity to ensure clean and sharp angles and undercuts and to provide good retention for the restoration.

formula
dental f. A formula devised to show the number and arrangement of teeth by means of letters and figures. In this formula I = Incisor; C = Canine; P = Premolar; M = Molar. The dental formula for the normal permanent dentition in man is I 2/2 C 1/1 P 2/2 M 3/3.
instrument f. Devised by G.V. Black as a means of differentiating different types and sizes of dental hand instruments. It consists of three figures representing three measurements: the width of the blade in 10ths of a millimetre; the length of the blade in millimetres; and the angle of the shaft in centigrades. (Where there is a fourth figure, in brackets after the first, this represents the angle of the cutting edge of the blade with its shaft in centigrades; it is usually seen on margin trimmers.)

formulary A collection of recipes or formulae for making up medicines.

fossa (*pl.* fossae) A shallow, irregular depression in a surface.
canine f. A depression on the external surface of the maxilla, immediately distal to the canine tooth socket.
central f. The shallow depression on the occlusal surface of a molar tooth.
condylar f., condyloid f. One of the two small depressions on the occipital bone, situated behind one of the condyles.
digastric f. 1. One of two depressions on the internal aspect of the body of the mandible on either side of the midline, providing the origin of the anterior belly of the digastric muscle. 2. Mastoid *notch.
glenoid f. Mandibular *fossa.
incisive f. 1. A depression on the maxilla behind the incisors. 2. A depression on the mandible below

the incisors, giving origin to the mentalis muscle. 3. A depression on the outer surface of the maxilla, giving origin to the depressor muscle of the nose.

infratemporal f. An irregular space on the skull, bounded by the zygoma and the ramus of the mandible, behind the maxilla.

jugular f. A depression in the petrous portion of the temporal bone, between the carotid canal and the stylomastoid foramen, for the jugular vein.

lingual f. A shallow depression found on the lingual surface of an incisor tooth.

mandibular f. The depression in the squamous portion of the temporal bone below the zygomatic process, in which the condyle of the mandible rests.

mastoid f. A depression on the lateral surface of the temporal bone, for the lateral sinus.

oral f. *Stomodeum.

palatine f. Incisive *fossa[1].

pterygoid f. A deep groove between the medial and lateral plates of the pterygoid process of the sphenoid bone.

pterygopalatine f. A small, funnel-like cleft between the pterygoid process of the sphenoid bone and the palatine bone and maxilla, on the lateral aspect of the skull and through which run the maxillary artery and the maxillary nerve; it also contains the pterygopalatine ganglion. *Also called* Bichat's fossa.

retromolar f. A depression lying between the anterior border of the ramus of the mandible and temporal crest.

scaphoid f. A depression in the lower surface of the medial pterygoid plate of the sphenoid bone, from which arises the tensor veli palatini muscle.

sphenomaxillary f. Pterygopalatine *fossa.

sublingual f. Sublingual *fovea.

submandibular f., submaxillary f. Submandibular *fovea.

suborbital f. Canine *fossa.

temporal f. The depression on the side of the cranium in which the temporal muscle lodges.

temporomandibular f. Mandibular *fossa.

triangular f. A shallow depression found on the occlusal surface of a molar or premolar, mesial or distal to the marginal ridges, and occasionally on the lingual surface of a maxillary incisor, close to the neck of the tooth, at the edge of the lingual fossa.

zygomatic f. Infratemporal *fossa.

Foster crown (F.W. Foster, fl. 1855. American dentist). A form of pivot tooth using a metal screw to secure it to the root canal.

Fournier's molars (J.A. Fournier, 1832-1914. French venereologist). Mulberry *molars.

fovea (*pl.* foveae) A small pit, depression or cup; used of depressions in the body, especially the fovea centralis of the retina.

palatine f. One of two pits situated on either side of the midline near the junction of the soft and hard palates; fovea palati.

pterygoid f. A depression on the anterior side of the neck of the mandible, the site of insertion of the external pterygoid muscle; fovea pterygoidea mandibulae.

sublingual f. A depression on the inner surface of the mandible, by the sublingual gland; fovea sublingualis.

submandibular f., submaxillary f. A depression on the inner surface of the mandible, by the submandibular gland, part of which may rest within it; fovea submandibularis.

foveate 1. Pitted. 2. Relating to or characterized by the presence of fovea.

foveola (*pl.* foveolae) A small fovea.

fracture A break, or the act of breaking, in a bone or cartilage.
articular f. One involving a joint surface on a bone.
comminuted f. A fracture in which the bone is broken into a number of pieces.
complex f. A fracture in which the break lines spread in different directions.
compound f. A fracture which is open externally.
depressed f. A fracture of the bones of the skull in which fragments have been depressed inwards.
direct f. A fracture at the point of injury or impact.
greenstick f. A fracture in which the bone is broken on one side but only bent on the other; seen in children.
indirect f. A fracture at a distance from the point of injury or impact.
Le Fort f. One of three main classes of fracture of the maxilla:
Class I: those affecting the alveolar process, the palate and the pterygoid processes, transversely.
Class II: a transverse fracture extending through the nasal bones, affecting the maxillary frontal process, the orbital plate, and descending through the maxillary antrum across to the pterygoid process; a pyramidal fracture.
Class III: those affecting the bridge of the nose and the orbit, the pyramidal processes of the maxilla and zygoma remaining attached; craniofacial disjunction.
open f. Compound *fracture.
pathological f. A fracture in bone which has been weakened by disease.
pyramidal f. *Le Fort fracture, Class II.
reduction of a f. The replacing of the displaced bone ends or fragments to the correct position.
simple f. A fracture which is not open externally.
spontaneous f. Pathological *fracture.

fraenulum, fraenum *See* frenulum, frenum.

fragilitas ossium *Osteogenesis imperfecta.

framework *In dentistry*, the metal skeleton of a denture or prosthesis on which the remaining portions are built up to produce a complete appliance.

Franceschetti syndrome (A. Franceschetti, b. 1896. Swiss ophthalmologist). Mandibulofacial *dysostosis.

Frankel appliance (R. Frankel, contemporary German orthodontist). A functional regulator; the only tissue-borne orthodontic appliance, with minimal contact with the teeth. The appliance is for the most part restricted to the vestibula, the buccal shields and lip pads reducing soft tissue pressure on the dentition and the lingual pad regulating the position of the mandible. It uses the oral and facial muscle forces to move teeth and generate arch expansion.

Frankfort plane, Frankfort horizontal plane A plane determined by the position of the two poria and the left orbitale, used in anthropology for orientating both living heads and skulls; adopted at the International Congress of Anthropologists, Frankfort-am-Main, 1884.

freeway space Interocclusal *clearance.

frenectomy Surgical excision of a frenum.

frenoplasty The surgical repositioning of an abnormally attached lingual frenum.

frenotomy Surgical relief of tongue-tie by cutting the lingual frenum; ankylotomy.

frenulum A small frenum.

frenulum labii inferioris The fold of mucous membrane attaching the lower lip to the mandibular gums below the central incisors.

frenulum labii superioris The fold of mucous membrane attaching the upper lip to the maxillary gums above the central incisors.

frenulum linguae The fold of mucous membrane attaching the under surface of the tongue to the floor of the mouth.

frenum A membranous fold supporting or limiting the movement of an organ.
buccal f. One of the folds of mucosa from the cheek to the alveolar process on either side of the oral cavity in the region of the canine tooth.
labial f. *Frenulum labii inferioris, *frenulum labii superioris.
lingual f. *Frenulum linguae.

frenum labiorum *Frenulum labii inferioris, *frenulum labii superioris.

frenum linguae *Frenulum linguae.

friable Easily crumbled.

Friteau's triangle (E. Friteau, b. 1867). A triangular area on the cheek having no branches of the facial nerve.

frog tongue *Ranula.

frontal Relating to the forehead; in front.

frontal bone One of the bones of the skull, forming the forehead.

frontal muscle Raises eyebrows and draws forward scalp. *See* Table of Muscles—frontalis.

frontal nerve Supplies the skin of the scalp. *See* Table of Nerves—frontalis.

fronto- Prefix signifying *forehead.*

frontomalar Relating to the frontal and the zygomatic (malar) bones.

frontomaxillary Relating to the frontal bone and the maxilla.

frontonasal Relating to the frontal and the nasal bones.

fronto-occipital Relating to the frontal and occipital bones.

frontoparietal Relating to the frontal and parietal bones.

frontotemporal Relating to the frontal and temporal bones.

frontotemporale The most anterior point of the temporal line at the zygomatic process of the frontal bone; a craniometric landmark.

frontozygomatic Relating to the frontal and zygomatic bones.

frugivorous Fruit-eating.

fulginous Of sooty or smoky appearance; used of a darkly coated tongue or mucous membrane.

fulguration Superficial tissue dehydration produced by a surgical electrode held slightly away from the tissue, causing sparking.

fungal Relating to a fungus.

fungicidal Relating to, having the properties of, a fungicide.

fungicide Any agent that destroys or inhibits the growth of a fungus or of fungi.

fungiform In the shape of a fungus.

fungistatic Inhibiting the growth of a fungus or of fungi; mycostatic.

fungoid Resembling a fungus.

fungous Relating to a fungus.

fungus (*pl.* fungi) 1. A class of plant organisms which includes moulds, mushrooms and toadstools. 2. A morbid growth of granulation tissue on the body.

fur A coating of epithelial scales and other matter found on the tongue in certain diseases or disorders.

furcal Forked.

furcation 1. The condition of being divided into prongs, or of being forked. 2. *In dentistry*, the area on a multirooted tooth where the roots divide.

furnace An apparatus by means of which metals or minerals may be treated with continuous and intense heat.

muffle f. Porcelain *furnace.

porcelain f. A type of oven used in dental ceramics, in which material may be heated without being directly exposed to the source of heat.

furrow A trench or groove.

mentolabial f. The horizontal groove just above the chin.

furuncle A *boil.

furunculosis The condition marked by crops of boils.

fusible Capable of being melted.

fusiform Spindle-shaped.

Fusiformis fusiformis, Fusiformis nucleatum **Fusobacterium nucleatum.*

fusion 1. The act or process of uniting or fusing together. 2. The state of being so fused. 3. *In dentistry,* the development of one tooth from two distinct tooth follicles; *also called* synodontia.

Fusobacterium A genus of the Bacteroidaceae family of bacteria, seen as slender spindle shapes, non-motile, Gram-negative and anaerobic.

F. fusiforme **Leptotrichia buccalis.*

F. nucleatum A species which has been found in deposits on teeth in a healthy mouth, but which is found in greater concentration in those with chronic periodontal disease.

F. polymorphum A variant of **F. nucleatum.*

F. plauti-vincenti **Leptotrichia buccalis.*

fusospirillosis, fusospirochaetosis Acute ulcerative *gingivitis.

G

g Abbreviation for *gram.*

G Gingival.

GA Gingivoaxial.

GBA Gingivobuccoaxial.

GLA Gingivolinguoaxial.

gm Abbreviation for *gram* (now rarely used).

gutt. Abbreviation for *gutta,* or *guttae*—a drop, or drops; used in prescription writing.

gag 1. To retch; to heave without vomiting. 2. A device to prevent the closure of the teeth during surgery, epileptic seizure, etc.

gag reflex Pharyngeal *reflex.

galea *In anatomy,* a general term for any helmet-like structure.

galea aponeurotica The aponeurosis connecting the separate parts of the occipitofrontal muscle. *See* Table of Muscles.

Galen's bandage (Claudius Galen, *c.* 130-200 AD. Greek physician and writer). A bandage used for head injuries in which each end is divided into three: the centre of the bandage is placed on the crown of the head, the two front strips fasten at the back of the neck, the two back strips fasten on the forehead, and the two side strips under the chin.

galvanism (L. Galvani, 1737-98. Italian physicist and physician).
dental g. The production of an electric current caused when two dissimilar metals used as restorations in the mouth come into contact; this can produce discomfort and even pain.

galvanocautery *Electrocautery.

ganglion 1. A knot or mass of nerve cells. 2. A tumour or swelling on an aponeurosis or on a tendon.
ciliary g. A small, flattened ganglion on the oculomotor nerve near the apex of the orbit; a peripheral ganglion of the parasympathetic nervous system.
cochlear g. A ganglion of the cochlear nerve, occupying the spiral canal of the modiolus.
genicular g., geniculate g. The ganglion on the intrapetrous section of the facial nerve in the facial canal, the point at which the nerve changes direction sharply; the ganglion of the facial nerve.
otic g. A peripheral ganglion of the parasympathetic nervous system, situated below the foramen ovale and connected functionally with the glossopharyngeal nerve; *also called* Arnold's ganglion.
pterygopalatine g. A ganglion in the pterygopalatine fossa, supplying sympathetic, facial and other nerves from the maxillary nerve and the intermedius nerve to the oral and nasal mucosa and the lacrimal glands; *also called* Bock's ganglion or Meckel's ganglion.
semilunar g. Trigeminal *ganglion.
sphenopalatine g. Pterygopalatine *ganglion.
spiral g. Cochlear *ganglion.
sublingual g. A nerve ganglion formed by fibres passing distally from the submandibular ganglion to the lingual nerve.
submandibular g., submaxillary g. A small ganglion on the hyoglossus muscle from which arises the nerve supply for the submandibular and sublingual glands from the maxillary nerve and intermedius nerve; *also called* Blandin's ganglion or Meckel's lesser ganglion.

trigeminal g. A ganglion in a recess of the dura mater from which arise the sensory fibres of the trigeminal nerve; *also called* Gasserian ganglion.
vestibular g. A ganglion on the vestibular nerve, within the internal auditory meatus, where the nerve fibres divide to supply the utricle, saccule and semicircular ducts.

For eponymous ganglia *see* under the name of the person first describing the ganglion.

ganglion *of the facial nerve* Genicular *ganglion.

gangosa Destructive ulceration affecting the nose, the hard palate and the nasopharynx; a late stage of yaws.

gangrene Necrosis of tissue due to failure of the arterial blood supply caused by injury or disease.

gangrenous Affected with gangrene.

ganoblast *Ameloblast.

Garretson's bandage (J.E. Garretson, 1828-95. American oral surgeon). A bandage used to immobilize the lower jaw; it is taken from above the forehead, crossing at the neck and fastening under the chin.

Gasserian ganglion (J.L. Gasser, fl. 1757. Austrian anatomist). Trigeminal *ganglion.

Gates crown (W.H. Gates, fl. 1875. American dentist). Almost identical with the *Bonwill crown; *also called* the Gates-Bonwill crown.

gauge Any instrument used to obtain measurements.
bite g. An instrument designed to aid in the establishment of a correct bite in prosthetic dentistry.
Boley g. A finely calibrated instrument used for intraoral measurements.

geisoma, geison The supraorbital prominence; the eyebrow ridge on the skull.

gel A colloid existing as a semisolid or gelatinous mass.
irreversible g. One converted from a sol, but which cannot be reconverted.

gelation 1. The process of change of a colloid from a sol to a gel. 2. Freezing.

geminate Twin; found in pairs.

gemination 1. The development of twins or pairs. 2. *In dentistry*, the development of two teeth from one follicle; they may be entirely separate or have only one pulp chamber and a groove or depression down the centre to mark the division. It is usually seen in the permanent upper anterior teeth. *Also called* schizodontia.
oliphyodontic g. A condition in which a primary tooth is fused to a permanent one.

genal Relating to the cheek.

general Affecting the body as a whole, or many parts; as opposed to *local*.

generic Relating to one genus.

genial Relating to the chin.

-genic Suffix signifying *productive of* or *producing*.

genio- Prefix signifying *chin*.

geniocheiloplasty Plastic surgery of both the chin and lower lip.

genioglossal Relating to the chin and the tongue.

genioglossus muscle One of the pair of extrinsic muscles on the under side of the tongue, which protrude and depress the tongue. *See* Table of Muscles—genioglossus.

geniohyoid Relating to the chin and the hyoid bone.

geniohyoid muscle The muscle that raises and draws forward the hyoid bone, with the jaw fixed. *See* Table of Muscles—geniohyoideus.

genion 1. The chin. 2. *In craniometry*, the apex of the mental protuberance.

genioplasty Plastic surgery of the chin.

genus In biological classification, the principal subdivision of a family, and itself dividing into species.

geny- Prefix signifying *jaw*.

genyantralgia Pain affecting the maxillary sinus (or antrum).

genyantritis Inflammation of the maxillary sinus (or antrum).

genyantrum The maxillary *sinus (or antrum).

genycheiloplasty Plastic surgery of both the cheek and the lip.

genyplasty Plastic surgery of the mandible.

geotrichosis Any infection caused by a species of *Geotrichum*.

Geotrichum A genus of yeast-like fungi, associated with bronchopulmonary and oral lesions.

geriodontics *Gerodontia, gerodontics.

germ 1. Any micro-organism, especially a pathogenic species. 2. A spore or seed. 3. The primitive embryo, or any part of it that will develop into a separate organ or part.
tooth g. The enamel organ, dental papilla and sac; the rudiments of the developing tooth.

germicidal Germ-destroying.

germinal Relating to germs.

gerodontia, gerodontics That branch of dentistry which is concerned with the care of old people.

gerodontic 1. Relating to gerodontics. 2. Relating to the effects of age on dental tissues.

ghost teeth *Odontodysplasia.

Gibson bandage (K.C. Gibson, 1849-1925. American dentist). A bandage for immobilizing the jaw and retaining the bone fragments in fracture of the mandible.

Gilmer splint (T.L. Gilmer, 1849-1931. American oral surgeon). Immobilization of a fractured mandible and restoration of normal occlusion by means of silver wire fastening upper to lower teeth.

gingiva (*pl.* gingivae) The gum tissue and mucous membrane surrounding the tooth and alveolar process.
attached g. That part of the gingiva which is attached both to the alveolar bone and to the cementum of a tooth.
free g. The closely adherent collar of gingiva around the neck of a tooth which also forms the outer wall of the gingival crevice.
marginal g. Free *gingiva.

gingival 1. Relating to the gingiva. 2. Relating to that wall of a tooth cavity which faces the gingival tooth surface.

gingival nerves Nerves that supply the gingiva. *See* Table of Nerves—gingivalis.

gingivalgia Neuralgic pain affecting the gums.

gingivectomy Surgical excision of the gum or of a gum lesion.

gingivitis Inflammation of the gingiva. Often used, inaccurately, to denote any form of gingival disease.
acute g. Gingival inflammation of sudden onset and short duration, without ulceration.
acute ulcerative g., acute necrotizing ulcerative g. An acute condition of the gingiva in which the predominant micro-organisms include *Bacteroides melanogenicus intermedius, Fusobacterium nucleatum*

and *Treponema vincentii*; it is characterized by necrosis of the papillae and subsequent involvement of the free gingiva. *Also called* Vincent's infection or Plaut-Vincent gingivitis. It may also spread to other parts of the mouth and throat as necrotizing ulcerative *gingivostomatitis and acute ulcerative *tonsillitis.

chronic g. Long-standing gingival inflammation, often associated with a build-up of plaque.

desquamative g. A chronic and diffuse inflammation of the gingiva, which develops greyish lesions which peel off exposing the red and sensitive tissue beneath.

expulsive g. Osteoperiostitis affecting a tooth or teeth, gradually expelling them from their sockets.

fusospirillary g., fusospirochaetal g. Acute ulcerative *gingivitis.

hyperplastic g. Gingival inflammation associated with chronic enlargement.

necrotizing ulcerative g. Acute ulcerative *gingivitis.

phagedenic g. Acute ulcerative *gingivitis.

plasma-cell g. A rare condition affecting the free and attached gingivae, which become bright red and oedematous, and which are infiltrated by large numbers of plasma cells.

pregnancy g. Gingivitis that is thought to be caused by the endocrine changes occurring during pregnancy; marked by hypertrophy and haemorrhage of the gums, and occasionally by tumour-like swelling.

proliferative g. Hyperplastic *gingivitis.

ulcerative g., ulceromembranous g. Acute ulcerative *gingivitis.

gingivo- Prefix signifying *gingiva*.

gingivoaxial Relating to the gingival and axial walls in the mesial or distal portion of a proximo-occlusal cavity.

g. angle. The angle formed at the junction of these walls; a *line* angle.

gingivobuccoaxial Relating to the gingival, buccal and axial walls in the mesial or distal portion of a proximo-occlusal cavity.

g. angle. The angle formed at the junction of these walls; a *point* angle.

gingivoglossitis Inflammation of both the gums and the tongue.

gingivolabial Relating to the gums and the lips.

gingivolinguoaxial Relating to the gingival, lingual and axial walls in the mesial or distal portion of a proximo-occlusal cavity.

g. angle. The angle formed at the junction of these walls; a *point* angle.

gingivopericementitis *Pyorrhoea alveolaris.

gingivoplasty Any method of eliminating periodontal pockets while preserving the natural outline of the gingiva as far as possible.

gingivosis Any degenerative condition affecting the gingiva.

gingivostomatitis Inflammation involving both the gingiva and the oral mucosa.

acute infectious g. Necrotizing ulcerative *gingivostomatitis.

allergic g. Gingivostomatitis due to hypersensitivity.

atypical g. Plasma-cell *gingivostomatitis.

herpetic g. A form of gingivostomatitis caused by infection with the herpes simplex virus, and characterized by inflammation, multiple vesicles and ulcers, and fever.

idiopathic g. Plasma-cell *gingivostomatitis.
necrotizing ulcerative g. An extension of acute ulcerative *gingivitis to the oral mucosa, with lesions that may involve the palate or pharynx, and characterized by pseudomembrane, ulceration and offensive odour. *Also called* Plaut's angina, pseudomembranous angina.
plasma-cell g. A condition of the oral mucosa which is characterized by inflammation of the lips, tongue and gingiva, associated with bleeding and diffuse plasma-cell infiltration.
streptococcal g. A form of gingivostomatitis associated with sore throat and caused by streptococcal infection.
white folded g. White sponge *naevus.

ginglymo-arthrodial Relating to a joint that is partly ginglymoid and partly arthrodial.

ginglymoid Resembling a ginglymus, or hinged joint.

ginglymus A hinged joint, allowing only a back and forward movement; a type of synovial joint.
helicoid g. Trochoid *joint.
lateral g. Trochoid *joint.

glabella The smooth prominence between the eyebrows.

glabrous Smooth and hairless.

gland An organ that produces secretion.
accessory parotid g. An anterior part of the parotid gland, which may be detached, found in about a third of the population.
anterior lingual g. A mixed salivary gland near the tip of the tongue, on its under surface; *also called* Blandin's gland or Nuhn's gland.
buccal g's. The mixed minor salivary glands of the buccal mucosa.
endocrine g. Any one of the ductless glands (adrenal, thyroid, etc.) supplying internal secretions to the body directly through the blood stream.
exocrine g. Any one of the glands, including salivary glands, which secrete through ducts which open on a body surface.
gingival g's. Pearly masses of epithelial cells found on the gums of infants; *also called* Serres' glands.
glossopalatine g's. Mucous glands situated behind the vallate papillae at the back of the tongue; term no longer used.
labial g's. Minor salivary glands situated below the surface of the labial mucous membrane.
lingual g's. Minor salivary glands of the tongue; *also called* Bauhin's glands.
mandibular g. Submandibular *gland.
molar g's. Those buccal glands opening through the buccinator muscle into the oral cavity in the region of the maxillary posterior molar teeth.
mucous g. One of the glands that form and secrete mucus.
palatine g's. Minor salivary glands situated at the back of the hard palate and in the soft palate.
parotid g. One of a pair of major salivary glands lying below the ear, between the ascending ramus of the mandible and the mastoid process.
retromolar g's. Molar *glands.
salivary g's. Major: any of the three pairs of large, saliva-secreting glands in the mouth: parotid, sublingual and submandibular; *minor*: the labial, buccal, molar, palatine and lingual saliva-secreting glands.
sebaceous g. One of the glands that secrete sebum.

seromucous g. Any gland that produces both serous and mucous secretion; a mixed salivary gland.
serous g. An exocrine gland, such as the parotid gland, which secretes a thin, watery, serous fluid.
staphyline g's. Palatine *glands.
sublingual g. One of a pair of major salivary glands forming a ridge on either side of the floor of the mouth, below the tongue; *also called* Rivinus' gland.
submandibular g., submaxillary g. One of a pair of major salivary glands lying on the inner edge of the mandible, in the region of the angle.
thyroid g. A large, ductless endocrine gland situated in front of the trachea, and consisting of two lateral lobes joined by an isthmus. It is made up of follicles lined with epithelium and secretes a colloid material.

For eponymous glands *see* under the personal name by which the gland is known.

glandular Relating to a gland.

Glaserian artery (J.H. Glaser, 1629-75. Swiss anatomist). A. tympanica anterior. *See* Table of Arteries.

Glaserian fissure (J.H. Glaser, 1629-75. Swiss anatomist). Petrotympanic *fissure.

glass-ionomer cement A translucent polyelectrolyte cement, composed of an aluminosilicate glass powder, which contains fluoride; it is used in restorations on anterior teeth, to fill pits and fissures, and as a base for other restorations.

glass polyalkenoate cement *Glass-ionomer cement.

glaze The shiny vitreous covering fused on to porcelain; *in prosthetic dentistry* this is used to give the effect of tooth enamel.

globular Relating to or resembling a globule.

globule A small, round mass.
dentine g's. Small, spherical bodies found in dentine during the mineralization process.

gloss-, glosso- Prefix signifying *tongue*.

-glossa Suffix signifying *tongue*.

glossagra Pain affecting the tongue.

glossal Relating to the tongue.

glossalgia Pain in the tongue.

glossanthrax Carbuncle, or anthrax, affecting the tongue.

glossauxesis The condition of having a swollen tongue.

glossectomy Total or partial excision of the tongue.

glossitis Inflammation of the tongue.
benign migratory g. Geographic *tongue.

glossocele Swelling of the tongue, and subsequent protrusion.

glossocoma Retraction of the tongue.

glossodesmus *Frenulum linguae.

glossodynamometer An instrument used to measure the ability of the tongue to resist pressure.

glossodynia Burning or painful condition of the tongue.

glossodynia exfoliativa *Moeller's glossitis.

glossoepiglottic, glossoepiglottidean Relating to the tongue and the epiglottis.

glossograph An instrument used to trace tongue movements during mastication or speech.

glossohyal Relating to the tongue and the hyoid bone.

glossoid Resembling a tongue.

glossolabial Relating to the tongue and the lips.

glossology 1. The science and study of the tongue and its diseases. 2. The definition and explanation of words.

glossolysis Paralysis of the tongue.

glossomantia Prognosis of a disease based on the appearance of the tongue.

glossoncus Any swelling of the tongue.

glossopalatine Relating to the tongue and the palate.

glossopalatine muscle M. palatoglossus. *See* Table of Muscles.

glossopalatine nerve N. intermedius. *See* Table of Nerves.

glossopathy Any disease of the tongue.

glossopexy An operation for the correction of glossoptosis by tying the base of the tongue to the front of the mandible with sutures, thus pulling the tongue well forward in the mouth.

glossopharyngeal Relating to the tongue and the pharynx.

glossopharyngeal muscle Part of constrictor pharyngis superior. *See* Table of Muscles—glossopharyngeus.

glossopharyngeal nerve The ninth cranial nerve, supplying the stylopharyngeus muscle and the parotid gland, and the mucosa of the tongue. *See* Table of Nerves—glossopharyngeus.

glossophytia Black *tongue.

glossoplasty Plastic surgery of the tongue.

glossoplegia Paralysis of the tongue.

glossoptosis Displacement of the tongue downwards.

glossopyrosis A burning sensation of the tongue.

glossorraphy Suturing of the tongue.

glossoscopy Diagnostic examination of the tongue.

glossospasm Spasm of the muscles of the tongue.

glossosteresis *Glossectomy.

glossotomy Incision of the tongue.

glossotrichia Hairy *tongue.

glottis The opening between the vocal cords.

glyco- Prefix signifying *sugar*.

glycoptyalism *Glycosialia.

glycosialia A condition in which sugar is present in the saliva.

glycosialorrhoea A condition in which there is excessive secretion of saliva containing sugar.

gnath-, gnatho- Prefix signifying *jaw*.

gnathalgia Neuralgic pain affecting the jaw.

gnathankylosis Ankylosis of the jaw.

gnathic Relating to the jaw.

gnathion 1. *In physical anthropology*, the lowest point on the median line of the mandible. 2. *In cephalometry*, the point at which the line bisecting the angle between the facial and mandibular planes crosses the outline of the mental symphysis as seen on a lateral skull radiograph.

gnathitis Inflammation of the jaws.

gnathodynamics The study of the physical forces involved in mastication.

gnathodynamometer An instrument used to record the force exerted in closing the jaws.

gnathodynia Pain in the jaw.

gnathology The study of the masticatory mechanism.

gnathoplasty Plastic surgery of the jaw or of the cheek.

gnathoplegia Paralysis of the muscles of the cheek.

gnathorrhagia Bleeding of the buccal mucosa or from the jaws.

gnathoschisis Congenital cleft of the jaw, as in cleft palate.

gnathospasmus *Trismus[1].

gnathostat 1. A device used to ensure the exact location of the jaws for purposes of photography, radiography or cephalometry. 2. A mechanical device used in orthodontics to orientate plaster casts so that there is a constant relationship between the Frankfort, mid-palatal and orbital planes.

gnathostatics A method of extraoral orthodontic diagnosis based on the craniometric relationship of the teeth to the rest of the skull.

gnathostomatics The physiology of the jaws and the mouth.

Goethe's bone (J.W. von Goethe, 1749-1832. German poet and anatomist). The *intermaxillary bone.

goitre Enlargement of the thyroid gland.
exophthalmic g. A condition associated with hyperthyroidism, and characterized by enlarged thyroid glands and exophthalmos; *also called* Graves' disease.
lingual g. Lingual *thyroid.

gold A soft, yellow metal, chemical symbol Au, used in dentistry for fillings and inlays.
crystal g., crystalline g. Mat *gold.
Dutch g. An alloy of zinc and copper.
mat g. Non-cohesive gold in the form of spongy crystals.
sponge g. Mat *gold.
white g. An alloy of gold with palladium, or with silver, platinum or nickel, these metals giving it a white or silvery appearance.

gomphiasis Looseness of the teeth.

gomphosis 1. Firm attachment of two bones without a movable joint. 2. The attachment between the bony tooth socket and the cementum of a tooth, which allows only limited movement.

Gongylonema A genus of nematode parasites found generally in domestic animals.

gongylonemiasis *of the mouth* Oral infestation with *Gongylonema*; occasionally found in humans.

gonio- Prefix signifying *angle*.

goniocheiloschisis Macrostomia; a transverse facial cleft.

goniocraniometry Measurement of the angles of the cranium.

goniometer An instrument used for measuring angles.

gonion 1. The outer tip of the angle of the mandible. 2. *In cephalometry*, the point on the shadow of the angle of the mandible located by bisecting the angle between the condylar and mandibular planes.

Gorlin-Chaudry-Moss syndrome (R.J. Gorlin, b. 1923. American oral pathologist; A.P. Chaudry, b. 1922. Indian-born American oral pathologist; M.L. Moss, b. 1923. American anatomist). Craniofacial dysostosis associated with micro-ophthalmia, ocular and dental anomalies, and patent ductus arteriosus.

Goslee tooth (H.J. Goslee, 1871-1930. American dentist). A porcelain tooth, attached to a metal base and readily interchangeable, used in cast bridge work.

Gottlieb's cuticle (B. Gottlieb, 1885-1950. Austrian dentist). *Gottlieb's epithelial attachment.

Gottlieb's epithelial attachment (B. Gottlieb, 1885-1950. Austrian dentist). The epithelial tissue attaching the gum to the tooth.

gouge A chisel with a hollowed or grooved blade for cutting or removing bone.

graft 1. A slip of tissue, such as skin, muscle or bone, or man-made bio-material, used to repair a defect by

implantation. 2. To attach such a slip of tissue in place.
allogenic g. *Allograft.
autogenous g. *Autograft.
homogenous g., homologous g. *Allograft.

Gram's method of staining (H.C.J. Gram, 1853-1938. Danish bacteriologist). A method for staining bacteria, first with aniline-gentian violet and then, after washing with alcohol, restaining with some other stain. Those bacteria that retain the first stain are called *Gram-positive*; those that decolourize with the use of alcohol are called *Gram-negative*.

granular Composed of granules.

granule A small grain or a particle.

granules, Fordyce's *Fordyce's spots.

granuloma A tumour composed of granulation tissue.
apical g. A localized mass of granulation tissue on or near the root of a tooth.
dental g. Apical *granuloma.
giant-cell g. A type of granuloma found in the jaws, most commonly in the tooth-bearing area of the mandible, in persons between 20 years and 30 years of age; it contains aggregations of multinuclear giant cells, and is frequently associated with bleeding. It may be found in bone (*central*) or in soft tissue (*peripheral*).
pyogenic g. A raised and circumscribed tumour-like lesion of the soft tissues, sessile or pedunculated, with a rough, ulcerated and necrotic surface, found in the gingiva, and characterized by acute inflammation, giving it a fiery red appearance; it bleeds easily and grows rapidly.

granulomatosis The development of multiple granulomas.

Graves' disease (R.J. Graves, 1797-1853. Irish physician). Exophthalmic *goitre.

Greene-Vermillion index (J.C. Greene, contemporary American public health dentist; J.R. Vermillion, contemporary American public health doctor). Simplified oral hygiene *index.

grinding Wearing away by rubbing with some abrasive substance.
spot g. The correction of occlusion by grinding down high areas on the teeth, fillings or prosthetic appliances, disclosed by articulating paper.

grinding-in The process of rectifying occlusal disharmony by grinding the occluding surfaces either of natural or artificial teeth.

groove A long, narrow channel or trough in any surface.
alveololingual g. A groove between the lower jaw and the tongue.
anterior palatine g. Incisive *canal.
developmental g. One of the grooves in the enamel surface of a tooth, marking the divisions of primary formation.
digastric g. Mastoid *notch.
infraorbital g. of the maxilla Infraorbital *sulcus.
labial g. A groove in the embryonic labial lamina which develops into the vestibule of the oral cavity.
labiomental g. Mentolabial *furrow.
mylohyoid g. Mylohyoid *sulcus.
nasopalatine g. A groove on the surface of the vomer in which lodge the nasopalatine nerve and vessels.
palatine g., palatomaxillary g. Greater palatine *sulcus of the palatine bone.
palatine g. of the maxilla Palatine *sulcus of the maxilla.
pterygopalatine g. 1. A groove on the ventral aspect of the pterygoid

process of the sphenoid bone. 2. A groove on the vertical portion of the palatine bone.

gubernaculum dentis The band of connective tissue attaching the dental sac of a permanent tooth to the surrounding oral mucosa.

Guerin's fracture (A.F.M. Guerin, 1816-95. French surgeon). *Le Fort fracture, Class I.

Guidi's canal (G. Guidi [V. Vidius], 1500-69. Italian anatomist and physician). Pterygoid *canal.

gum 1. Sticky secretion from certain trees. 2. *In dentistry,* the *gingiva.

gum rash *Strophulus.

gumboil *Parulis.

gumma A tertiary syphilitic lesion in the form of a soft, rubbery tumour composed of granulation-like tissue.

gummatous Relating to a gumma.

gun

amalgam g. *Amalgam carrier.

Gunning splint (T.B. Gunning, 1813-89. American dentist). An interdental splint, like a solid double dental plate, used in fracture of the mandible.

gustation The sense of taste, or the act of tasting.

gustatory Relating to the sense of taste.

gustatory artery A. lingualis. *See* Table of Arteries.

gutta Latin for *a drop*; used in prescription writing, and abbreviated *gutt.*

gutta-percha The dehydrated product of the juice of certain sapotaceous trees. It is a plastic substance, used *in dentistry* for temporary fillings, in root canal treatment, and so on.

guttural Relating to the throat.

Gysi's articulator (A. Gysi, fl. 1936. Swiss dentist). An apparatus used in the construction of artificial dentures, with which all possible movements of the mandible and the condyles can be reproduced.

H

H Chemical symbol for hydrogen.

HBV Hepatitis B virus.

HCl Chemical symbol for hydrochloric acid.

h.d. Abbreviation for *hora decubitus*—at bedtime (lit. *at the hour of bed*); used in prescription writing.

Hg Chemical symbol for mercury.

HIV Human immunodeficiency virus; AIDS is the clinical consequence of infection with this virus.

h.s. Abbreviation for *hora somni*—at bedtime (lit. *at the hour of sleep*); used in prescription writing.

habit Any learned response, which is repeated frequently in a given situation.
oral h. One that can affect the occlusion; examples are thumb sucking and tongue thrust.

haem-, haemato-, haemo- Prefix signifying *blood.*

haemangioameloblastoma A form of ameloblastoma containing many blood vessels.

haemangioendothelioma *Angiosarcoma.

haemangioma A benign hamartoma arising from blood vessels.
ameloblastic h. *Haemangioameloblastoma.
arterial h. Capillary *haemangioma.
capillary h. A form of haemangioma consisting of closely-packed collections of thin-walled capillaries; found in the mucosa of the lips and mouth.
cavernous h. A form of haemangioma consisting of large, blood-filled cavernous vascular canals.

haemangiopericytoma A tumour arising from the cells surrounding the capillaries and small arteries.

haemartoma Old term for *haemangioma.

haematemesis Vomiting of blood.

haematogenous 1. Blood-produced. 2. Blood-producing.

haematoma A swelling caused by the extravasation of blood into the tissues.
eruption h. Eruption *cyst.

haematostatic *Haemostatic.

haemodia The condition of having abnormally sensitive teeth.

haemophilia An hereditary defect of the blood-clotting mechanism, appearing in the male but transmitted through the female.

haemophiliac A sufferer from haemophilia.

Haemophilus A genus of parasitic, rod-shaped organisms, Gram-negative, non-motile and aerobic or facultatively anaerobic, occurring on the mucous membrane.

haemoptysic Relating to or characterized by haemoptysis.

haemoptysis The presence of blood in the sputum, caused by bleeding in the upper respiratory tract or the lungs.

haemorrhage Internal or external loss of blood due to injury or other damage to a blood vessel.

haemorrhagenic Causing bleeding.

haemorrhagic Relating to or affected by haemorrhage.

haemorrhoid
lingual h. Swelling of the veins at the root of the tongue.

haemostasis 1. The arrest of bleeding. 2. The checking of the blood circulation at any point.

haemostat 1. An agent used to inhibit bleeding by applying it directly to the wound or the site of the bleeding. 2. Haemostatic *forceps.

haemostatic 1. Relating to the arrest of bleeding. 2. An agent used in haemostasis.

haemostyptic *Haemostatic.

halitosis Foetid-smelling breath.

Haller's ansa (A. von Haller, 1708-77. Swiss anatomist). The loop formed below the stylomastoid foramen between the glossopharyngeal nerve and the lingual branch of the facial nerve.

Haller's circle (A. von Haller, 1708-77. Swiss anatomist). Circulus arteriosus halleri. *See* circulus vasculosus nervi optici.

hamartoma A tumour-like mass of superfluous tissue, the result of faulty development of tissues or cells.

hamate Hook-shaped.

Hamilton's bandage (F.H. Hamilton, 1813-86. American surgeon). A special bandage consisting of straps of linen webbing attached to a leather thong.

Hammond splint 1. An orthodontic splint used for repositioning a tooth or teeth. 2. A double archwire fixed to the teeth and used to immobilize a jaw fracture.

hamular, hamulate 1. Shaped like a hook. 2. Relating to a hamulus.

hamulus A hook-shaped process on a bone.

pterygoid h. A hook-like descending process of the medial pterygoid plate of the sphenoid bone.

Hanau's equation (R.L. Hanau, contemporary American dentist). An algebraic formula used in the setting up of an anatomical articulator. It provides for the simulation of the Bennett movement by relating the angular rotation (V) of the condylar path about a vertical axis to its rotation (H) about a horizontal axis. $V = H/8 + 12$ where V is the deviation from the sagittal plane and H the deviation from the coronal plane, measured in degrees.

'hand-foot-mouth' disease Vesicular *stomatitis with exanthem.

handpiece The hand-held device, incorporating a chuck, into which various rotary or reciprocating instruments for cutting or cleaning the tooth may be fitted; it is connected to the dental engine and may be belt-driven or air-driven. Depending upon the angle of the shaft to that of the instrument, the handpiece may be described as *straight*, *right-angle*, or *contra-angle*.

air turbine h. Turbine *handpiece.

contra-angle h. One that has two or more bends in the shaft; designed to reach areas of the oral cavity where access is limited.

right-angle h. One in which the rotary instrument is held at right angles to the shaft.

straight h. One in which the rotary instrument is held directly in line with the shaft.

turbine h. One incorporating an air-driven rotor.

Hannover's intermediate membrane (A. Hannover, 1814-94. Danish anatomist). An acellular layer of material in a developing mammalian tooth separating developing cementum from root dentine and from the ameloblasts. In the fully formed root it is represented by an acellular layer lying between the dentine and the cementum.

Hansen's disease (G.H.A. Hansen, 1841-1912. Norwegian bacteriologist and physician). *Leprosy.

haphalgesia A condition in which intense pain is felt from a slight touch.

hapl-, haplo- Prefix signifying *simple, single.*

haplodont Having teeth with simple, smooth conical crowns and simple roots.

Hapsburg jaw Mandibular prognathism, similar to the hereditary condition that affected the Hapsburg dynasty.

Hapsburg lip The over-developed lower lip often accompanying Hapsburg jaw.

hare-lip Congenital fissure of one or both sides of the upper lip.

hare-lip needle A cannula which is introduced into the wound during an operation for hare-lip, and held in place by a figure-of-eight suture.

Hartley-Krause operation (F. Hartley, 1857-1913. American surgeon; F.V. Krause, 1857-1937. German surgeon). An operation for the relief of facial neuralgia by excision of the Gasserian ganglion. Devised, independently, by both Hartley and Krause.

Hartman's solution (L.L. Hartman, 1893-1951. American dentist). A solution of thymol, sulphuric ether and ethyl alcohol used to desensitize dentine.

hatchet A hand instrument with a sharp, straight blade in the same plane as the handle; it may be single bevelled or bibevelled, and is used for chipping away tooth structure and smoothing cavities.

enamel h. A type of chisel with a contra-angled shaft giving it a hatchet form.

haustus Latin for *a draught*; used in prescription writing, generally with *fiat*, abbreviated *f.h.* (fiat haustus).

Hawley retainer (C.A. Hawley, 20th century American dentist). A horseshoe-shaped plate with clasps to the premolars and a labial wire from the lingual surface of the incisors; the most commonly used orthodontic removable retaining appliance.

head 1. The uppermost part of the body, containing the special sensory organs and the brain. 2. The upper end of a bone, especially of a long bone. 3. Implant *abutment.

headcap 1. A plaster cap used with metal jaw splints in fracture of the jaw or of the facial bones. 2. *Headgear.

headgear *In orthodontics*, a webbing or plastic strapping harness which fits over the patient's head and is used to supply attachment for extra-oral traction.

healing coping *Cover screw.

Heath's operation (C. Heath, 1835-1905. English surgeon). An operation for ankylosis treated by dividing the ascending rami of the mandible with a saw; performed within the mouth.

Heck's disease (J.W. Heck, b. 1923. American dentist). Focal epithelial *hyperplasia.

hect-, hecto- Prefix signifying *one hundred.*

helcoid Ulcer-like.

helcosis The condition of having ulcers; ulceration.

helix *In anatomy*, the convex margin of the pinna of the ear.

hem-, hemato-, hemo- For words with these prefixes *see* those beginning with haem-, haemato-, haemo-.

hemi- Prefix signifying *half*, or *one side* (right or left) of a body, organ or part.

hemiageusia, hemigeusia Loss or absence of a sense of taste in one side of the tongue only.

hemialgia Pain affecting one half of an organ or part, or one side of the body only.

hemiatrophy Atrophy affecting one half of an organ or part, or one side of the body only.

hemidesmosome A structure found on the basal surface of an epithelial cell, the attachment site between the cell and the underlying membrane; one half of a desmosome.

hemifacial Relating to or affecting one side of the face only.

hemigeusia *See* hemiageusia.

hemiglossal Relating to or affecting one side of the tongue only.

hemiglossectomy Surgical removal of one side of the tongue.

hemiglossitis Inflammation affecting one side of the tongue only.

hemiglossoplegia Paralysis affecting one side of the tongue only.

hemignathia The condition of having only half a jaw.

hemihypermetria Abnormal extension or protrusion of one half of a part.

hemihyperplasia Hyperplasia affecting only one side or one half of an organ or part.

hemihypertrophy Hypertrophy affecting one side or one half of a body, an organ, or a part.

hemihypogeusia *Hemiageusia.

hemilingual Relating to or affecting one side of the tongue only.

hemimacroglossia Abnormal development and size of one side of the tongue.

hemimandibulectomy The surgical removal of one side of the mandible.

hemimaxillectomy The surgical removal of one side of the maxilla.

hemipalatolaryngoplegia Paralysis affecting the muscles on one side of the soft palate and the larynx.

hemiplegia Paralysis affecting one side of the body.
facial h. Paralysis affecting one side of the face only.
faciolingual h. Paralysis affecting one side of the face and the tongue.

hemisection, hemisectomy 1. Cutting in two, or bisection. 2. *In dentistry*, the surgical division of a multi-rooted tooth through the furcation so that one damaged or diseased root may be removed, together with the associated crown area.

hemiseptum The remaining part of an interdental septum after either the mesial or the distal part has been destroyed by a lesion.

hemo- *See* haemo-.

hepatitis Inflammation of the liver.
acute infective h. A generally benign form of hepatitis caused by hepatitis A virus, and characterized by fever, jaundice and liver enlargement.
homologous serum h. Serum *hepatitis.
infective h. Any form of hepatitis caused by a specific virus or occurring in an infective disease.
serum h. A form of hepatitis caused by hepatitis B virus and spread by blood transfusion or contaminated instruments, especially syringes; it is very similar to acute infective hepatitis, but may be fatal in the acute stage.

herbivorous Grass- and herb-eating.

Herbst appliance (E. Herbst, fl. 1930. German orthodontist). The only fixed functional orthodontic appliance; maxillary and mandibular splints are fixed to the teeth and the splints are joined by a pin and tube apparatus which controls the position of the mandible; used in treatment of Angle's Class II malocclusion. *Also called* pin and tube appliance.

hereditary Relating to heredity.

heredity The transmission of a characteristic from parent to child, or to later generations.

Hering's nerve (H.E. Hering, 1866-1948. German physiologist). The carotid sinus branch of the glossopharyngeal nerve.

herpangina An infection of the oral cavity caused by Coxsackie virus A and characterized by sore throat, headache and temperature, with small vesicles on the tongue and pharynx which later become ulcerated.

herpes An acute inflammatory skin infection, of viral origin, and characterized by vesicles which appear in clusters.

herpes labialis Cold sores or blisters occurring on the lips; often associated with fever.

herpes simplex Herpes vesicles affecting the mucous membranes in particular, and developing on the borders of the lips and nostrils.

herpes zoster An acute viral infection characterized by inflammation of sensory ganglia, and an eruption of vesicular lesions on the skin of the areas supplied by the affected nerve or nerves.

herpetic Relating to herpes.

herpetiform Herpes-like; used of an eruption generally resembling herpes.

Hertwig's sheath (W.A.O. Hertwig, 1849-1922. German anatomist). Epithelial root *sheath.

hetero- Prefix signifying *different, other.*

heterocellular Formed of different types of cells.

heterodont Having teeth that have different forms; as opposed to *homodont.*

heterogeneous Consisting of different substances; as opposed to *homogeneous.*

heterogenous Derived from different species; as opposed to *homogenous.*

heterograft *Xenograft.

heteroplasia Formation of tissue abnormal either in structure or in position.

heterostomy The condition of having an asymmetrical mouth.

heterotopic Occurring in a place other than normal.

heretotransplant *Xenograft.

heterotrophic Relating to organisms which require a complex source of carbon for nourishment and growth; as opposed to *autotrophic.*

hex-, hexa- Prefix signifying *six.*

hiatal Relating to a hiatus.

hiation Yawning.

hiatus Any gap, opening or fissure.
buccal h. A transverse facial cleft.
ethmoidal h. *Hiatus semilunaris.
facial h., h. of facial canal *Hiatus of canal for greater petrosal nerve.
h. of canal for greater petrosal nerve The opening in the petrous portion of the temporal bone leading to the facial canal, containing the greater petrosal nerve, and also a branch of the middle meningeal artery.

h. of canal for lesser petrosal nerve The small opening in the petrous portion of the temporal bone through which passes the lesser petrosal nerve.
maxillary h., h. of maxillary sinus The opening on the inner surface of the maxilla, joining the nasal cavity and the maxillary sinus.

hiatus semilunaris A long, narrow and curved depression in the middle meatus of the nose; it leads to paranasal air sinuses: the *superior* opening draining the frontal sinus and the *inferior* (maxillary hiatus) leading to the maxillary sinus.

Highmore, antrum of (N. Highmore, 1613-85. English anatomist). Maxillary *sinus.

highmoritis Inflammation of the antrum of Highmore, the maxillary sinus.

hilar Relating to a hilum.

hilum (*pl.* hila) A pit or opening in an organ, generally where the vessels or ducts enter.

hilus *See* hilum.

hingebow Adjustable axis *facebow.

Hirschfeld canal (I. Hirschfeld, 1881-1965. American dentist). Nutrient *canal.

Hirschfeld's nerve (I. Hirschfeld, 1816-76. Polish anatomist). A lingual branch of the facial nerve which goes to form Haller's ansa.

hirudiniasis Infestation of the mouth and the upper respiratory tract by leeches.

histo- Prefix signifying *tissue*.

histochemistry The use of known chemical and physical reactions to identify chemical substances within the tissues; a branch of histology.

histogenesis The embryonic development of tissues.

histologic, histological Relating to histology.

histology The study of the anatomy and physiology of tissues and cells using microscopic techniques.

histopathological Relating to histopathology.

histopathology The study of minute structural changes in diseased tissue; histological pathology.

histoplasmosis A generalized fungal infection caused by *Histoplasma capsulatum*, with nodular, ulcerative or vegetative lesions frequently seen on the lips, tongue, palate and mucous membrane; *also called* Darling's disease.

hoe A hand instrument similar to a hatchet, with the cutting edge of the blade at right angles to the handle.
periodontal h. An instrument used for removing calculus and other deposits from the tooth surface.

holistic An approach to treatment that takes into consideration the whole person, not just the disease or condition.

hollow 1. A depression or concavity. 2. Descriptive of an empty container.

homalocephalus A person having a flat head.

homaluranus A person having an unusually flat palatal arch.

homo- Prefix signifying *same, like*.

homodont Having teeth all of the same form; as opposed to *heterodont*.

homogeneous Of one kind or substance; as opposed to *heterogeneous*.

homogenous Derived from one species, and being therefore similar; as opposed to *heterogenous*.

homograft *Allograft.

homologous Having the same or corresponding structure or position, but not necessarily similar in function.

homotransplant *Allograft.

hood
tooth h. Dental *operculum.

hood crown A half-cap crown covering the lingual, approximal and occlusal surfaces of a tooth.

hook *In dentistry,* a curved or bent device of wire or other flexible material used to catch round a tooth to provide either support or anchorage for traction.

hora decubitus Latin for *at bedtime* (lit. *at the hour for bed*); used in prescription writing, and abbreviated *h.d.*

hora somni Latin for *at bedtime* (lit. *at the hour of sleep*); used in prescription writing, and abbreviated *h.s.*

hormion The point of attachment of the vomer and the sphenoid bone, between the alae of the vomer; a craniometric landmark.

horn A pointed protuberance or projection.
pulp h. One of the horn-like projections of the pulp chamber into the crown of a tooth.

Horner's teeth (W.E. Horner, 1793-1853. American dentist). Incisor teeth with horizontal grooves caused by enamel deficiency.

Hotchkiss's operation (L.W. Hotchkiss, 1859-1926. American surgeon). An operation for the removal of buccal carcinoma, involving the excision of a portion of the mandible, sometimes of the maxilla, and plastic repair of the cheek from the neck tissues.

How crown (W.S. How, fl. 1883. American dentist). A porcelain-faced crown attached by means of four pins bent round a post in the tooth root, the exposed parts being built up with amalgam.

Howland-Perry crown An improved form of the *Mack crown, having better retention.

Howship's lacuna (J. Howship, 1781-1841. English surgeon). Resorption *lacuna.

Hullihen's acutenaculum (S.P. Hullihen, 1810-57. American dentist). A type of needle-holder used in cleft palate surgery.

humectant 1. Moistening. 2. Any moistening agent.

Humphry's operation (Sir G.M. Humphry, 1820-96. English surgeon). An operation for excision of a mandibular condyle.

Hunter's glossitis (W. Hunter, 1861-1937. English physician). Ulcerative glossitis occurring in pernicious anaemia.

Hunter-Schreger bands *Schreger's lines *in enamel.*

Hutchinson's incisors (Sir Jonathan Hutchinson, 1828-1913. English physician). Permanent incisors having narrow and notched incisal edges; found in congenital syphilis.

hydrargyrum *Mercury.

hydro- Prefix signifying *water.*

hydrocolloid A type of dental impression material; a viscous colloid sol which is converted into a rigid and insoluble gel; it may be *reversible* or *irreversible.*

hydrocyst A cyst whose contents are of a watery nature; an obsolete term.

hydro-flo technique A term originated by E.O. Thompson, American dentist, to designate a technique of cavity preparation in which the field of operation is constantly irrigated in a stream of warm water, and the water removed from the mouth by vacuum suction.

hydroglossa *Ranula; an obsolete term.

hydropic *Oedematous; an obsolete term.

hydrostomia A condition characterized by constant dribbling from the mouth; *hypersalivation.

hydrous Containing water.

hygiene Principles and practice of general and personal cleanliness for the promotion of health and prevention of disease.
dental h. Oral *hygiene.
mouth h. Oral *hygiene.
oral h. Principles of hygiene as applied to the mouth, to ensure cleanliness of the teeth and promote healthy gingiva.

hygienic Relating to hygiene.

hygienist
dental h. A dental auxiliary trained to perform certain preventive operations, such as scaling and polishing the teeth, to teach oral hygiene, and to apply topical fluorides and pit and fissure sealants, under the direction of a dentist.

hygro- Prefix signifying *moisture*.

hygroma A swelling caused by fluid surrounding an inflamed bursa, or distending a sac or cyst.

hyo- Prefix signifying *U-shaped*; *in anatomy* denotes some relationship with the *hyoid* arch or bone.

hyobasioglossus The basal portion of the hyoglossal muscle.

hyoglossal Relating to the hyoid bone and the tongue.

hyoglossus muscle One of the pair of extrinsic muscles that draw down the sides of the tongue. *See* Table of Muscles—hyoglossus.

hyoid artery A. infrahyoidea and A. suprahyoidea. *See* Table of Arteries.

hyoid bone U-shaped bone forming the arch between the larynx and the base of the tongue; it supports the tongue and provides attachment for some of the facial muscles.

hyomandibular 1. Relating to the hyoid and mandibular arches in the embryo. 2. Relating to the cartilaginous portion of the hyoid arch in fish.

hypalgesia Reduced sensibility to pain.

hypanisognathism The condition of having the maxillary teeth broader than the mandibular teeth, causing a lack of correspondence between the jaws.

hypanisognathous Relating to or characterized by hypanisognathism.

hyper- Prefix signifying 1. *excessive, exaggerated*; 2. *above* (in anatomy or zoology).

hyperaemia Excess of blood causing localized congestion.

hyperaesthesia Increased, abnormal sensitivity to pain.

hyperalgesia The condition of being excessively sensitive to pain.

hyperalveolism A condition in which the alveolar process is too high in relation to the base of the jaw; it may be *maxillary* or *mandibular*.

hyperbrachycephalic Showing an extreme degree of brachycephaly; having an exceptionally broad head.

hypercalcification Excessive deposition of calcium salts in any normally calcified tissue.

hypercementosis Over-development of cementum on tooth roots.

hyperdontia The condition of having supernumerary teeth present in the mouth.

hyperdontogeny *Hyperodontogeny.

hyperemia *See* hyperaemia.

hyperfunction Abnormal, excessive functioning.

hypergenia A condition in which an otherwise normal chin is too high in relation to the rest of the facial skeleton.

hypergeusia Abnormally acute sense of taste.

hyperhidrosis Excessive sweating.

hyperkeratosis linguae Black *tongue.

hyperodontogeny The condition of developing supernumerary teeth, or even a complete third dentition.

hyperorthognathous Relating to or characterized by hyperorthognathy.

hyperorthognathy Excessive orthognathia; having a very low gnathic index.

hyperostosis Bone hypertrophy; exostosis.

hyperplasia Over-development of an organ or tissue, due to increased production of cells.
cementum h. *Hypercementosis.
chronic perforating h. Internal root *resorption.
denture h. Denture-induced *hyperplasia.
denture-induced h. Hyperplasia of the mucous membrane in the buccal and labial sulcus, caused by persistent irritation from poorly fitting dentures.
fibrous gingival h. Gingival *fibromatosis.
fibrous inflammatory h. Denture-induced *hyperplasia.
focal epithelial h. Hyperplasia affecting the labial and lingual mucosa, and sometimes the floor of the mouth, palate and buccal mucosa, and characterized by soft, sessile papules, especially on the lower lip; the condition is usually seen in children and adolescents, and its course may be prolonged. *Also called* Heck's disease.
gingival h. Enlargement of the gingiva, generally non-inflammatory; it may be drug-induced in those on long-term anticonvulsant therapy with phenytoin.
inflammatory fibrous h. Denture-induced *hyperplasia.
inflammatory papillary h. A lesion most commonly seen in the palate, and characterized by small, soft, bright red papillae; almost always observed in patients with poorly fitting dentures, and rarely in dentate patients.
papillary h., papilliferous h. Inflammatory papillary *hyperplasia.

hyperplastic Relating to or affected by hyperplasia.

hyperptyalism *Hypersalivation.

hypersalivation Excessive secretion of saliva.

hypersensitivity *Allergy.

hypersialosis *Hypersalivation.

hypertaurodontism A severe form of *taurodontism in which there is no division of the tooth roots.

hypertelorism An abnormal distance between any two organs or parts.
ocular h. A craniofacial deformity characterized by enlargement of the sphenoid bone, great breadth across the bridge of the nose, and resulting width between the eyes.

hypertension Exceptionally high tension, especially abnormally high blood pressure.

hypertensive Relating to hypertension.

hyperthyroidism A condition caused by abnormal hyperfunction of the thyroid gland, characterized by weight loss, weakness and nervousness, and often by exophthalmic goitre.

hypertrophic Relating to or characterized by hypertrophy.

hypertrophy An abnormal increase in the size of an organ or part due to enlargement of its constituent cells.
cementum h. *Hypercementosis.

hypnodontics The application of hypnosis to dentistry.

hypnosis Sleep, or a trance state, especially one induced artificially by verbal suggestion or concentration upon some object.

hypnotic 1. Relating to hypnosis. 2. Inducing sleep.

hypnotism The process of inducing sleep or a trance.

hypo- Prefix signifying 1. *deficient, lacking*; 2. *below* (in anatomy and zoology).

hypoaesthesia Lessened sensitivity to pain.

hypoalveolism A condition in which the alveolar process is not high enough in relation to the base of the jaw; it may be *maxillary* or *mandibular*.

hypobranchial Below the branchial arches.

hypocalcification Defective development resulting in an insufficient deposit of calcium salts in any normally calcified tissue.

hypocondylar Below a condyle.

hypocone The distolingual cusp on a maxillary molar tooth.

hypoconid The distobuccal cusp on a mandibular molar tooth.

hypoconule The fifth, distal cusp of a maxillary molar tooth.

hypoconulid The fifth, distal cusp of a mandibular molar tooth.

hypodermic Under the skin.

hypodontia Congenital absence of several teeth; often, inaccurately, called partial anodontia.

hypofibrinogenaemia A form of fibrinogenaemia in which the fibrinogen content of the blood is low.

hypofunction Deficient or diminished function.

hypogenia A condition in which an otherwise normal chin is too low in relation to the rest of the facial skeleton.

hypogeusia Diminution of the sense of taste.

hypoglossal Underneath the tongue.

hypoglossal nerve The twelfth cranial nerve, supplying the muscles of the tongue. *See* Table of Nerves—hypoglossus.

hypoglossiadenitis Inflammation of the sublingual glands.

hypoglossitis Inflammation of the sublingual tissues.

hypoglottis 1. The under part of the tongue. 2. *Ranula.

hypognathous Having a protruding mandible.

hypomicrognathic Having an abnormally small lower jaw; extreme micrognathism.

hypo-ostosis Bone hypoplasia.

hypopharynx The lower or laryngeal part of the pharynx; an obsolete term.

hypophyseal, hypophysial Relating to an hypophysis; more specifically, relating to the pituitary gland.

hypophysis An outgrowth, especially used of the pituitary body.

hypoplasia Under-development of an organ or tissue.
enamel h. *Amelogenesis imperfecta.

hypoplastic Relating to hypoplasia.

hypoptyalism *Hyposalivation.

hyposalivation Reduced secretion of saliva.

hyposiagonarthritis Inflammation affecting the temporomandibular joint.

hyposialadenitis Inflammation of the submandibular salivary glands.

hyposialosis *Hyposalivation.

hypostomatous A zoological term for those animals which have the mouth on the lower side.

hypostomia An extreme form of microstomia, the mouth being merely a slit opening into a pharyngeal sac.

hypostosis Deficient bone development.

hypotelorism An abnormally decreased distance between two organs or parts.

hypotension Abnormally low tension, especially abnormally low blood pressure, often seen in shock.

hypotensive Relating to hypotension.

hypothyroidism Deficient thyroid secretion, or the condition this produces.

hypsi- Prefix signifying *high.*

hypsibrachycephalic Having an exceptionally broad and high skull.

hypsicephalic Having an abnormally high skull.

hypsistaphylic, hypsistaphyline Having an abnormally high and pointed palatal arch.

hypsistenocephalic Having an abnormally high and narrow skull, with mandibular prognathism and prominent facial bones.

hypsocephalous *Hypsicephalic.

hypsodont Having teeth with long crowns and short roots; seen in herbivorous animals.

I

I 1. Chemical symbol for iodine. 2. Symbol for *permanent* incisor.

id. Abbreviation for *idem*—the same; used in prescription writing.

IL Incisolingual.

ILa Incisolabial.

in. Abbreviation for *inch*.

in d. Abbreviation for *in dies*—daily; used in prescription writing.

IP Incisopulpal.

-iasis Suffix signifying *diseased condition.*

iatrogenic Produced by the action of a doctor, or of medical treatment.

-ic Suffix signifying *relating to*.

ichor The thin, watery discharge from a wound or an ulcer.

ichorous Relating to ichor.

ichthyosis linguae *Leukoplakia (*linguae*).

idem Latin for *the same*; used in prescription writing and abbreviated *id.*

idio- Prefix signifying *self, distinct*; used in medicine it signifies *self-produced.*

idiopathic Self-originated, primary, relating to idiopathy.

idiopathy Any spontaneous or primary pathological condition, with no apparent external cause.

idiosyncrasy *In medicine*, reaction to a particular drug in therapeutic doses in a manner not necessarily related to its pharmacological properties.

imbalance Lack of equilibrium; in an unbalanced state.

imbrication *In dentistry*, the overlapping of anterior teeth within the same arch.

imbrication line One of the grooves in the surface of tooth enamel, marking the edges of the lines of Retzius.

immature Not yet fully developed; unripe.

immune Protected against or resistant to a specific disease.

immunity Natural or acquired resistance to specific diseases or poisons.

immunization The process or the method of rendering immune.

immuno- Prefix signifying *immune*.

immunology The study of immunity.

impacted Wedged in or confined.

impaction The condition of being tightly wedged.

imperforate Congenitally closed; applied to a structure that would normally be open.

impermeable Not permitting a passage, especially of fluid.

impervious Not affording a passage, particularly of fluid.

implant 1. To insert into the body or to graft, as in plastic surgery. 2. Any device or tissue that is inserted, partially or totally, under the body tissues.

blade endosseous i. A flat, blade-shaped design of implant, most commonly metal, inserted into a surgically prepared vertical channel in bone, used for the treatment of partial edentulousness and generally in the posterior oral segment; it may be vented - i.e. have openings through which tissue can grow. *Also called* plate-form endosseous implant.

dental i. Any device that is implanted under the oral tissues of the jaws, with some part protruding

into the mouth; it is used for the support and retention of appliances or prostheses. Dental implants may be classified by position, material or design.
endodontic i. A metal pin or post extending through the root canal into the periapical bone to lengthen and strengthen a pulpless tooth.
endodontic endosseous i. A metal pin or rod inserted through the prepared root canal into the periapical bone to stabilize a mobile tooth.
endosseous i. *In dentistry,* an implant inserted into a residual bony ridge, either alveolar and/or basal bone, as a base for a prosthesis; mostly constructed of metal, but may be coated with some inert material.
endosteal i. Endosseous *implant.
interdental i. One that uses natural teeth as abutments.
mucosal i. Intramucosal *insert.
oral i. Any biomaterial or appliance surgically inserted into either bone or soft tissue for cosmetic or functional purposes.
plate-form endosseous i. Blade endosseous *implant.
ramus frame endosseous i. A combination type of mandibular implant, consisting of a framework resting on the chin, the main part above the gum tissue and a blade implant inserted into the anterior border of the ramus; it is used to support an overdenture.
root-form endosseous i. A type of implant that goes vertically into bone; usually conical or cylindrical, it may be hollow or screw or a combination.
submersible endosseous i. An endosseous implant having a removable head and neck to allow healing and maturation of the implant site in isolation from the oral cavity before placement of any prosthesis.
subperiosteal i. A framework, conforming to the bone surface of the jaw, more commonly the mandible, inserted below the mucoperiosteum, and having abutments exposed in the mouth on which bridges, dentures etc. may be fixed; it is used to support some type of overdenture in the completely edentulous.
transendodontic i. A form of endodontic endosseous *implant: a specially designed rod inserted into the root canal.
transmandibular i. A form of transosseous *implant.
transosseous i. One that penetrates the full thickness of the bone; used exclusively in the lower jaw and inserted from below: it generally supports a removable prosthesis. The two main types are the mandibular staple *bone plate and the transmandibular *implant.
transosteal i. Transosseous *implant.
transradicular i. A form of endodontic endosseous *implant; a specially designed rod inserted into the bone through the root canal.

implant abutment That part of an oral implant which protrudes through the gingiva into the mouth, and on which a denture is supported.

implant dentistry That branch of dentistry concerned with the design and use of prostheses involving some form of oral implant surgically inserted into hard or soft tissue within the mouth.

implant denture An artificial denture supported by a framework fastened to the alveolar process beneath the periosteum, and having protruding abutments.

implant interface The area of contact between an implant and the host site; it may be either fibrous integration by the imposition of collagenous tissue or osseo-integration where there is direct contact with the bone.

implant prosthodontics That branch of restorative dentistry which follows the placement of an implant or implants.

implantation 1. The operation of grafting. 2. The transfer of a sound tooth to replace one extracted, or to fill an artificial socket. 3. The placing of some foreign substance within the body tissues for restoration purposes.

implantodontics, implantodontology Implant *dentistry.

implantology The science and practice of placing implants within the body.
dental i. Implant *dentistry.
oral i. Implant *dentistry.

impression 1. Any dent or hollow in a soft substance. 2. A negative likeness or mould of an object obtained in a plastic substance, from which a model may be cast—e.g. the impression obtained of the teeth and the mouth, prior to the construction of dentures.

impression compound A plastic material used for taking dental impressions, and composed of fatty acids, shellac, glycerin, and some form of filler, such as talc or plaster of Paris. The actual composition of individual compounds is treated as a trade secret.

impression coping *Cover screw.

impression tray A metal receptacle in which wax or plastic impression material is placed when taking mouth impressions.

in dies Latin for *daily*; used in prescription writing, and abbreviated *in d.*

in vitro Within glass; referring to observations made in a test-tube or culture dish; as opposed to *in vivo*.

in vivo Within a living organism; as opposed to *in vitro*.

in- Prefix signifying 1. *in, on, towards*; 2. *not*.

inankyloglossia A condition in which the tongue is incapable of movement; tongue-tie.

inborn Formed or developed *in utero*; innate.

inception Beginning.

inch A unit of measurement of length, one-twelfth of a foot.

incidence The number of cases of a disease appearing in a given place over a given period of time.

incipient Beginning to develop, coming into existence.

incisal Cutting.

incisal edge *of a tooth* The edge that cuts, the biting edge of an incisor or canine.

incision (pronounced *in-sizh-un*) A wound or cut in body tissue, or the act of making such a cut. 2. The cutting action of the incisor teeth.

incision (pronounced *in-siz-i-on*) The line of intersection between the median plane and the mandibular occlusal plane.

incisive 1. Capable of cutting. 2. Relating to the incisor teeth.

incisivus labii inferioris Part of the orbicularis oris muscle, extending from the area of the mandibular canine to the angle of the mouth.

incisivus labii superioris Part of the orbicularis oris muscle, extending from the area of the maxillary canine to the angle of the mouth.

incisolabial Relating to the incisal edge and the labial surface of an anterior tooth.

incisolingual Relating to the incisal edge and the lingual surface of an anterior tooth.

incisoproximal Relating to the incisal edge and either the distal or mesial surface of an anterior tooth.

incisor classification *See under* malocclusion.

incisor tooth A cutting tooth in the centre of the dental arch. There are two incisors in each quadrant in both the primary and the permanent dentition in man, one *central* and one *lateral*.

incisura *See* notch.

inclination The tilt of a tooth away from the vertical, in any direction.

inclusion *In dentistry*, the embedding of a tooth in the alveolar bone to such an extent that it cannot erupt.

inclusion cyst Any cyst arising from epithelial residues within connective tissue; in bone such cysts occur along lines of fusion.

increment The amount of increase within a given period.

incrustation The formation of a crust.

incus One of the small bones in the ear, shaped like an anvil, and often so called.

indentation 1. A dent, pit, or depression. 2. The condition of being serrated, or notched.

index (*pl.* indexes, or indices) 1. The forefinger. 2. A number or formula expressing the ratio between two dimensions of a part, used especially in craniometry. 3. A number or formula expressing the degree of involvement in a diseased state, for purposes of comparison, as for example in periodontal surveys.

alveolar i. Gnathic *index.

calculus i. See oral hygiene index.

cephalic i. The ratio of cranial breadth (× 100) to cranial length which gives an indication of the shape and size of a head.

Community Periodontal Index of Treatment Needs An index (CPITN) designed for the WHO, to assess treatment needs rather than periodontal status; it may be used for epidemiological surveys or oral health screening of individuals. Examination, using the WHO ball-pointed periodontal probe, is based on three maxillary and three mandibular sextants within the mouth, excluding the third molars. For surveys certain index teeth in each sextant are scored, and for individual screening the worst finding for all teeth in a sextant, recording 0 for no sign of disease, 1 for gingival bleeding, 2 for supragingival or subgingival calculus, 3 for pathological pocketing from 4mm to 6mm, and 4 for pocketing of 6mm or over. Treatment needs are recorded as 0 = no treatment; I = improvement in personal oral hygiene (Code 1); II = I + scaling (Codes 2 & 3); III = I + II + complex treatment (Code 4).

cranial i. Cephalic *index.

debris i. See oral hygiene index.

dental i. The ratio of dental length (× 100) to basinasal length; *also called* Flower's index.

facial i. The ratio of facial length (× 100) to facial width which gives an indication of the shape and size of a face.

gingival i. An index (GI) for assessing the quantity and severity of gingival disease in individual mouths. The gingiva around each tooth is scored as four separate areas, and the total score divided by 4. The index value is obtained by dividing the sum of the tooth scores by the number of teeth present.

gingival periodontal i. An index for measuring gingival and periodontal status in an individual mouth by scoring gingival health in each arch on the basis of one anterior and two posterior segments, the highest score within a segment being taken as the score for that segment, on a scale of 0-3; periodontal health is similarly scored for pocket depth on a scale of 0-6 and for presence of debris or calculus on a scale of 0-3. In each score the final value is obtained by dividing the total by the number of segments.

gnathic i. The ratio of facial length (× 100) to basinasal length which gives an indication of the shape and size of a jaw.

morphologic face i. A craniometric index: the ratio of basion—nasion distance (× 100) to bizygomatic breadth.

oral hygiene i. A quantitative index (OHI) for assessing oral hygiene within groups. The scores are derived from a debris index (DI) and a calculus index (CI) measuring on a numeric scale the amount of debris and calculus on both the buccal and lingual surfaces of teeth in three segments of each arch.

oral hygiene i., simplified A similar index (OHI-S) to OHI, but with fewer surfaces examined and a shorter scoring scale. The value is calculated from the sum of the totals of the debris index and the calculus index, divided by 6. *Also called* Greene-Vermillion index.

oral status and intervention i. An index (OSI) adopted by WHO and FDI as a convenient means of classifying oral health and treatment procedures, on a scale from 0 (healthy) to 9 (requiring complicated, invasive and costly care intervention). It attempts to provide improved communication between policymakers, the community, dental educators and the dental profession.

i. of orthodontic treatment need This index (IOTN) has two components: an assessment of the aesthetic impairment, based on dental casts and black and white photographs, and scored on a scale of 1 (most acceptable) to 10 (least acceptable) compared with 10 standard colour photographs; and a dental health component (DHC) evaluating the degree of malocclusion on a scale of 1 (no need for treatment) to 5 (very great need), only the worst occlusal feature being scored.

PMA i. An index for measuring gingivitis by scoring the interdental papillae (P), marginal gingiva (M) and attached gingiva (A) for presence (1) or absence (0) of inflammation. The total scores for each arch are then added together to give the index value. *Also called* Schour-Massler index.

palatal i. The ratio of palatal width (× 100) to palatal length which gives an indication of the shape and size of a palate; *also called* palatine index or palatomaxillary index.

palatine i., palatomaxillary i. Palatal *index.

periodontal disease i. A quantitative index (PDI) of periodontal state in individuals or groups, assessed on the examination of six teeth, three in each arch, with scoring of 0-3 for gingival inflammation only, and 4-6 for inflammation with pocketing; *also called* Russell index.

periodontal i. A quantitative index (PI) for assessing the degree of gingival and periodontal disease in individual mouths. The scores range from 0 (for no disease present) to 8 (for advanced destruction and loss of function), and the value is derived from the sum of the individual scores divided by the total number of teeth present. *Also called* Ramfjord index.

plaque i. An index for assessing the amount of plaque in individuals or groups. This may be based on the use of a disclosing rinse or tablets, scoring the plaque revealed on a scale of 0-5, on all teeth other than 3rd molars; the final value is given by dividing the sum of the scores for all teeth by the number of teeth present. Another method of assessment examines the tooth surface at the circumference of the gingival margin on a scale of 0-3, again dividing the total score by the number of teeth present.

retention i. An index for assessing the potential of the tooth surfaces in an individual to retain food debris, etc. Each tooth is scored round the gingival margin, in four areas, on a scale of 0-3, based on the presence of calculus and carious cavities and on the state of the margins of any restorations; each score is divided by 4 and the sum of all the scores is divided by the number of teeth present.

index, Flower's Dental *index.

index, Greene-Vermillion Simplified oral hygiene *index.

index, Ramfjord Periodontal *index.

index, Russell Periodontal disease *index.

index, Schour-Massler PMA *index.

indigenous Native, especially to a particular country or area.

indolent 1. Sluggish. 2. Painless.

induced 1. Brought on by an outside agency. 2. Artificially produced.

induction *In embryology*, the interaction between derivatives of different germ layers that leads to the formation of structures and organs as, for example, the mouth, the jaws and the teeth.

indurated Hardened.

induration 1. The state of being hard, or the process of becoming hard. 2. An area of hard tissue.

inert Not active; having no action.

infancy ring A line marking the arrested mineralization of tooth enamel, formed at about 12 months.

infection The communication of disease by the invasion of body tissue by specific pathogenic micro-organisms.

infection, Vincent's Acute ulcerative *gingivitis.

infectious, infective Relating to or caused by infection.

inferior Situated below; applied in anatomy to structures nearer the feet; as opposed to *superior*.

inferior sagittal sinus A venous sinus joining the great cerebral vein to form the straight sinus. *See* Table of Veins—sinus sagittalis inferior.

inferolateral Situated below and on one side.

inferomedian Situated below and in the middle.

inferoposterior Situated both below and behind.

infiltrate 1. To pass into a cell or tissue or intercellular space, e.g. fluid or cells. 2. The substance thus passed.

infiltration 1. A process by which a substance or fluid enters a cell or tissues, or intercellular space; it may be either an abnormal amount of a substance normally present or some foreign substance. 2. The condition produced by this process.

infiltration anaesthesia Local anaesthesia produced by the infiltration of an anaesthetic agent into the surrounding tissue.

inflammation The reaction of living tissue to injury. *Acute* inflammation is marked by redness, pain, heat and swelling; *chronic* inflammation combines infiltration with inflammatory cells and reparative processes.

inflammatory Relating to or characterized by inflammation.

inflation Distention with a gas, especially air.

infra- Prefix signifying *beneath, within.*

infrabulge *Undercut².

infraclusion A form of malocclusion in which the occluding surfaces of the teeth are below the normal occlusal plane; often due to ankylosis.

infracondylism Deviation of the mandibular condyles in a downward direction.

infradentale The lowest point on the midline of the mandible on the alveolar margin, between the central incisors.

infrahyoid Below the hyoid bone.

infrahyoid artery Branch from the superior thyroid artery, supplying the thyrohyoid muscle. *See* Table of Arteries—infrahyoidea.

inframandibular Below the mandible.

inframaxillary Below the jaw.

infra-occlusion *Infraclusion.

infraorbital Lying beneath the floor of the orbit.

infraorbital artery Branch of the maxillary artery, supplying the upper lip, side of the nose, lower eyelid and lacrimal sac. *See* Table of Arteries—infraorbitalis.

infraorbital nerve Sensory nerve supply to the lower eyelid, skin and mucosa of the nose, upper lip and maxillary teeth. *See* Table of Nerves—infraorbitalis.

infraplacement Downward displacement of a tooth.

infrastructure The basic framework of any structure, as, for example, the skeleton.

infrastructure *of an implant* That part below the soft tissues and providing retention.

infratemporal Below the temporal bone.

infratemporale A craniometric point on the great wing of the sphenoid bone, below the temple.

infratrochlear nerve Supplies the skin over the bridge of the nose. *See* Table of Nerves—infratrochlearis.

infraversion *Infraclusion.

ingestion The act of absorbing any substance, such as food, into the body.

Ingrassia's wing (G.F. Ingrassia, 1510-80. Italian anatomist). The lesser wing of the sphenoid bone.

inhalation anaesthesia General anaesthesia induced by the inhaling of gaseous or volatile liquid anaesthetic agents.

inhale To draw breath into the lungs.

inial Relating to the inion.

inion The most prominent point in the midline on the posterior occipital protuberance; a craniometric landmark.

injection 1. The forcing, under pressure, of a liquid into some part or tissue of the body. 2. The liquid injected.

inlay A type of tooth filling which is cast to fit the prepared tooth cavity and cemented in position; inlays are usually of gold or porcelain.

innervation 1. The nerve supply or distribution of an organ or part. 2. The supply of nerve stimulus to a part.

innocent Benign; not malignant.

innominate artery Brachiocephalic trunk. *See* Table of Arteries—truncus brachiocephalicus.

innominate vein V. brachiocephalica. *See* Table of Veins.

inoperable Not able, or suitable, to be treated by surgery.

inorganic 1. Without organs. 2. Not of organic origin, or relating to substances not of organic origin. 3. *In chemistry*, relating to substances that do not contain carbon, with the exception of carbonates and cyanides.

inostosis The process by which bony tissue is re-formed to replace tissue that has been destroyed.
cementum i. A pathological thickening of cementum developing inwards into the dentine.

insalivation The moistening of food with saliva.

inscription The main part of a prescription, containing the details of ingredients and quantities to be used.

insectivorous Insect-eating.

insert
intramucosal i. A metal stud attached to a denture and fitting into a prepared pocket in the oral mucosa to improve retention.

insertion 1. The act of placing something in, of implanting. 2. *In anatomy*, the point of attachment of a muscle to the part which it moves.

insidious Unperceived, coming on gradually and stealthily.

inspection Examination by eye of the body or any of its parts.

inspissation The process of thickening of body fluids by evaporation of readily vaporizing parts.

instrument A small tool, device or implement.
cone-socket i. One in which the shank and blade or nib are separate from the handle, and screw into it.
dental i. Any one of the many different types of device used either hand-held or in a handpiece in the practice of dentistry.
double-ended i. One that has a blade or nib at both ends of the handle.
long-handled i. One which has the handle, shank and blade made from one piece of metal.
rotary i. Any instrument, hand operated or power operated, which works by rotation; for example, burs.

instrument formula Devised by G.V. Black as a means of differentiating different types and sizes of dental hand instruments. It consists of three figures representing three measurements: the width of the blade in 10ths of a millimetre; the length of the blade in millimetres; and the angle of the shaft in centigrades. (Where there is a fourth figure, in brackets after the first, this represents the angle of the cutting edge of the blade with its shaft in centigrades; it is usually seen on margin trimmers.)

instrumentation The use of instruments in treatment.

intaglio Carving in hard material; used of carving on a dental model in the construction of a denture.

integument The skin.

integumentary Relating to the integument, or skin.

inter- Prefix signifying *between, within.*

interalveolar Between alveoli.

interarticular Within a joint; between articular surfaces.

intercavernous sinus One of two sinuses joining the cavernous sinuses, and forming a ring round the pituitary fossa. *See* Table of Veins—sinus intercavernosus.

intercellular Between the cells in tissue.

intercondylar Between condyles.

intercuspation The interlocking of the cusps on the posterior teeth of one jaw into the corresponding fissures in the teeth of the other jaw in occlusion.

interdental Between the teeth.

interdentale The point in the midline between the central incisors on the tip of the alveolar septum; that in the maxilla is called *i. superius* and that in the mandible *i. inferius*.

interdentium The space between two adjacent teeth.

interdigitation *Intercuspation.

interference

cuspal i. The contact of a cusp with an opposing tooth, preventing contact of other cusps.

interfrontal Between the two halves of the frontal bone.

interglobular Between or among globules.

intergonial Between the angles of the mandible, or gonia.

interior Inside, situated within, an organ, part or cavity.

interlabial Between the lips.

intermaxilla The *intermaxillary bone.

intermaxillary Between the maxillae; as opposed to *intramaxillary*.

intermaxillary bone One of several small bones in the centre of the upper jaw in the foetus, which become fused in adult life; *also called* Goethe's bone.

intermediate 1. Placed in between. 2. *In dentistry*, any non-conducting substance used to line a tooth cavity before it is filled either with gold or amalgam, to protect the pulp.

intermediofacial nerve N. facialis. *See* Table of Nerves.

intermedius nerve Supplies the glands of the nose and mouth, and the taste-buds. *See* Table of Nerves.

intermittent Occurring at intervals, with periods of cessation; as opposed to *continuous*.

internal Inside.

internarial Between the nostrils.

interocclusal Between the occlusal surfaces of opposing teeth.

interosseous Occurring between bones.

interpolation Surgical tissue transplantation.

interproximal Between approximated surfaces.

interradicular Situated between roots.

interstitial Relating to or situated within the interstices of a part or of tissue.

intertriginous Chafed; affected by chafing of the skin.

intervascular Situated between vessels.

intra- Prefix signifying *within*.

intra-arterial Within an artery.

intra-articular Within a joint.

intrabuccal Within the cheek, or within the oral cavity.

intracellular Occurring within a cell or cells.

intracoronal Within the tooth crown.

intracranial Within the cranium.

intralingual Within the tongue.

intramaxillary Within one jaw; as opposed to *intermaxillary.*

intramedullary Within the bone marrow.

intramembranous Within a membrane.

intramuscular Within a muscle or muscles.

intranarial Within the nostril.

intranasal Within the nose.

intraoral Within the oral cavity.

intraosseous Within a bone.

intrastitial Within the tissue cells or tissue fibres.

intrathecal Within a sheath.

intratracheal Within the trachea.

intravascular Within a vessel or vessels.

intravenous Within or into a vein.

intraventricular Within a ventricle.

intrinsic Situated within, or relating solely to one part; as opposed to *extrinsic.*

intrusion The condition of a tooth having been thrust down into its socket; it may be caused by a pathological condition or it may be part of orthodontic treatment.

intubation The introduction of a tube through the mouth or the nose, to allow air, gas or vapour to pass into the lungs.

invaginate To fold back one part of a tube or other tissue so that it is enclosed within another part of itself, as in a sheath.

inversion A turning inward or a state of being turned inwards.

inversion *of a tooth* The condition of a tooth that erupts with the root uppermost.

invest To pack in investment material, as in the construction of artificial dentures.

investment, investment material 1. Any refractory setting material used to enclose the wax pattern of dentures, crowns or inlays preparatory to casting; it forms the mould from which these are later cast. 2. Any material used to surround and support metal units during soldering.

involucrum A sheath; particularly the new bone sheath that forms about a sequestrum.

involution A turning or rolling inwards.
buccal i. The inward folding of the ectoderm in the embryo which forms the stomodeum.

iontophoresis Therapeutic treatment by the electrical introduction of ions into the body tissues.

ipsilateral side *In prosthetic dentistry,* the *working side.

iron A metallic element, chemical symbol Fe; hard, ductile and malleable.

irradiation Exposure to radiation; used of treatment with infra-red, ultra-violet or gamma rays or with x-rays.

irrigation The process of washing out, as of a cavity with a stream of water.

irritant 1. Causing irritation. 2. An agent that causes irritation.

irritation 1. The act of stimulating. 2. A condition of over-excitement and hypersensitivity.

irritation point In the testing of vital tooth pulp with an electric current, the average reading at which, on application of the current, a tingling sensation is felt, but before pain is produced.

ischaemia Deficiency in the blood supply to a part or an organ; it may be due to constriction, contraction or blocking of the arteries.

ischaemic Relating to or affected by ischaemia.

ischemia *Ischaemia.

iso- Prefix signifying *same, equal.*

isocellular Composed of equal-sized or similar cells.

isodont Having teeth of the same shape and size.

isognathous Having jaws of the same shape and size.

isograft A graft derived from one member of a pair of monozygotic twins and transplanted to the other.

isomorphous Having the same form.

iter dentium The passage through which a permanent tooth erupts.

-itis Suffix signifying *disease, inflammation.*

ivory Dentine, especially the bone-like substance of the tusks of elephants, walrus, etc.

J

jacket crown A porcelain or acrylic veneer crown which is placed over the prepared remains of a vital natural tooth.

jackscrew An old term for an orthodontic appliance that expanded the dental arch by means of a screw in a threaded socket.

Jackson appliance, Jackson crib (V.H. Jackson, 1850-1929. American dentist). An orthodontic skeleton wire appliance, passing round both the buccal and lingual surfaces of all the teeth in one arch, and joined at intervals to keep it firmly in place. It is used as a foundation to which additions may be made to apply pressure to any given tooth or teeth.

Jackson's paralysis; Jackson-Mackenzie syndrome (J.H. Jackson, 1835-1911. English neurologist; Sir S. Mackenzie, 1844-1909. English physician). *Mackenzie's syndrome.

Jacob's ulcer (A. Jacob, 1790-1874. Irish ophthalmic surgeon). A rodent ulcer affecting the face and eyelid.

Jacobson's nerve (L.L. Jacobson, 1783-1843. Danish anatomist and physician). The *tympanic nerve.

Jadassohn-Tièche naevus (J. Jadassohn, 1863-1936. German dermatologist; and M. Tièche). Blue *naevus.

jaquette A root planing instrument, used for the removal of subgingival calculus, and for smoothing root surfaces by the removal of the surface layer of cementum.

jaw The mandibular or maxillary facial process.
accessory j's. A developmental defect in which segments of the maxilla and/or the mandible are replicated to a greater or lesser extent; teeth, when present, are supernumerary in form.
big j. *Actinomycosis.
Hapsburg j. Mandibular prognathism, similar to the hereditary condition that affected the Hapsburg dynasty.
lower j. The *mandible.
lumpy j. *Actinomycosis.
parrot j. The facies associated with severe protrusion of the maxilla and the consequent abnormal relation of the anterior teeth.
phossy j. Jaw necrosis caused by phosphorus poisoning.
pipe j. A painful condition of the jaw caused by constant carrying of a tobacco pipe in the mouth.
upper j. The *maxilla.
wolf j. Bilateral cleft extending through the palate, jaw and lip.

jaw clonus reflex *Jaw jerk reflex.

jaw jerk reflex Clonic contraction of the muscles of mastication and upward jerking of the mandible, produced by a downward blow on the relaxed and open jaw. Observed in sclerosis of the lateral columns of the spine.

jaw prop An appliance for holding the jaws open during an operation performed under general anaesthesia.

jaw protrusion 1. *Prognathism. 2. Mandibular *protraction of the jaws.

jaw winking Movement of the lower jaw causing an involuntary movement of the eyelids.

jaw-bone The *mandible.

jet injector A form of syringe without a needle, which can be used to inject small quantities of solution in the form of a fine, high-pressure jet.

Johnson band (J.E. Johnson, 1888-1969. American orthodontist). A form of band which is adjusted with pliers to fit the tooth.

Johnson twin wire arch (J.E. Johnson, 1888-1969. American orthodontist). An orthodontic archwire made up of two thin stainless-steel wires in parallel, fastened to attachments on bands cemented to the teeth and used to correct misalignment of teeth within the dental arch.

joint 1. The place of connection between two bones, allowing of more or less movement; an articulation. 2. The place at which two parts of any structure are connected.
arthrodial j. Plane *joint.
ball and socket j. Spheroidal *joint.
bar j. *In prosthetic dentistry*, a device on a bar attachment designed to permit movement between two parts of a prosthesis.
biaxial j. One in which movement is possible in two of the three perpendicular planes.
bilocular j. A type of synovial joint divided into two cavities by an intra-articular disc; the temporomandibular joint is a bilocular joint.
butt j. A joint created by joining two structures end to end; in dentistry, for example, the joint between an abutment and a restoration.
cartilaginous j. One in which two bones are connected by a solid plate or band of cartilage; a synchondrosis.
condyloid j., condylar j. A biaxial ball and socket type of synovial joint.
diarthrodial j. Synovial *joint.
false j. *Pseudarthrosis.
fibrocartilaginous j. *Symphysis.
fibrous j. Any joint or join connected with fibrous tissue, for example, a *suture*.
ginglymus j. *Ginglymus.
gliding j. Plane *joint.
ligamentous j. *Syndesmosis.
mandibular j. Temporomandibular *joint.
multiaxial j. One in which movement is possible in all three planes.
pivot j. Trochoid *joint.
plane j. A uniaxial type of synovial joint in which the apposing bone surfaces are almost flat.
rotary j. Trochoid *joint.
saddle j. A biaxial type of synovial joint in which the apposing bone surfaces are saddle-shaped.
spheroidal j. A multiaxial type of synovial joint in which one bone end is ball-shaped and fits into a socket in the apposing bone.
synarthrodial j. Fibrous *joint.
synovial j. A freely movable joint in which there is a cavity between the apposing bones, whose surfaces are covered with articular cartilage; the joint cavity is enclosed by a capsular ligament, the inner aspect of which is lined by synovial membrane which secretes a lubricating fluid (synovium) into the cavity. Some synovial joints, such as the temporomandibular joint, also have a fibrocartilaginous disc dividing the cavity into two.
temporomandibular j. A synovial joint between the mandible and the temporal bone; one of the pair of articulating joints of the jaw.
trochoid j. A uniaxial synovial joint in which the end of one of the two bones is enclosed by a fibrous cuff in which it can rotate.
uniaxial j. One in which movement is possible in only one plane.

unilocular j. A synovial joint with only one joint cavity.

Jourdain's disease (A.L.B. Jourdain, 1734-1816. French physician). *Pyorrhoea alveolaris.

jugal Relating to a jugum, or yoke; especially relating to the zygomatic bone.

jugal bone The malar or zygomatic bone.

jugale The craniometric point at the angle of the maxillary and masseteric edges of the zygomatic bone.

jugomaxillary Relating to the zygomatic bone and the maxilla.

jugular Relating to the neck.

jugular nerve Communicating branch from the superior cervical ganglion to the vagus nerve. *See* Table of Nerves—jugularis.

jugular veins The veins receiving blood from the veins of the brain, face and neck. *See* Table of Veins—jugularis.

jugum A yoke or yoke-like process; ridge connecting two points.

jumping the bite The forcible movement forward of a retruded mandible to obtain normal occlusion and correct crossbite.

junction The area of joining or meeting between two or more organs.

amelodentinal j. The line marking the join between the enamel and the dentine.

cementodentinal j. Dentinocemental *junction.

cemento-enamel j. The line where the cementum of the root joins the enamel of the crown; the cervix of the tooth.

dentinocemental j. The line marking the fusion between dentine and cementum.

dentinoenamel j. Amelodentinal *junction.

dentogingival j., dentinogingival j. Epithelial *attachment.

mucogingival j. The line at which the alveolar mucous membrane and the attached gingiva unite.

juxta- Prefix signifying *near* or *adjoining*.

juxtangina Inflammation of the muscles of the pharynx.

K

k Abbreviation for *kilo-* or *thousand.*

K 1. Chemical symbol for potassium. 2. Symbol for Kelvin.

kg Symbol for *kilogram.*

Kaposi's sarcoma (M. Kaposi-Kahn, 1837-1902. Austrian dermatologist). A malignant tumour containing blood vessels, lymph vessels or fibrous tissue and blood pigment; secondary lesions may occur on the tongue, buccal mucosa and lower lip.

Kazanjian's operation (V.H. Kazanjian, 1879-1974. Armenian-born American plastic and maxillofacial surgeon). A variant of vestibuloplasty, using localized pedicle flaps of mucosa based at the lip or at the crest of the alveolar ridge.

kebocephaly *See* cebocephaly.

kelectome An instrument used to remove specimens of tissue from a tumour for examination.

keloid A fibrous hyperplastic scar growth on the skin.

keloid *of the gums* Gingival *fibromatosis.

Kelvin scale (W. Thomson, Lord Kelvin, 1824-1907. Scottish physicist). An absolute temperature scale, corresponding to Celsius, but with freezing point at 273.15 K and boiling point 373.15 K.

Kennedy bar (E. Kennedy, 1883-1952. American dentist). Continuous bar *retainer.

Kennedy classification (E. Kennedy, 1883-1952. American dentist). A classification of partially edentulous arches and partial dentures. It is based on the location of the edentulous areas within the arch in relation to the remaining natural teeth.

Class I: Edentulous area posterior to remaining natural teeth—bilateral.

Class II: Edentulous area posterior to remaining natural teeth—unilateral.

Class III: Edentulous area between remaining anterior and posterior natural teeth, either unilateral or bilateral.

Class IV: Single edentulous area, anterior to remaining natural teeth and crossing the midline.

kephal- *See* cephal-

keratin An insoluble protein which forms the basis of all horny tissue: *hard* keratin is found in nails and hair; *soft* keratin forms part of the upper layer of the skin.

keratinize To become or to be made horny.

keratinous 1. Relating to or containing keratin. 2. Horny.

keratinogenesis, keratogenesis The development of horny tissue.

keratocyst 1. Primordial *cyst. 2. Odontogenic *keratocyst.

odontogenic k. A bony cyst of the jaws, with its lumen filled with keratin, usually found in the region of the third molar and ramus of the mandible; it may be unilocular or multilocular.

keratogenous Promoting or causing the growth of horny material.

keratoid Horn-like.

keratolysis Exfoliation of the horny layer of the epidermis.

keratolytic 1. Relating to keratolysis. 2. An agent causing keratolysis.

keratomycosis linguae Black *tongue.

keratosis 1. A general term for epithelial lesions showing excess keratin. 2. Any condition characterized by the presence of such lesions.
sublingual k. Keratosis of the floor of the mouth, which shows precancerous potential.

keratosis labialis A condition characterized by horny patches on the mucosa of the lips.

keratosis linguae *Leukoplakia (*linguae*).

keroid *Keratoid.

Kesling appliance (H.D. Kesling, 1901-1979. American orthodontist). A type of soft occlusal splint designed to treat bruxism by maintaining a specific relationship between the mandible and the maxilla.

Kesling spring (H.D. Kesling, 1901-1979. American orthodontist). A type of spring used in fitting an orthodontic appliance, to obtain spacing between teeth for the placing of bands.

key An old instrument used for extracting teeth; so called because of its resemblance to a door-key.
torquing k. An instrument used in orthodontics to connect edgewise brackets to rectangular archwires.

kine-, kino- Prefix signifying *movement.*

kinetic Relating to or producing motion.

Kingsley's splint (N.W. Kingsley, 1829-1913. American dentist). A vulcanized oral splint, made to a model of the fractured jaw with the fracture reduced, and having wires at each end extending outside the mouth to be attached to a headband.

kiotome A knife used for surgical removal of the uvula.

kiotomy Surgical removal of the uvula.

Klein's muscle (E.E. Klein, 1844-1925. Hungarian histologist). *Krause's muscle.

knife A cutting instrument, varying in size and shape, used in surgery and anatomy.

knitting The process of repair of a bone fracture.

knot 1. A small solid mass of cells or of tissue. 2. The fastening of two ends of cord or suture by interlacing them so that they cannot easily come apart.
enamel k. An aggregation of epithelial cells at the base of the enamel organ, which have not yet differentiated into stellate reticulum.

knurl A small knob or protuberance, especially on instrument handles to ensure a firm grasp.

Kocher's operation (E.T. Kocher, 1841-1917. Swiss surgeon). A operation for excision of the tongue through an incision running from the mastoid process to the hyoid bone and to the symphysis of the mandible.

Kölliker's dental crest (R.A. von Kölliker, 1817-1905. Swiss anatomist). Dental *crest.

kolyseptic Checking septic processes.

Koplik's spots (H. Koplik, 1858-1927. American physician). Small, whitish spots on the mucous membrane of the mouth in the early stages of measles; *also called* Filatov's spots.

Korff's fibres (K. von Korff, b. 1867. German anatomist). Precollagenous fibres of the dental pulp, which pass between the odontoblasts in developing dentine and undergo a collagenous change, becoming incorporated in the dentine matrix.

koronion *See* coronion.

Koyter's muscle (V.Koyter, 1534-1600. Dutch anatomist). The corrigator supercilii muscle. *See* Table of Muscles.

Krause's muscle (K.F.T. Krause, 1797-1868. German anatomist and surgeon). The lip muscle; *also called* Klein's muscle.

Krause's operation (F.V. Krause, 1857-1937. German surgeon). *Hartley-Krause operation.

Krimer's operation (J.F.W. Krimer, 1795-1834. German surgeon). An operation for closure of a palatal fissure by means of wide mucoperiosteal flaps sutured at the median line.

Krompecher's tumour (E. Krompecher, 1870-1926. Hungarian pathologist). A rodent *ulcer.

Kuhnt's operation (H. Kuhnt, 1850-1925. German ophthalmologist). An operation for treatment of frontal sinus disease by the removal of the anterior wall and the curetting of the mucous membrane.

L

l Symbol for *litre*.

L Lingual.

l. Abbreviation for *left*.

La Labial.

LA Linguoaxial.

LaC Labiocervical.

LAC Linguoaxiocervical.

LaG Labiogingival.

LAG Linguoaxiogingival.

LaI Labioincisal.

LaL Labiolingual.

lb Abbreviation for *libra*—a pound.

LC Linguocervical.

LD Linguodistal.

LG Linguogingival.

LI Linguoincisal.

LM Linguomesial.

LO Linguo-occlusal.

LP Linguopulpal.

labial 1. Relating to the lips. 2. That surface of a tooth which is towards the lips.

labial artery Branch of the facial artery, supplying the lips and nasal septum; two branches: inferior and superior. *See* Table of Arteries—labialis.

labial nerves Supply the skin of the lips and cheek. *See* Table of Nerves—labialis.

labio- Prefix signifying *lips*.

labioalveolar Relating to the lips and the alveolar process.

labiocervical *Labiogingival.

labiodental Relating to the lips and the teeth.

labiogingival Relating to the labial and gingival walls of a mesial, distal or proximo-incisal cavity in an incisor or a canine.

l. angle The angle formed at the junction of these walls; a *line* angle.

labioglossolaryngeal Relating to the lips, the tongue and the larynx.

labioglossopharyngeal Relating to the lips, the tongue and the pharynx.

labiogression The condition of having the anterior teeth forward of their normal position in the dental arch.

labio-incisal Relating to the labial surface and the incisal edge of an anterior tooth.

labiolingual Relating to both the lips and the tongue.

labiomental Relating to the lips and the chin.

labiomycosis Any fungal disease of the lips.

labionasal Relating to the lips and the nose.

labiopalatine Relating to the lips and the palate.

labioplacement Displacement of a tooth labially.

labioplasty *Cheiloplasty.

labiotenaculum An instrument used for holding the lip during surgical procedures.

labioversion The state of being labially displaced; used of a tooth.

labium (*pl.* labia) A lip.

labium leporinum *Hare-lip.

labrale A cephalometric soft-tissue landmark representing the most prominent part on either lip; that of the upper lip is known as *labrale superior* and that of the lower as *labrale inferior*.

labyrinth The inner ear.

labyrinthine artery Supplies the internal ear; *also called* internal auditive or auditory artery. *See* Table of Arteries—labyrinthi.

laceration 1. A tear or a wound made by tearing. 2. The act of tearing.

lacrimal Relating to tears (lacrimae).

lacrimal artery Supplies the cheek, eyelid, eye muscle, and lacrimal gland. *See* Table of Arteries—lacrimalis.

lacrimal bone A very thin bone on the upper anterior portion of the orbit, articulating with ethmoid, frontal and maxillary bones.

lacrimal nerve Supplies the skin about the lateral commissure of the eye. *See* Table of Nerves—lacrimalis.

Lactobacillus The type genus of the Lactobacillaceae family of bacteria, Gram-positive rods, non-sporing, non-motile and anaerobic or facultatively aerobic, capable of producing lactic acid and carbon dioxide from carbohydrates.

lacuna (*pl.* lacunae) A gap, space or depression; a defect. *In dental anatomy*, lacunae are spaces containing cementoblasts.
absorption l. Resorption *lacuna.
resorption l. One of the absorption spaces in bone, semilunar hollows which are, or have been, occupied by osteoclasts; *also called* Howship's lacuna.

laevocondylism Deviation to the left of the mandibular condyles.

lagocheilus, lagostoma *Hare-lip.

Lain's disease (E.S. Lain, 1876-1970. American dermatologist). Burning of the tongue and the soft tissues of the mouth due to electrogalvanism caused by the use of dissimilar metals in dental restorations.

lambda The junction of the lambdoid and sagittal sutures, the site of the posterior fontanelle; a craniometric landmark.

lamella (*pl.* lamellae) A thin leaf or scale.
enamel l. One of the flat, organic bands running transversely through the enamel of a tooth.

lamellar Relating to a lamella.

lamina (*pl.* laminae) A thin, flat plate or layer.
buccal l., buccogingival l. Vestibular *lamina.
dental l. The ridge of thickened epithelium along the margin of the gum in the embryo, from which is formed the enamel organ.
dentogingival l. Dental *lamina.
vestibular l. The oral ectoderm which later divides to form the vestibule of the oral cavity.

lamina dentalis Dental *lamina.

lamina dura *In dentistry*, a thin layer of cortical bone lining the tooth socket, important on x-rays, where it shows up as a continuous thin white line.

laminagraphy *Tomography.

laminated Composed of thin layers or laminae.

lamination The make-up of a structure composed of various thin layers of material.

lancet A knife-like instrument used to cut soft tissues.

lancinating Shooting, tearing or sharply cutting; used to describe pain.

Land's crown (C.H. Land, 1847-1922. Canadian-born American dentist). A very early type of porcelain jacket crown.

laniary Dagger-like; used to describe a form of canine tooth.

lapis dentalis Dental *calculus.

laryngeal Relating to the larynx.

laryngeal artery Supplies the larynx; two branches: inferior and superior. *See* Table of Arteries—laryngea.

laryngeal nerves Supply the larynx and cricothyroid; *also called* N. laryngeus. *See* Table of Nerves—laryngealis.

laryngo- Prefix signifying *larynx*.

laryngopharyngitis sicca Inflammation and dryness of the mucous membranes of the larynx and pharynx. Part of the complex known as *Sjörgen's syndrome*.

laryngospasm Spasmodic contraction of the larynx.

larynx The organ of voice production; a musculocartilaginous structure situated between the trachea and the pharynx.

latent 1. Potential. 2. Concealed.

lateral Relating to a side; as opposed to *medial* or *central*.

latero- Prefix signifying *at the side* or *towards the side*.

lateroalveolism A condition in which the alveolar process is in a lateral position in relation to the base of the jaw; it may be *maxillary* or *mandibular*.

laterodetrusion The movement of the mandible at the start of mastication, being backwards, downwards and sideways.

laterogenia A condition in which the chin is shifted laterally.

laterognathism Asymmetry of the chin caused by either over-development or under-development of one side of the mandible compared with the other, or by trauma or disease.

lateromandibulism A condition in which the mandible, although both halves have the same dimensions, is shifted laterally.

lateromaxillism A condition in which the maxilla, of normal size, is positioned laterally.

lateroretrusion Any backward and sideways movement of the mandible, especially during mastication.

laterotrusion The movement of the mandible to left or right during mastication.

lavage 1. The washing out or irrigation of some organ. 2. To wash out.

Lawrence crown (H. Lawrence, fl. 1849. American dentist). Identical with the *Foster crown.

layer A sheet of material or tissue of uniform thickness.
adamantine l. *Enamel.
ameloblastic l. A cell layer, derived from the enamel epithelium, from which tooth enamel develops.
basement l. Basement *membrane.
enamel l. Ameloblastic *layer.
odontoblastic l. The layer of cells lining the pulp cavity and sending fibres into the dentine.
prickle-cell l. The stratum germinativum of the epidermis or squamous epithelium, excluding basal cells.
submantle l. A fine layer of interglobular dentine just below the mantle dentine.
subodontoblastic l. A transparent layer of connective tissue cells inside the odontoblast layer of the tooth pulp; *also called* Weil's basal layer.

Le Fort fracture (L.C. Le Fort, 1829-93. French surgeon). One of three main classes of fracture of the maxilla:
Class I: those affecting the alveolar process, the palate and the pterygoid processes, transversely.
Class II: a transverse fracture extending through the nasal bones, affecting the maxillary frontal process, the orbital plate, and descending through the maxillary antrum across to the pterygoid process; a pyramidal fracture.
Class III: those affecting the bridge of the nose and the orbit, the pyramidal processes of the

maxilla and zygoma remaining attached; craniofacial disjunction.

lead A soft, grey-blue metal, chemical symbol Pb, which has poisonous salts; it is much used in alloys and solder.

lead line A bluish line on the edge of the gums, seen in lead poisoning; *also called* Burton's line.

leiomyoma A benign myoma composed of smooth muscle fibres.

leiomyosarcoma A rare malignant form of leiomyoma.

length

arch l. The distance between the most posterior teeth on one side and those on the other, measured round the arch.

basialveolar l. The distance from the basion to the prosthion at the lower end of the intermaxillary suture.

basinasal l. The distance from the basion to the nasion.

dental l. The distance from the mesial surface of the first premolar to the distal surface of the last molar in one quadrant of the maxillary arch.

lenitive Soothing, demulcent.

lenticel A small circular and biconvex (lens-shaped) gland, especially one found at the base of the tongue.

lentula A flexible spiral instrument used to carry sealer into the root canal.

leontiasis ossea Hypertrophy of the cranial bones, particularly the maxillae and the facial bones, giving the face a lion-like expression.

leotropic Relating to an anticlockwise spiral—i.e. one turning from right to left.

leprosy A chronic granulomatous infection caused by *Mycobacterium leprae*, with oral lesions on the tongue, lips and palate and sometimes gingival hyperplasia; *also called* Hansen's disease.

lepto- Prefix signifying *small, fine, weak*.

leptocephalic Having an abnormally small or narrow skull.

leptodontous Having abnormally slender teeth.

leptomicrognathous The condition of having a slight degree of micrognathia; having a slightly undersized jaw.

leptoprosopic Having a high and narrow or thin face.

Leptospira A genus of the Leptospiraceae family of bacteria, seen as motile coils, Gram-negative, aerobic, able to survive in water, and with some parasitic strains.

leptostaphyline Having a narrow palate.

Leptotrichia A genus of the Bacteroidaceae family, bacterial organisms seen as straight or curved threads, unbranched and with rounded or pointed ends, Gram-negative, anaerobic on first isolation and non-motile; found in the oral cavity in man.

L. buccalis The type species, a non-pathogenic organism found in the oral cavity, especially in dental plaque; *also called* Vignal's bacillus.

lesion A wound or injury, or a patch of disease on the skin; a morbid change in tissue function.

leucaemia *See* leukaemia.

leukaemia A disease affecting the blood-forming organs, frequently fatal; it is characterized by an increase of abnormal leukocytes in the blood and marked changes in the spleen, bone marrow, and lymphatic glands.

leuko- Prefix signifying *white* or *colourless*.

leukocyte One of the white cells found in blood, produced by bone marrow and in the lymph nodes, and part of the body's defence mechanism.

leukoedema A condition of the buccal mucosa resembling leukoplakia, and characterized by a whitish film over the mucous membrane associated with intracellular oedema.

leukokeratosis mucosae oris *Leukoplakia (*buccalis*).

leukokeratosis nicotina palati A form of leukoplakia found in smokers, and characterized by inflammation of the palatal mucosa, followed by the appearance of multiple whitish nodules, and later by keratinization and thickening of the palatal epithelium.

leukoma 1. A whitish opacity of the cornea. 2. *Leukoplakia (*buccalis*).

leukopenia An abnormal reduction in the number of leukocytes in the blood.

leukoplakia White thickened patches which develop on the tongue (*linguae*), the gums, the palate, and the buccal mucous membrane (*buccalis*); sometimes tend to malignancy. L. buccalis *also called* Bazin's disease.

levator muscles Muscles that raise or pull upwards. *See* Table of Muscles.

levocondylism *See* laevocondylism.

lichen planus An inflammatory skin disease characterized by a flat, papular eruption; in the mouth the lesions may appear on the buccal mucosa, the tongue, or, more rarely, on the lips.

lichenoid 1. Lichen-like. 2. A condition of the tongue found in the young and characterized by whitish spots surrounded by yellow rings.

ligament A tough band of fibrous tissue connecting bones or supporting vessels.
alveolodental l. Periodontal *ligament.
capsular l. *Capsule[1].
periodontal l. The layer of fibrous tissue surrounding the root of the tooth, attached to the cementum, the alveolar bone and the free gingiva and supporting the tooth in its socket.
sphenomandibular l. An accessory ligament of the temporomandibular joint, running from the spine of the sphenoid bone to the lingula of the mandible.
stylomandibular l. An accessory ligament of the temporomandibular joint, running from the styloid process of the temporal bone to the angle of the mandible.
temporomandibular l. The ligament that helps prevent displacement of the mandibular condyle; it is a thickening of the joint capsule and its fibres pass from the lateral aspect of the articular eminence to the posterior aspect of the neck of the condyle.

ligature 1. A cord or wire for tying vessels. 2. *In orthodontics*, a wire or thread used to fasten a tooth to an appliance or to another tooth. 3. The act of tying with a cord or thread.

limbus alveolaris The free margin of the alveolar process.

line Any streak, long thin mark, or boundary.
accretion l's. Incremental *lines.
ala-tragal l. The line from the lower border of the ala of the nose to the upper border of the tragus of the ear.
alveolar l. In craniometry, a line from the prosthion to the nasion.

alveolobasilar l. In craniometry, a line from the prosthion to the basion.
alveolonasal l. Alveolar *line.
basialveolar l. In craniometry, the line joining the basion and the alveolar point.
basinasal l. In craniometry, a line from the basion to the nasion.
blue l. Lead *line.
calcification l's. Incremental *lines.
cervical l. The line formed at the cemento-enamel junction.
copper l. A line, which may be greenish or purple, on the edge of the gums, seen in copper poisoning; *also called* Corrigan's line.
facial l. *Camper's line.
gingival l. Gingival *margin.
imbrication l. One of the grooves in the surface of tooth enamel, marking the edges of the enamel striae of Retzius.
incremental l. One of the lines said to show the laminar structure of dentine and enamel in a tooth.
lead l. A bluish line on the edge of the gums, seen in lead poisoning; *also called* Burton's line.
mylohyoid l. A ridge on the inner surface of the mandible, running from the ascending ramus to the chin, to which the mylohyoid muscle and the superior constrictor pharyngis are attached.
nasal l. The line or furrow that runs on either side from the alae of the nose to the angles of the mouth; *also called* de Salle's line.
nasobasilar l. Basinasal *line.
nasolabial l. A line joining the edge of the nose to the angle of the mouth on the same side.
neonatal l. An incremental line in the dentine and the enamel of a tooth formed *in utero,* marking the development of the tooth structure at the time of birth.
oblique l. of the mandible A ridge on the external surface of the mandible running upwards from the mental tubercle to become the anterior border of the ramus.

line angle An angle formed at the junction of two tooth surfaces or of two cavity walls; line angles are named according to the surfaces or walls that form them.

line of occlusion A term used by Angle to denote the line joining areas of contact of the teeth in normal occlusion.

linea alba buccalis A thickened whitish line on the buccal mucosa, at the level of the occlusal plane, from the corner of the mouth to the posterior teeth, thought to be the result of slight trauma.

linear Relating to or resembling a line.

liner Any material used on the inner surfaces of a cavity or container for protection or insulation.
cavity l. Material used in dentistry to protect and insulate the tooth tissues after the excavation of caries before the placing of a restoration in a prepared cavity.

lingua The tongue.

lingua fraenata *Ankyloglossia.

lingua plicata Fissure of the tongue.

lingua villosa nigra Black *tongue.

lingual Pertaining to the tongue.

lingual artery Supplies the sublingual gland, and the tongue, tonsils and epiglottis. *Also called* gustatory artery. *See* Table of Arteries—lingualis.

lingual muscles *inferior and superior*: M. longitudinalis inferior and M. longitudinalis superior.
transverse and vertical: M. transversus linguae and M. verticalis linguae. *See* Table of Muscles.

lingual nerve Supplies the mucosa of the anterior portion of the tongue and the floor of the mouth. *See* Table of Nerves—lingualis.

lingual quinsy *See* quinsy.

linguale The point at the upper end of the mandibular symphysis on the lingual surface.

linguiform Tongue-shaped.

lingula mandibulae The thin and sharp lower edge of the inferior dental foramen.

linguo- Prefix signifying *tongue*.

linguo-axial Relating to the lingual and axial walls in the mesial or distal portion of a proximo-occlusal cavity.
l. angle The angle formed at the junction of these walls; a *line* angle.

linguocclusal *Linguo-occlusal.

linguocervical *Linguogingival.

linguoclination Tilting of a tooth in a lingual direction.

linguodental Relating to both the tongue and the teeth.

linguodistal 1. Distal and towards the tongue. 2. Relating to the lingual and distal surfaces of a tooth, or to the lingual and distal walls in the step portion of a proximo-occlusal cavity.
l. angle The angle formed at the junction of these walls; a *line* angle.

linguogingival 1. Relating to the tongue and the gums. 2. Relating to the lingual and gingival walls of a mesial, distal or proximo-incisal cavity, or in the step portion of a proximo-occlusal cavity.
l. angle The angle formed at the junction of these walls; a *line* angle.

linguo-incisal Relating to the lingual surface and the incisal edge of an anterior tooth.

linguomesial Relating to the lingual and mesial surfaces of a tooth, or to the lingual and mesial walls in the step portion of a proximo-occlusal cavity.
l. angle The angle formed at the junction of these walls; a *line* angle.

linguo-occlusal Relating to the lingual and occlusal surfaces of a molar or premolar, or to a cavity affecting those surfaces.

linguopapillitis Inflammation and ulceration of the papillae of the tongue.

linguoplacement Displacement of a tooth lingually.

linguopulpal Relating to the lingual and pulpal walls of an occlusal cavity, or of the step portion of a proximo-occlusal cavity.
l. angle The angle formed at the junction of these walls; a *line* angle.

linguoversion The position of a tooth which is inclined inwards towards the tongue.

lip One of the fleshy outer edges of the mouth.
cleft l. *Hare-lip.
double l. Superfluous tissue and mucous membrane below the red margin of the lips.
Hapsburg l. The over-developed lower lip often accompanying Hapsburg jaw.
hare-l. See hare-lip.

lip bumper A type of myofunctional appliance, acting on teeth in one arch only.

lip fissure *Hare-lip.

lip furrow band Vestibular *lamina.

lip plumper The labial flange on a denture or obturator built up to hold the cheeks and lip in their normal position.

lipo- Prefix signifying *fat*.

lipocyte A fat cell.

lipofibroma A tumour composed of both fatty and fibrous tissue.

lipoid Resembling fat.

lipoma A benign tumour composed of fat cells.

lipomatoid Resembling a lipoma.

lipomatosis Excessive localized accumulations of fat in the tissues.

lipomatous Relating to or resembling a lipoma.

lipomyoma A tumour composed of both fatty and muscular tissue.

liposarcoma A rare malignant form of lipoma.

liquefaction The change to a liquid state.

Liston's operation (R. Liston, 1794-1847. Scottish surgeon). An operation for excision of the maxilla.

lithiasis Calculus formation within the body.

litho- Prefix signifying *calculus*.

livid Of a leaden colour; black and blue; discoloured, as from congestion or contusion.

Lizar's operation (J. Lizar, c. 1787-1860. Scottish surgeon). An operation for excision of the maxilla by a curved incision from the angle of the mouth to the zygoma.

load
occlusal l. The force exerted on the posterior teeth during mastication.

lobe 1. A rounded part or projection of an organ, marked off by fissures or constrictions. 2. A primary division in the formation of the tooth crown.

lobular Relating to lobes or lobules.

lobulated Composed of lobes or lobules.

lobule A small lobe, or one of the divisions of a lobe.

local Restricted to or affecting one part or area only; as opposed to *general*.

lock *In orthodontics*, the device used to fasten a wire appliance to the band on a tooth.
bite l. A device that can be attached to the bite rims of a denture to retain them in the same position out of the mouth as they occupied in it.

lockjaw 1. *Trismus^2. 2. A common term for *tetanus.

locular Relating to or characterized by loculi.

loculus (*pl.* loculi) A space or small cavity.

Logan crown (M.L. Logan, 1844-85. American dentist). A porcelain crown, having a concave base, and attached to the tooth by means of a platinum post baked into the porcelain.

Logan's bow An apparatus used in cleft lip surgery after suturing to hold the two parts of the lip forward until they heal in that position, and to prevent tension on the sutures.

longissimus capitis muscle Extends the vertebral column; *also called* M. trachelomastoideus. *See* Table of Muscles.

longissimus cervicis muscle Extends spinal column; *also called* M. transversus colli. *See* Table of Muscles.

longitudinal muscles Paired intrinsic muscles of the tongue which change its shape; *also called* lingual muscles. *See* Table of Muscles—longitudinalis.

longus capitis muscle Controls movement of head and neck. *See* Table of Muscles.

longus cervicis muscle M. longus colli. *See* Table of Muscles.

longus colli muscle Flexes vertebral column; *also called* M. longus cervicis. *See* Table of Muscles.

lophodont Having the crowns of the teeth in the form of ridges or crests.

loupe A convex, magnifying lens.
binocular l's. A set of magnifying lenses mounted in spectacle frames.

Ludwig's angina (W. F. von Ludwig, 1790-1865. German surgeon). A rare but severe form of cellulitis affecting the floor of the mouth, and spreading to the pharynx.

lues *Syphilis.

luetic Relating to syphilis.

lug *In dentistry,* a projection from a prosthetic appliance which fits into a prepared seat in an abutment and acts as support and retention.

Luken's band A band having the clamps on the buccal side.

lumen The space within the walls of a tube.

lupus erythematosus An inflammatory autoimmune disease, affecting the connective tissue and blood vessels; it takes many different forms, some of which produce oral and facial lesions.

lupus vulgaris A common and severe form of skin and subcutaneous tuberculosis, characterized by red-brown nodules, with ulceration and scarring; it affects the face, and may also affect the oral mucosa.

luting agent A form of thin, fine-grained cement used to retain crowns, inlays, etc.

luxation 1. *Dislocation. 2. *In dentistry,* the separation of a tooth from its socket due to injury.

lycostoma Cleft *palate.

lymph Clear fluid found in the lymphatic vessels; it is derived from the tissues and the blood and carries blood proteins from the liver, fats from the intestines and foreign antigens, lymphocytes and excess tissue fluid through the body system.

lymph node One of the many small filtering organs found in clusters along the lymphatic vessels, through which the lymph is drained and which produce lymphocytes.

lymphadenitis Inflammation of the lymph nodes.

lymphadenopathy Any disease affecting the lymph glands. Often used to describe the signs of swelling and tenderness of lymph glands elicited during diagnostic investigation.

lymphangioendothelioma A form of lymphangioma with a concentration of endothelial cells.

lymphangioma A benign tumour composed of newly-formed lymphatic vessels.
capillary l. A form of lymphangioma containing small lymphatic vessels; occurring in the region of the head and neck.
cavernous l. A form of lymphangioma consisting of cavernous lymphatic spaces; it is the most common type of lymphangioma, usually found on the tongue, but also found on the buccal mucosa and the palate.
cystic l. A cystic growth containing lymphatic material; found in the neck, and more common in children than in adults.

lymphangiosarcoma A malignant *lymphangioendothelioma.

lymphangitis Inflammation of the lymph vessels.

lymphatic 1. Relating to lymph. 2. One of the vessels containing lymph.

lymphocyte One of the spherical motile cells, produced by the lymph nodes, which are the principal cells involved in immune reactions.

lymphoepithelioma A form of squamous cell carcinoma affecting the tonsils and pharynx; an anaplastic tumour containing lymphocytes and carcinomatous tissue.

lymphoid Resembling lymph or lymphatic cells.

lymphoma Any tumour composed of lymphoid tissue.

lymphomatoid Resembling a lymphoma.

lymphomatosis The development of multiple lymphomas.

lymphomatous Resembling or relating to a lymphoma.

lymphosarcoma A malignant mesenchymal tumour with proliferation of lymphocytes.

Lyon forceps (J. A. Lyon, 1882-1955. American physician). Bone forceps with heavy jaws, used especially in excision of maxillary bone.

lysozyme A basic protein found in saliva, tears, etc.

lyssa Lingual *septum.

M

m Symbol for *metre*.

M Abbreviation for *permanent* molar.

m. Abbreviation for *misce*—mix; used in prescription writing.

man. Abbreviation for *mane*—in the morning; used in prescription writing.

MB Mesiobuccal.

MBO Mesiobucco-occlusal.

MBP Mesiobuccopulpal.

MC Mesiocervical.

MD Mesiodistal.

m. et sig. Abbreviation for *misce et signa*—mix and label; used in prescription writing.

m. ft. Abbreviation for *mistura fiat*—let a mixture be made; used in prescription writing.

mg Symbol for *milligram*.

MG Mesiogingival.

MI Mesioincisal.

MID Mesioincisodistal.

mil. Abbreviation for *millilitre*.

misc. Abbreviation for *misce*—mix; used in prescription writing.

mist. Abbreviation for *mistura*—a mixture; used in prescription writing.

ml Symbol for *millilitre*.

ML Mesiolingual.

MLa Mesiolabial.

MLaI Mesiolabioincisal.

MLaP Mesiolabiopulpal.

MLI Mesiolinguoincisal.

MLP Mesiolinguopulpal.

mm Symbol for *millimetre*.

MO Mesio-occlusal.

MOD Mesio-occlusodistal.

mod. praesc. Abbreviation for *modo praescripto*—in the manner directed; used in prescription writing.

mor. sol. Abbreviation for *more solito*—in the usual way; used in prescription writing.

MP Mesiopulpal.

maceration The softening of a substance by soaking in a liquid.

Mack crown (C.H. Mack, fl. 1872. American dentist). A hollow porcelain crown held in position by being cemented on to pins screwed into the root canal.

Mackenzie's syndrome (Sir S. Mackenzie, 1844-1909. English physician). Paralysis affecting the tongue, soft palate, and vocal fold on one side; *also called* Jackson's paralysis or Jackson-Mackenzie syndrome.

macro- Prefix signifying *enlargement*.

macroalveolism A condition in which the alveolar process is too large in relation to the rest of the facial skeleton; it may be *maxillary* or *mandibular*.

macroblepharia The condition of having abnormally large eyelids.

macrocephalic Having an abnormally large head.

macrocheilia The condition of having abnormally large lips.

macrocheilitis Swelling and inflammation of the lips.

macrodontia, macrodontism The condition of having abnormally large teeth; it is an hereditary condition. *Also called* megalodontia.
relative m. The condition in which the teeth are too large in relation to the dental arches.

macrogenia A condition in which the chin is too large in relation to the rest of the facial skeleton.

macrogingivae 1. Gingival *hyperplasia. 2. Gingival *fibromatosis.

macroglossia The condition of having a large, over-developed tongue.

macrognathia The condition of having an abnormally large mandible or maxilla.

macrolabia *Macrocheilia.

macromandibulism A condition in which the body of the mandible is proportionately too large for the rest of the facial skeleton.

macromaxillism A condition in which the maxilla is proportionately too large for the rest of the facial skeleton.

macroplasia Abnormal growth of tissue or of a part.

macroscopic Visible without the aid of a microscope.

macrosis Excessive development.

macrostomia The condition of having an abnormally large mouth.

macrotooth A tooth of abnormally large size.

macula (*pl.* maculae) *See* macule.

macular Relating to or characterized by macules.

maculation 1. The development of macules. 2. The condition of being spotted.

macule A circumscribed patch of discoloration on the skin.
oral melanotic m. A small, solitary and well-circumscribed pigmented lesion which may be found on the lower lip, gingiva, buccal mucosa or hard palate.

maculopapular Having the characteristics of both a macule and a papule.

madescent Moist.

Magill band (W.E. Magill, fl. 1871. American dentist). A plain band, cemented to the tooth and used in the fixation of an expansion arch or other orthodontic appliance.

Magitot's disease (E. Magitot, 1833-97. French dentist). *Periodontoclasia.

magma 1. A paste, or other amorphous pulpy mass. 2. *In pharmacy*, a suspension of a precipitate in water.

magnification Apparent increase in size, especially by the use of lenses, as in a microscope.

maintainer Anything designed to keep the existing state of an object, or of objects in relation to each other.
space m. A passive orthodontic appliance used to prevent overcrowding of teeth or closure of a space into which a tooth is expected to erupt; it may be *fixed*, *removable* or *fixed-removable* (that is, removable only by the dentist).

makro- *See* macro-

mal- Prefix signifying *faulty* or *impaired.*

mala The cheek.

malacia A morbid softening of the tissues or of other parts.

malacotic Relating to malacia; used particularly of the teeth.

malalignment 1. Any condition in which the teeth are outside the line of the dental arch. 2. In the treatment of fractures, denotes a poor join between the two ends of the broken bone.

malar Relating to the cheek, or to the cheek-bone.

malar bone The *zygomatic bone or cheek-bone.

malar nerve N. zygomaticofacialis. *See* Table of Nerves.

Malassez's rests (L.C. Malassez, 1842-1909. French physiologist). Epithelial cell *rests.

maldevelopment Impaired or abnormal development.

maleruption Eruption of a tooth out of its normal position.

malformation Impaired formation, deformity.

malfunction *Dysfunction.

malignant Virulent, and becoming increasingly so; threatening life, as of a lesion or tumour of uncontrolled growth, producing metastases.

malinterdigitation Faulty occlusion of the teeth.

malleable Able to be hammered out into thin sheets, one of the properties of a metal.

mallet, automatic Mechanical *condenser.

malocclusion Any deviation from the normal occlusion of the teeth, resulting in impaired function.

Angle's classification of malocclusion:

Class I. Relative position of the dental arches, mesiodistally, normal, with malocclusions usually confined to the anterior teeth.

Class II. Retrusion of the lower jaw, with distal occlusion of the lower teeth.

Division 1a. Narrow upper arch, with lengthened and prominent upper incisors, lack of nasal and lip function. Mouth-breathers.

Division 1b. Same as *a*, but with only one lateral half of the arch involved, the other being normal. Mouth-breathers.

Division 2a. Slight narrowing of the upper arch; bunching of the upper incisors, with overlapping and lingual inclination; normal lip and nasal function.

Division 2b. Same as *a*, but with only one lateral half of the arch involved, the other being normal; normal lip and nasal function.

Class IIIa. Protrusion of the lower jaw, with mesial occlusion of the lower teeth; lower incisors and cuspids lingually inclined.

Class IIIb. Same as *a*, but with only one lateral half of the arch involved, the other being normal.

buccal segment classification: A classification of anteroposterior relationships according to the relationships of the mandibular buccal teeth to the maxillary buccal teeth.

Class I. Normal anteroposterior relationship.

Class II. Mandibular teeth at least one-half cusp width distal to their correct relationship with the maxillary teeth.

Class III. Mandibular teeth at least one-half cusp width mesial to their correct relationship with the maxillary teeth.

incisal classification: A classification based on the anteroposterior incisor relationship.

Class I. The lower incisor edges occlude with or lie immediately below the cingulum plateau (middle part of the palatal surface) of the upper central incisors.

Class II. The lower incisor edges lie posterior to the cingulum plateau of the the upper incisors.

Class III. The upper central incisors are retroclined. The overjet is usually minimal but may be increased.

skeletal classification: A classification based on the relationship between the deepest points in the incisor segment of the maxilla and of the mandible.

Class I: Basal bone of the mandible is normal in relation to the maxilla.

Class II: Basal bone of the mandible is post-normal to the maxilla.

Class III: Basal bone of the mandible is pre-normal to the maxilla.

malomaxillary Relating to both the malar (zygomatic) bone and the maxilla.

maloplasty Plastic surgery of the cheek.

malposition Any deviation from the normal position; used particularly of a tooth that is out of occlusion or out of the line of the arch.

malpractice Improper or injurious treatment in medicine or dentistry.

malrelation Abnormal or faulty relation of two connected or contacting parts, as in malocclusion of the teeth.

malturned Abnormally turned, used of a tooth that is rotated on its long axis so that it is in an abnormal position.

mamelon One of three rounded prominences on the incisal edge of a newly-erupted incisor.

mandible The bone of the lower jaw.

mandibular Relating to the mandible.

mandibular nerve Supplies the muscles of mastication and the mucosa of the cheek, floor of the mouth and front of the tongue. *See* Table of Nerves—mandibularis.

mandibulofacial Relating to both the mandible and the facial bones.

mandibuloglossus A variant portion of the genioglossus muscle, which extends to the side of the tongue from the posterior border of the mandible.

mandibulomarginalis A variant portion of the platysma muscle, which extends forward over the angle of the mandible from the mastoid process.

mandibulopharyngeal Relating to the mandible and the pharynx.

mandrel A spindle or shaft for holding a tool for rotation; used with a dental engine to hold polishing discs, etc.

manducation *Mastication.

manducatory Relating to mastication.

mane Latin for *in the morning*; used in prescription writing and abbreviated *man.* or *m.*

manipulation Skilful use of the hands, especially in treatment.

mantle dentine The thin, superficial outer layer of dentine.

manual 1. Relating to the hand. 2. Performed by hand, as opposed to *mechanical*.

manudynamometer An apparatus that measures the force of thrust of an instrument.

marble bone disease *Osteopetrosis.

margin A border or edge.

alveolar m. The top edge of the bone forming the tooth sockets.

cavosurface m. The edge of a cavity with the tooth surface.

gingival m. The unattached edge of the gingiva at the necks of the teeth.

infraorbital m. of the maxilla The rounded edge of the orbital surface of the maxilla, which forms a segment of the orbit.

lacrimal m. of the maxilla The posterior border of the frontal process of the maxilla, articulating with the lacrimal bone.

lingual m. The edge of the tongue, which is in contact with the teeth and the gingiva.

marginal Relating to a margin.

marrow The soft tissue found in the canals and interstices of bones.

marsupialization An operation for the evacuation of a cyst and the suturing of its walls to the edges of the wound, the cavity closing by granulation; used where complete extirpation is not possible.

Maryland bridge A bridge in which the abutments are bonded to the acid-etched surfaces of the supporting teeth. Although the teeth undergo little preparation, the fitting surfaces of the metal abutments are etched to improve the mechanical retention of the bonding agent.

masking *In dentistry,* an opaque covering for the metal portions of a restoration or prosthesis.

Mason's detachable crown (W.L. Mason, fl. 1896. American dentist). A crown having a removable porcelain facing on a post and collar base.

masseter The muscle that raises the mandible in mastication. *See* Table of Muscles.

masseteric Relating to the masseter muscle.

masseteric artery Supplies the deep surface of the masseter muscle. *See* Table of Arteries—masseterica.

masseteric nerve Motor and sensory nerves for the masseter muscle and temporomandibular joint. *See* Table of Nerves—massetericus.

massodent An instrument used for massaging the gums.

mastication The act of chewing.

masticatory Relating to mastication.

masticatory system Those oral structures involved in mastication.

mastoid 1. A thick process of the temporal bone. 2. Relating to the mastoid process.

mastoid artery Supplies the dura mater, lateral sinuses and mastoid cells. *See* Table of Arteries—mastoidea.

mastoidale The lowest point on the mastoid process; a craniometric landmark.

materia alba A soft, white or creamy deposit on the teeth, building up over underlying plaque, and made up of food debris and dead epithelial cells; it can be rinsed off with a spray.

materia medica The science of drugs and their sources, preparations and uses.

matrix 1. Intercellular tissue. 2. A mould used in casting. 3. The female portion of a precision attachment.
amalgam m. *Matrix band.
dentine m. The intercellular connective tissue of which dentine is composed; it is organic in the early stages of development but is later mineralized.
enamel m. The organic secretion of the ameloblasts within which the inorganic enamel crystallites are laid down.
organic m. Enamel *matrix.

matrix band *In dentistry*, a thin band of metal used to provide a temporary tooth wall to support a filling.

maxilla (*pl.* maxillae) One of the two bones that form the upper jaw; generally, however, the singular term is used to denote the upper jaw as a whole.

maxillary Relating to the maxilla.

maxillary artery Supplies the mandibular alveolar process, cheek muscles, etc. *Also called* internal maxillary artery. *See* Table of Arteries—maxillaris.

maxillary nerve Supplies the skin of the upper part of the face, maxillary teeth, and mucosa of nose, cheeks and palate, as well as meninges. *See* Table of Nerves—maxillaris.

maxillate Possessing jaws.

maxillectomy Excision of the maxilla.

maxillitis Inflammation of the maxilla or of a maxillary gland.

maxillodental Relating to the maxilla and the teeth.

maxillofacial Relating to the maxilla and other facial processes.

maxillofrontale The craniometric point at which the frontomaxillary suture meets the lacrimal crest; one of a pair.

maxillojugal Relating to the maxilla and the cheek.

maxillolabial Relating to the maxilla and the lip.

maxillomandibular Relating to both the maxilla and the mandible.

maxillopalatine Relating to the maxilla and the hard palate.

maxillopharyngeal Relating to the maxilla and the pharynx.

maxillotomy Surgical sectioning of the maxilla; maxillary osteotomy.

maxilloturbinal The inferior nasal concha, or turbinate bone.

maximum The greatest, or most, of anything; as opposed to *minimum*.

meatus A passage, canal or orifice.
acoustic m. Auditory *meatus.
auditory m. The canal within the ear, running from the concha to the tympanic membrane (*external*); and from the tympanic membrane through the petrous bone, giving passage to the facial and auditory nerves and the internal auditory artery (*internal*).
nasal m. One of the spaces below each of the conchae in the lateral wall of the nasal cavity; each is named after the concha to which it belongs: *inferior, middle* and *superior*.

meckelectomy Surgical removal of the pterygopalatine ganglion (Meckel's ganglion).

Meckel's cartilage (J.F. Meckel, *the younger*, 1781-1833. German surgeon). The cartilage forming the first branchial arch in the foetus.

Meckel's ganglion (J.F. Meckel, *the elder*, 1714-74. German anatomist). 1. Pterygopalatine *ganglion. 2. Submandibular *ganglion (lesser ganglion of Meckel).

mecocephalic *Dolichocephalic.

medial Towards the midline; internal.

median Situated in the centre, or on the midline of the body.

medical Relating to medicine.

medicament Any medicinal substance.

medicinal 1. Relating to a medicine. 2. Possessing healing attributes.

medicine 1. The study and treatment of diseases, especially treatment without recourse to surgery. 2. Any drug used for the treatment of a disease.

medicodental Relating to both medicine and dentistry.

medio- Prefix signifying *middle*.

mediofrontal Relating to the middle of the forehead.

mediopalatine Relating to the centre portion of the palate.

medium *See* culture medium.

medulla *Marrow.

mega- Prefix signifying *great, enlarged*.

megadont A person with abnormally large teeth.

megadontia, megadontism *Macrodontia, macrodontism.

megadontic Relating to megadontism.

megaglossia *See* megaloglossia.

megagnathous Having a large jaw; macrognathic.

megalo- Prefix signifying *large*, especially *abnormally large*.

megalocephaly 1. The condition of having an abnormally large head. 2. *Leontiasis ossea.

megalodontia *Macrodontia, macrodontism.

megaloglossia A form of macroglossia, due to hypertrophy of the tongue muscle.

-megaly Suffix signifying *abnormal enlargment*.

megaprosopous Having an abnormally large face.

Méglin's palatine point (J.A. Méglin, 1756-1824. French physician). The point at which the descending palatine nerve emerges from the palatomaxillary canal.

melano- Prefix signifying *melanin* or *black*.

melanoameloblastoma Melanotic neuro-ectodermal *tumour of infancy.

melanocytoma
dermal m. Blue *naevus.

melanodontia, infantile *Odontoclasia[1].

melanodontoclasia *Odontoclasia[1].

melanofibroma Blue *naevus.

melanoglossia Black *tongue.

melanoma A malignant tumour composed of cells pigmented with melanin, and characterized by its black colour.
benign mesenchymal m. Blue *naevus.

melanoplakia Patchy pigmentation of the oral mucous membrane, associated with stomatitis, jaundice and other diseases.

melanotrichia linguae Black *tongue.

melitis Inflammation of the cheek.

melitoptyalism The condition in which the secretion of saliva contains glucose.

Melkersson-Rosenthal syndrome (E.G. Melkersson, 1898-1932. Swedish physician; C. Rosenthal, contemporary German physician). A childhood syndrome manifesting itself in a diffuse swelling of the lips, recurrent facial paralysis and fissured tongue; there may also be palatal leukoplakia, gingival thickening and macroglossia.

melo- Prefix signifying *cheek*.

meloncus Any tumour of the cheek.

meloplasty Plastic surgery of the cheek.

meloschisis A facial cleft.

Melotte's metal (G.W. Melotte, 1835-1915. American dentist). A soft alloy of bismuth, lead and tin, which is used in dentistry.

membrana adamantina Reduced enamel *epithelium.

membrana eboris The membrane surrounding the tooth pulp, composed of the remains of odontoblasts; an obsolete term.

membrane A thin layer of tissue lining a cavity, covering a part, or separating two adjacent cavities.
adamantine m. Reduced enamel *epithelium.
alveolodental m. Periodontal *ligament.
basement m. An extracellular layer that separates the epithelium from the connective tissue of most organs.
buccopharyngeal m. That area of the primitive embryo which later develops into the mouth and the pharynx.
enamel m. Reduced enamel *epithelium.
hyoglossal m. That part of the oral mucous membrane which connects the hyoid bone to the tongue.

mucous m. The membrane containing mucous glands, which lines those passages and cavities of the body which communicate with the exterior.
periodontal m. Periodontal *ligament.
subepithelial m. Basement *membrane.
submucous m. A layer of connective tissue lying between the mucous membrane and the lower tissue structures; in the mouth it is found in the region of the soft palate.
synovial m. A membrane secreting synovial fluid, which covers the articulating surfaces and ligaments of a joint.

membranous Relating to or characteristic of a membrane.

meningeal artery Branches from various arteries supplying the dura mater, cranium and trigeminal ganglion. *See* Table of Arteries—meningea.

meningeal artery, accessory A. pterygomeningea. *See* Table of Arteries.

meningeal nerves Supplying the meninges. *See* Table of Nerves—meningeus.

meniscectomy Surgical removal of the interarticular disc, for example from the temporomandibular joint.

meniscus *In anatomy,* a crescent-shaped structure, particularly an interarticular disc of fibrocartilage.

mensa An old term for the occlusal surface of a molar tooth.

mental 1. Relating to the mind. 2. Relating to the chin.

mental artery Supplies the lower lip and chin. *See* Table of Arteries—mentalis.

mental nerve Supplies skin of chin and lower lip. *See* Table of Nerves—mentalis.

mentalis muscle Protrudes lower lip and wrinkles skin of chin; *also called* M. levator menti. *See* Table of Muscles.

mento- Prefix signifying *chin.*

mentolabial Relating to the chin and the lip.

mentolabial muscle M. depressor labii inferioris. *See* Table of Muscles.

menton The lowest point on the outline of the symphysis menti seen on a lateral skull radiograph which has been orientated with the Frankfort plane horizontal. It is equivalent to the anthropological point *gnathion[1].

mentum The chin.

mercurial Relating to mercury.

mercuric Relating to mercury as a bivalent element.

mercurous Relating to mercury as a univalent element.

mercury A metallic element, chemical symbol Hg, a silver-white and shining fluid at normal temperatures. It is only soluble in nitric acid, and partially soluble in boiling hydrochloric acid. It combines both as a univalent and a bivalent element.

mero- Prefix signifying *part.*

mesal *Mesial.

mesaticephalic *Mesocephalic.

mesenchyma, mesenchyme The embryonic connective tissue formed from the mesoderm.

mesenchymal Relating to, or derived from, the mesenchyma.

mesial In the region of, nearer to, the midline. *In dentistry,* nearer to the midline within the dental arch.

mesio- Prefix signifying *towards the midline* or *mesial.*

mesioangular Relating to any mesial angle.

mesiobuccal Relating to the mesial and buccal surfaces of a tooth or the mesial and buccal walls of an occlusal cavity in a molar or premolar.
m. angle The angle formed at the junction of these walls; a *line* angle.

mesiobuccocclusal *Mesiobucco-occlusal.

mesiobucco-occlusal Relating to the mesial, buccal and occlusal surfaces of a tooth.

mesiobuccopulpal Relating to the mesial, buccal and pulpal walls of an occlusal cavity, or in the step portion of a proximo-occlusal cavity in a molar or premolar.
m. angle The angle formed at the junction of these walls; a *point* angle.

mesiocclusal *Mesio-occlusal.

mesiocclusodistal *Mesio-occluso-distal.

mesiocervical *Mesiogingival.

mesioclination Mesial tilting of a tooth.

mesioclusion A form of malocclusion in which the mandibular teeth occlude anterior to the maxillary teeth.

mesiodens A supernumerary tooth, often unerupted, found in the upper jaw between the central incisors.

mesiodistal Relating to the mesial and distal surfaces of a tooth.

mesiogingival Relating to the mesial and gingival walls of a buccal or lingual cavity in a molar or premolar.
m. angle The angle formed at the junction of these walls; a *line* angle.

mesiogression With the teeth forward of their normal position in the dental arch.

mesio-incisal Relating to the mesial and incisal surfaces of an incisor or canine, or to a cavity affecting these surfaces.

mesio-incisodistal Relating to the mesial, incisal and distal surfaces of an incisor or canine, or to a cavity affecting those surfaces.

mesiolabial Relating to the mesial and labial surfaces of a tooth, or to the corresponding walls in the step portion of a proximo-incisal cavity.
m. angle The angle formed at the junction of these walls; a *line* angle.

mesiolabio-incisal Relating to the mesial and labial surfaces and the incisal edge of an anterior tooth.

mesiolingual Relating to the mesial and lingual surfaces of a tooth, or to the mesial and lingual walls of an occlusal cavity in a molar or premolar.
m. angle The angle formed at the junction of these walls; a *line* angle.

mesiolinguocclusal *Mesiolinguo-occlusal.

mesiolinguo-occlusal Relating to the mesial and lingual surfaces and the incisal edge of an anterior tooth.

mesiolinguopulpal Relating to the mesial, lingual and pulpal walls of an occlusal cavity, or in the step portion of a proximo-occlusal cavity.
m. angle The angle formed at the junction of these walls; a *point* angle.

mesio-occlusal Relating to the mesial and occlusal surfaces of a tooth, or to the mesial and occlusal walls of a buccal or lingual cavity in a molar or premolar.
m. angle The angle formed at the junction of these walls; a *line* angle.

mesio-occlusodistal Relating to the mesial, occlusal and distal surfaces of a molar or premolar, or to a cavity affecting these surfaces.

mesiopulpal Relating to the mesial and pulpal walls of an occlusal cavity in a molar or premolar.
m. angle The angle formed at the junction of these walls; a *line* angle.

mesiopulpolabial Relating to the mesial, pulpal and labial walls of a cavity in an incisor or canine.
m. angle The angle formed at the junction of these walls; a *point* angle.

mesiopulpolingual Relating to the mesial, pulpal and lingual walls in the step portion of a proximo-incisal cavity.
m. angle The angle formed at the junction of these walls; a *point* angle.

mesioversion The position of a tooth that is inclined towards the median line.

mesoblast *Mesoderm.

mesocephalic Having a cephalic index of between 75.0 and 79.9; having a head with a moderate relationship between its greatest length and breadth.

mesoconch Having an orbit of medium height.

mesoconid The central distal cusp on a mandibular molar.

mesocranic *Mesocephalic.

mesodens *Mesiodens.

mesoderm The middle germinal layer in the primitive embryo.

mesodont Having medium-sized teeth.

mesognathion The hypothetical lateral portion of the premaxilla.

mesognathous Having a slightly projecting jaw, with a gnathic index between 98 and 103.

mesophryon The *glabella.

mesoprosopic Having a medium-width face.

mesostaphyline Having a palate of medium width, with a palatal index between 80.0 and 84.9.

mesostyle A small cusp or fold of enamel between the paracone and the metacone on the buccal surface of a maxillary molar.

metabolic Relating to metabolism.

metabolism The physical and chemical changes in the tissues by which a living body is maintained and energy generated.

metacone The distobuccal cusp of a maxillary molar.

metaconid The mesiolingual cusp of a mandibular molar.

metaconule A small cusp between the metacone and the protocone on the maxillary teeth of animals.

metal Any element having the following properties: hardness, ductility, malleability, lustre, fusibility, good conduction of heat and electricity.
cliche m. A fusible alloy of tin, lead, antimony and bismuth.
queen's m. An alloy composed of tin and antimony.

metallic Relating to a metal.

metaplasia The alteration of tissue from one form to another.
atypical m. *Dysplasia.

metaplasia *of pulp* A degenerative condition in which the tooth pulp has lost its power to form dentine, and has become merely connective tissue.

metastasis The transfer of a disease or of a tumour from a primary focus to other, unconnected, parts of the body, due to the transfer of the pathogenic organisms or of the tumour cells.

metastatic Relating to metastasis.

metastyle A small cusp on the lingual side of a maxillary molar or premolar, just posterior to the metacone.

meter 1. A measuring device. 2. To measure out; especially in medicine and dentistry related to the continuous flow of intravenous drugs. 3. *See* metre.

-meter Suffix signifying *measuring device.*

metodontiasis 1. The permanent dentition. 2. Faulty tooth development or eruption.

metopic Relating to the forehead.

metopion A craniometric point between the frontal eminences on the midline of the forehead.

metre The basic unit of length in the metric system, about 39.3 inches.

metric system The most commonly used system of weights and measures, based on multiples of ten and one hundred. The basic units are the metre (length), the gram (weight or mass) and the litre (capacity). Multiples of these basic units are designated by the prefixes deca- 10, hecto- 100, and kilo- 1000; fractional units are designated by corresponding prefixes deci- 1/10, centi- 1/100, and milli- 1/1000.

micro- Prefix signifying *small, extremely small.* 2. Used in medicine to signify *abnormally small.*

microaerophilic Requiring only minute traces of free oxygen for growth; used of micro-organisms.

microalveolism a condition in which the alveolar process is too small in relation to the rest of the facial skeleton; it may be *maxillary* or *mandibular.*

microbe Any micro-organism, but used particularly of pathogenic bacteria.

microbial Relating to microbes.

microbiology The study of micro-organisms.

microcephalic Having an abnormally small head.

microcheilia The condition of having abnormally small lips.

Micrococcaceae A family of cocci; spherical cells divided in more than one plane, Gram-positive, aerobic or facultatively anaerobic.

Micrococcus A genus of the Micrococcaceae family of bacteria, Gram-positive, non-motile and aerobic, with the cells grouped in irregular clusters.

M. pneumoniae **Streptococcus pneumoniae.*

micrococcus One of the completely separate type of cocci. *See* coccus.

microdentism *Microdontia, microdontism.

microdontia, microdontism The condition of having abnormally small teeth; a developmental disorder which may involve all teeth, a few teeth or only a single tooth.

relative m. The condition in which the teeth are too small in relation to the dental arches.

microdontic Relating to microdontia.

microgenia A condition in which the chin is too small in relation to the rest of the facial skeleton.

microglossia The condition of having a small, under-developed tongue.

micrognathia Congenital hypoplasia of the mandible or of the maxilla.

microleakage *In restorative dentistry,* a term used for the passing of fluids, micro-organisms or ions between the restoration and the adjacent cavity walls.

micromandible, micromandibulare 1. An extremely small mandible. 2. The condition of having an extremely small mandible.

micromandibulism A condition in which the body of the mandible is proportionately too small for the rest of the facial skeleton; it may give a 'bird face' appearance.

micromaxillism A condition in which the maxilla is proportionately too small in both width and length for the rest of the facial skeleton.

micromotor A miniature electric motor which can be coupled directly to a handpiece.

micro-organism Any form of plant or animal life visible only under the microscope.

microscope An instrument used for magnifying minute objects.

microscopic Minute, visible only through a microscope.

microscopy Observation and examination with a microscope.

Microspironema **Treponema.*

microstomia The condition of having an abnormally small mouth.

microtia The condition of having an abnormally small external ear.

microtooth A tooth of abnormally small size.

migration *of a tooth* Gradual spontaneous movement of a tooth, seen in advanced periodontal disease.

Mikulicz's aphthae (J. von Mikulicz-Radecki, 1850-1905. Polish surgeon). *Periadenitis mucosa necrotica recurrens.

Mikulicz's disease (J. von Mikulicz-Radecki, 1850-1905. Polish surgeon). Chronic swelling of the lacrimal and salivary glands due to the replacement of glandular by lymphoid tissue.

milk teeth Primary *teeth.

Miller's elevator An instrument designed with a slightly curved shank, allowing the blade to pass between the distal root of a second molar and the crown of a third molar; used in the removal of impacted lower third molars.

milli- Prefix signifying *one-thousandth.*

milling-in The process of perfecting the occlusion of dentures by rubbing them together, either in the mouth or in an articulator, with an abrasive between the occluding surfaces.

mimesis The imitation by one disease of another.

mineralization The addition of minerals or mineral salts to the body.

Mirault's operation (G. Mirault, 1796-1879. French surgeon). 1. An operation for plastic repair of unilateral hare-lip by means of a flap turned down at one side and attached on the opposite side. 2. An operation for excision of the tongue, in which the lingual arteries are tied off first.

mirror A highly polished, reflective surface.

dental m. A small mirror designed for use in the mouth.

mouth m. Dental *mirror.

misce Latin for *mix*; used in prescription writing, and abbreviated *misc.* or *m.*

miscible Capable of being mixed.

mistura Latin for *a mixture*; used in prescription writing, and abbreviated *mist.* or *m.*

mitosis Indirect division of cells, the typical method of cell reproduction; karyokinesis.

mitotic Relating to or characterized by mitosis.

mobility *In dentistry,* the looseness of a tooth; pathologically the excessive movement of a tooth or teeth as a result of periodontal disease.

model A reproduction in metal or plastics made from an impression of an object; a cast.

modiolus A point near the corner of the mouth at which several of the facial muscles intersect.

modo praescripto Latin for *in the manner directed*; used in prescription writing, and abbreviated *mod. praesc.*

Moeller's glossitis (J.O.L. Moeller, 1819-87. German surgeon). Chronic superficial inflammation and excoriation of the tongue, spreading to the palate and cheeks, and marked by smoothness and burning pain; *also called* glossodynia exfoliativa.

molar, molar tooth One of the back, grinding teeth. There are two in each quadrant in the primary dentition and three in each quadrant in the permanent dentition in man.
mulberry m's. Small dome-shaped permanent first molars, with the cusps close together and affected by enamel hypoplasia; a developmental defect seen in congenital syphilis. *Also called* Moon's molars or Fournier's molars.

molar glands Mixed glands near the openings of the parotid ducts.

molariform In the shape of a molar.

molarion The point of the most distal cusp on either side of the mandibular arch.

molars, Fournier's Mulberry *molars.

molars, Moon's Mulberry *molars.

mold *See* mould.

monangled, monoangled *Of an instrument*: having only one angle in the shank.

Monilia **Candida.*

moniliasis *Candidiasis.
oral m. Infection of the mouth with *Candida albicans*; may be a precancerous condition when chronic.

mono- Prefix signifying *one, single.*

monobloc Myofunctional *appliance.

monococcus A single coccus, one not united in pairs, chains or groups.

monodont Having only a single tooth.

monofluor-phosphate A chemical complex, containing fluoride, used in toothpaste and as a topical application for the prevention of dental caries.

monolocular Having only one cavity; applied to synovial joints.

monomaxillary Relating to or affecting one jaw only.

monomer Any substance composed of single molecules. Frequently applied to substances capable of undergoing polymerization.

mononuclear Having only one nucleus.

monophyodont Having only one, permanent, set of teeth.

monoradicular Having only one root.

monostotic Affecting only one bone.

Monson's curve (G.S. Monson, 1869-1933. American dentist). *See* curve of Monson.

Moon's molars (H. Moon, 1845-92. English surgeon). Mulberry *molars.

Moorehead's retractor (F.B. Moorehead, 1875-1947. American oral surgeon). A type of instrument for drawing back the edges of wounds, used in dental surgery.

Morand's foramen (S.F. Morand, 1697-1773. French surgeon). The caecal *foramen of the tongue.

Moraxella A genus of the Neisseriaceae family of microorganisms, Gram-negative and aerobic; divided into two subgenera: *Moraxella*, seen as rods, often short and plump, and *Branhamella*, seen as small cocci, either single-cell or paired.

morbid Relating to or affected with disease.

morbus gallicus *Syphilis.

mordacious Biting, caustic or pungent.

mordant Any substance used to fix dyes or stains.

more solito Latin for *in the usual way*; used in prescription writing, and abbreviated *mor. sol.*

morphologic, morphological Relating to morphology.

morphology The study of the forms and structure of living organisms.

Morrison crown (W.N. Morrison, 1842-96. American dentist). A gold shell crown, formed by an axial band with a swaged occlusal cap; *also called* Beers' crown.

morsal Occlusal; relating to the masticating surface of a molar or premolar.

mortar A bell- or urn-shaped vessel in which drugs are ground or crushed with a pestle.

motile Capable of spontaneous movement.

mottling The condition of a surface marked by spots or patches of a different colour or of a different shade; *in dentistry* applied particularly to enamel affected by chronic endemic fluorosis.

mould 1. The growth or deposit produced by certain types of fungi. 2. The hollow shape in which something is cast or fashioned. 3. To model or cast an object in such a hollow shape.
acrylic m. A stent used in oral plastic surgery to secure an intraoral skin graft.

mouth 1. The entrance to any canal or body cavity. 2. The oral cavity, containing the teeth and the tongue.
tapir m. A condition characterized by loose, thickened lips, and caused by atrophy of the orbicularis oris muscle.
trench m. 1. Acute ulcerative *gingivitis. 2. Acute ulcerative *stomatitis.
white m. *Thrush.

mouth guard An appliance worn in the mouth to protect the teeth from injury during sporting activities such as boxing, rugby football, etc.

mouth hygiene Oral *hygiene.

mouth mirror Dental *mirror.

mouth prop Jaw *prop.

mouth-breathing Habitual respiration through the mouth instead of through the nose.

mouthwash Any medicated solution used for rinsing the mouth, either for cleansing or for treating diseases of the oral mucosa.

muciferous Mucus-secreting.

mucilage 1. A sticky paste used as a vehicle in pharmacy or as a demulcent. 2. A natural gum dissolved in plant juices, occurring in plants.

mucilaginous Relating to or having the characteristics of mucilage.

mucin The chief constituent of mucus, a mixture of glycoproteins soluble in water but precipitated in alcohol or acids.

mucin plaque Acquired *pellicle.

mucinous Relating to or characterized by mucin.

muco- Prefix signifying *mucus*, or *mucous membrane*.

mucocele 1. Distention of an organ or vessel caused by an accumulation of mucus. 2. A circumscribed, bluish mucous swelling, with a tendency to recur, arising from an abnormal accumulation of mucous secretion; most commonly found in the lower lip.

mucocutaneous Relating to the mucous membrane and the skin.

mucodermal Relating to the mucous membrane and the skin.

mucodermatitis Inflammation affecting a mucous membrane.

mucoepidermoid Relating to the mucous membrane and the epidermis.

mucogingival Relating to the mucous membrane and the gingiva.

mucoid Mucus-like.

mucomembranous Relating to the mucous membrane.

mucoperiosteum Periosteum having a mucous covering, as in the auditory apparatus.

mucopurulent Containing both mucus and pus.

mucormycosis *Phycomycosis.

mucosa The mucous membrane.
alveolar m. The mucous membrane lining the vestibule of the mouth.

mucosal Relating to the mucous membrane.

mucositis Inflammation of the mucous membrane.
chemotherapy m. Oral lesions producing a burning sensation, areas of redness and possibly ulceration, the ulcers becoming numerous and large; relatively infrequent side-effect of chemotherapy.
migratory m. *Stomatitis areata migrans.
radiation m. Characteristic diffuse inflammatory change in the mucosa produced by radiation therapy.

mucous Relating to mucus.

mucus The viscid secretion of the mucous glands, covering the mucous membrane.

muffle furnace Porcelain *furnace.

mulberry molars Small dome-shaped permanent first molars, with the cusps close together and affected by enamel hypoplasia; a developmental defect seen in congenital syphilis. *Also called* Moon's molars or Fournier's molars.

muller A flat-bottomed pestle, used to grind drugs on a slab.

multi- Prefix signifying *many.*

multicellular Composed of numerous cells.

multicusped *Multicuspidate.

multicuspidate Having several cusps, as on a posterior tooth.

multidentate Having many teeth, or many tooth-like projections.

multilocular Containing many cells or small cavities.

multinuclear Having several nuclei.

multirooted Having several roots; used of molar teeth.

Mummery's fibres (J.H. Mummery, 1847-1926. English dentist). Nerve fibrils in developing dentine.

mummification *of dental pulp* Removal of previously devitalized pulp to the level of the pulp chamber floor, and the treatment of the radicular portion to render it inert.

muscle A contractile organ by means of which movement is produced in an animal organism.
articular m. One attached to the membrane of a synovial joint and inserted into the capsule.
extrinsic m. One having its origin in a different organ or part from its insertion.
intrinsic m. One in which both the origin and insertion are in the same organ or part.

involuntary m. Any muscle that contracts of itself, and is not under the control of the will.
skeletal m. The type of muscle tissue connected with the bony skeleton; striated muscle.
smooth m. Muscle consisting of spindle-shaped, unstriped fibres; involuntary muscle is usually of this type.
sphincter m. One that surrounds and closes a natural opening.
striated m. Muscle in which the fibres have cross-striations; voluntary muscle is usually of this type.
striped m. Striated *muscle.
unstriated m. Smooth *muscle.
unstriped m. Smooth *muscle.
voluntary m. Any muscle directly controlled by the will.

For specific muscles of the head and neck *see* Table of Muscles.

muscle, Koyter's M. corrugator supercilii. *See* Table of Muscles.

muscular Relating to or characterized by muscle.

muscular artery Supplies the muscles of the eye. *See* Table of Arteries—muscularis.

musculature The system of muscles in the body, or in any one part of it.

musculocutaneous, musculodermic Relating to both muscle and skin.

musculomembranous Relating to both muscle and membrane.

mush bite Squash *bite.

Mycobacteriaceae A family of parasitic rod-shaped organisms of the order Actinomycetales.

Mycobacterium The type genus of the Mycobacteriaceae family of bacteria, seen as non-motile slender rods, sometimes branching; aerobic and considered to be Gram-positive.

mycocide *Fungicide.

mycosis A disease caused by a fungus.

mycostatic *Fungistatic.

mycotic Relating to any fungal disease or mycosis.

mycteric Relating to the nasal cavity.

myelogenic, myelogenous Produced by the bone-marrow cells.

myeloid Relating to bone marrow.

myeloma A tumour arising from, and composed of, bone-marrow cells.

mylo- Prefix signifying *molar*.

mylodus An old term for a molar tooth.

mylohyoid Relating to the mandibular molars and the hyoid bone.

mylohyoid muscle Assists in raising hyoid bone and depressing mandible during swallowing. *See* Table of Muscles—mylohyoideus.

mylohyoid nerve Supplies the mylohyoid muscle and the anterior belly of the digastric muscle. *See* Table of Nerves—mylohyoideus.

mylopharyngeal muscle Part of constrictor pharyngis superior. *See* Table of Muscles–mylopharyngeus.

myo- Prefix signifying *muscle*.

myoblast One of the cells from which muscle fibres develop.

myoblastoma A benign tumour, usually called *granular cell* myoblastoma, once thought to be composed of primitive myoblasts, now of disputed origin; it may occur on the skin and mucous membrane, or in the gastrointestinal tract. The oral cavity is commonly affected, especially the gingiva and the lateral and dorsal surfaces of the tongue.

myofascial Relating to the muscle fascia.

myofunctional Relating to muscle function.

myoid Muscle-like.

myology The study of muscle and muscles.

myoma A tumour derived from or composed of muscle tissue. If it is smooth muscle it is called a *leiomyoma*, and if it is striated muscle a *rhabdomyoma*.

myomatosis The development of multiple myomas.

myomatous Relating to or resembling a myoma.

myositis Inflammation affecting voluntary muscle.

myositis ossificans A condition of the muscles, tendons and ligaments, in which bone is irregularly deposited in the affected site; it may be *progressive*, which is thought to be an hereditary disease, or *traumatic*, occurring at the site of an injury. The masseter muscle and the temporal muscle may be affected, leading to difficulty in opening the mouth.

myotomy The surgical cutting of a muscle.

myxadenitis Inflammation affecting a mucous gland or glands.

myxadenitis labialis *Cheilitis glandularis.

myxo- Prefix signifying *mucus, mucous, mucoid.*

myxochondroma A tumour composed of both mucous tissue and cartilage tissue.

myxofibroadenoma *Adenofibroma.

myxofibroma *Myxoma.

myxoid Mucus-like.

myxoma A benign tumour composed of mucous connective tissue.
odontogenic m. A tumour of the tooth-bearing parts of the jaws composed of myxoid tissue; it may be locally malignant.

myxorrhoea A copious flow of mucus.

N

N Chemical symbol for nitrogen.

Na Chemical symbol for sodium.

NAD Abbreviation for *no appreciable disease; nothing abnormal discovered.*

NaF Chemical symbol for sodium fluoride.

Ni Chemical symbol for nickel.

noct. Abbreviation for *nocte*—at night; used in prescription writing.

noct. maneq. Abbreviation for *nocte maneque*—at night and in the morning; used in prescription writing.

n.p.o. Abbreviation for *nil per os*—nothing by mouth.

NTP Abbreviation for *normal temperature and pressure.*

NYD Abbreviation for *not yet diagnosed.*

naevoid Naevus-like, resembling a naevus.

naevoxantho-endothelioma A condition characterized by hard yellow nodules which appear on the skin in infants; most commonly seen on the face and extremities.

naevus 1. A birth mark; a developmental pigmented area of the skin or mucous membrane. 2. A benign tumour of the melanogenic system; it may be *pigmented* or *non-pigmented.*

blue n. A benign blue-black melanotic tumour, seen as a small, sharply-defined nodular growth on the face, and also on the forearms and hands, most frequently in childhood; *also called* Jadassohn-Tièche naevus.

oral epithelial n. White sponge *naevus.

white sponge n. A naevus affecting the oral and nasal mucosa, characterized by white spongy lesions of thickened folded mucous membrane; it is thought to be an hereditary condition.

naevus cavernosus Cavernous *haemangioma.

naevus flammeus A congenital capillary haemangioma, most common on the cutaneous surface of the face or neck, and darkish red in colour; *also called* port-wine stain.

Nance's leeway space The difference between the space occupied by the primary canine and two molars and that occupied by the permanent canine and premolars on each side of the dental arch.

nano- Prefix signifying *abnormally small.*

nanocephalous Having an abnormally small head.

nanoid Dwarf-like.

nape The back of the neck, the nuche.

narcosis A state of profound unconsciousness or stupor, produced by a drug.

narcotic 1. Relating to narcosis. 2. Any agent that produces narcosis and relief of pain. 3. Any person addicted to narcotics.

naris (*pl.* nares) A nostril.

nasal Relating to the nose.

nasal arteries Supply the nasal cavity and septum and the adjacent sinuses. *See* Table of Arteries—dorsalis nasi (*also called* nasi externa) and nasalis posterior lateralis.

nasal bone One of the two small bones which make up the bridge of the nose.

nasal muscle M. nasalis, pars alaris and M. nasalis, pars transversa. *See* Table of Muscles.

nasal nerves Supply the skin and mucosa of the nose. *See* Table of Nerves—nasalis.

nasal vein, external The vein draining the side of the nose. *See* Table of Veins—nasalis externa.

nasion The midpoint of the frontonasal suture. *In cephalometrics* it is both a *soft tissue* landmark: the deepest point of the depression at the root of the nose below the forehead; and a *hard tissue* landmark: the most anterior point of the frontonasal suture, seen on a lateral skull radiograph.

nasitis Inflammation of the nasal mucous membrane.

Nasmyth's membrane (A. Nasmyth, d. 1848. Scottish dental surgeon). 1. Primary enamel *cuticle[1]. 2. Reduced enamel *epithelium. 3. Primary enamel cuticle and reduced enamel epithelium.

naso- Prefix signifying *nose*.

nasoantral Relating to the nose and the maxillary antrum.

nasobronchial Relating to the nose and the bronchi.

nasobuccal Relating to the nose and the cheek.

nasobuccopharyngeal Relating to the nose, the cheek and the pharynx.

nasociliary Relating to the nose and the eye and eyebrow.

nasociliary nerve Supplies the eyeball, skin and mucosa of the nose and eyelid, and the ethmoidal and sphenoidal air sinuses. *See* Table of Nerves—nasociliaris.

nasofrontal Relating to the nose and the frontal bone.

nasolabial Relating to the nose and the lip.

nasolabialis A slip of muscle from M. orbicularis oris, attaching the upper lip to the nasal septum.

nasolacrimal 1. Relating to the nasal and lacrimal bones. 2. Relating to the nose and the lacrimal apparatus.

nasomaxillary Relating to the nasal processes and the maxilla.

nasomental Relating to the nose and the chin.

naso-oral Relating to the nose and the mouth.

nasopalatine Relating to the nose and the palatine processes.

nasopalatine artery A. sphenopalatina. *See* Table of Arteries.

nasopalatine nerve Supplies the mucosa of the hard palate and the nose; *also called* nerve of Cotunnius or nerve of Scarpa. *See* Table of Nerves—nasopalatinus.

nasopharyngeal 1. Relating to both the nose and the pharynx. 2. Relating to the nasopharynx.

nasopharynx That part of the pharynx which extends above the soft palate.

nasospinale A point at the base of the anterior nasal spine, the midpoint on a line connecting the lowest points on the margin of the nasal aperture on each side.

natural Not artificial, abnormal or pathological.

nausea A feeling of sickness, or a tendency to vomit.

nauseous Relating to or producing nausea.

neck 1. That part of the body connecting the head and the upper part of the trunk. 2. Any narrowed or constricted portion at the junction of two parts. 3. The narrowed junction between the enamel and the cementum of a tooth; the tooth cervix.

neckstrap An apparatus fitting round the neck and used to provide attachment for extraoral traction to an orthodontic appliance.

necrobiosis Gradual deterioration of cells, leading finally to their death.

necrobiotic *Necrotic.

necrosis Death of a circumscribed area of tissue.
dental n. Tooth decay.
infectious oral n. *Cancrum oris.

necrotic Relating to or characterized by necrosis.

necrotizing Causing or producing necrosis.

needle A sharp-pointed instrument, used to suture or to puncture tissue.
aspirating n. A long, hollow needle used to withdraw fluid from a cavity.
hare-lip n. A cannula introduced into the wound during an operation for hare-lip, and held in place by a figure-of-eight suture.
hypodermic n. A form of hollow needle used with a syringe for injections.
suture n. A sharp-pointed and generally curved needle with an eye for thread, used for surgical suturing.

needle culture Stab *culture.

nefrens Having no teeth; an obsolete term.

Neisseria (A.L.S. Neisser, 1855-1916. German physician). A genus of the Neisseriaceae family of bacteria, Gram-negative, parasitic, non-motile and aerobic cocci, found in the mucous membrane in mammals.

Neisseriaceae A family of either coccal or rod-shaped aerobic, Gram-negative bacteria.

neo- Prefix signifying *new.*

neoblastic Relating to, or arising from, new tissue.

neonatal Relating to the newborn.

neonate A newborn infant.

neoplasia The process of development of a neoplasm.

neoplasm An abnormal mass of tissue, the growth of which exceeds and is unco-ordinated with that of the normal tissues, and persists in the same excessive manner after cessation of the stimuli which evoked the change (Willis).

neoplastic Relating to or characteristic of a neoplasm.

nepiology That branch of paediatrics relating to infants and young children.

nerve A cord-like bundle of fibres which transmits sensations or impulses for movement from one part of the body to another.
afferent n. Any nerve receiving and transmitting impulses from the periphery to the centre.
autonomic n. Any nerve of the autonomic nervous system.
cranial n. Any one of twelve pairs of peripheral nerves arising directly from the brain stem. *See* Table of Nerves—craniales.
efferent n. Any nerve carrying impulses from the centre to the periphery.
intrinsic n. Any nerve supplying impulses to the muscles, glands, or mucous membranes of an organ or part.
motor n. Any of the nerves whose impulses produce movement in the organism.
parasympathetic n. Any nerve of the parasympathetic part of the autonomic nervous system, concerned with the detailed and general functioning of the glands and viscera in normal circumstances.

peripheral n. Any nerve whose distribution is to the skin; loosely used of any branch of the central nervous system.
secretory n. Any efferent nerve whose stimulation increases activity in the gland to which it is distributed.
sensory n. An afferent nerve, transmitting sensations of pain, touch, etc., to the central nervous system from the periphery.
somatic n. One of the nerves supplying voluntary muscles, tendons, joints, skin, and parietal serous membranes.
sympathetic n. Any nerve of the sympathetic part of the autonomic nervous system, concerned with the functioning of glands and viscera during stress.
vasomotor n. Any nerve that controls the calibre of blood or lymph vessels; it may be a *vasodilator* or a *vasoconstrictor*.

nerve, Jacobson's *Tympanic nerve.

nerve of Arnold (F. Arnold, 1803-90. German anatomist). N. auricularis. *See* Table of Nerves.

nerve of Cotunnius (D. Cotugno (Cotunnius), 1736-1822. Italian anatomist). The *nasopalatine nerve.

nerve of Cruveilhier (J. Cruveilhier, 1791-1874. French pathologist). An occasional branch of the facial nerve.

nerve of Scarpa (A. Scarpa, 1747-1832. Italian anatomist and surgeon). N. nasopalatinus. *See* Table of Nerves.

nerve of the pterygoid canal Supplies the lacrimal glands and the glands of the nose and palate. *See* Table of Nerves—canalis pterygoidei.

nerve of Vidius (V. Vidius (G. Guido), d. 1569. Italian anatomist and physician). N. canalis pterygoidei. *See* Table of Nerves.

nervous 1. Relating to a nerve. 2. Relating to the condition of nervousness.

nervous system
autonomic n.s. That part of both the central nervous system and the peripheral nervous system which controls the involuntary efferent nerves and afferent nerves located in internal organs and concerned with visceral function.
central n.s. The brain and the spinal cord.
peripheral n.s. The twelve pairs of cranial nerves and the thirty-one pairs of spinal nerves which convey information to and from the central nervous system throughout the body.

Neubauer's artery (J.E. Neubauer, 1742-77. German anatomist). A. thyroidea ima. *See* Table of Arteries.

Neumann's sheath (E.F.C. Neumann, 1834-1918. German pathologist). Partially mineralized tissue lining the dentinal tubules; *also called* dentinal sheath.

neural Relating to a nerve or nerves.

neuralgia Recurrent spasmodic attacks of severe pain affecting areas supplied by a sensory nerve at any point along its course or at the nerve-ending.
trigeminal n. Severe unilateral paroxysmal pain affecting areas of the face supplied by the trigeminal nerve, sometimes associated with involuntary contraction of the facial muscles on the affected side.

neuralgic Relating to or affected with neuralgia.

neurectomy Surgical excision of a nerve.

neurilemmoma A slow-growing and benign tumour of the tissue of the nerve sheath, occasionally found in the mouth, maxillary sinus and salivary glands.

neuritis Inflammation of a nerve.

neuro- Prefix signifying *nerve*.

neurofibroma A benign tumour arising from the nerve-fibre cells.

neurofibromatosis An hereditary disease characterized by the presence of neurofibromas. It may affect the oral and buccal mucosa, palate and jaws. *Also called* von Recklinghausen's disease.

neuroid Nerve-like.

neurology The study of the nervous system and the treatment of its diseases.

neuroma A tumour arising from or composed of nerve cell tissue.
traumatic n. A tumour-like nodule of nerve fibres occurring at the site of amputation of a nerve, for example, on the mental nerve near to the mental foramen.

neuromuscular Relating to both nerves and muscles.

neuropathy Any disease affecting the nerves or nervous tissue.

neurospasm Spasmodic twitching due to nerve spasm.

neurotomy Cutting of a nerve.

neurotropic Attracted to or having an affinity for nervous tissue.

neutral Neither acid nor alkali.

neutralize To make neutral or inert.

neutrocclusion Angle Class I *malocclusion.

nevus *See* naevus.

newborn Recently born, applied to infants in their first two or three days of life.

niche *In anatomy,* a depression or recess in an otherwise smooth and even surface.
enamel n. One of a pair of funnel-shaped depressions in the dental lamina of a developing tooth.

nickel A silver-white metal, chemical symbol Ni, with properties very similar to those of iron.

nidal Relating to a nidus.

nidus (*pl.* nidi) A focal point of infection.

nigrities linguae Black *tongue.

nitric Relating to nitrogen as a bivalent element.

nitro- Prefix signifying *nitrogen*, or *nitrogen dioxide*.

nitrogen A colourless and odourless gas, chemical symbol N, existing free in the atmosphere. It is an important constituent element in all animal and vegetable matter.

nitrogenous Containing nitrogen.

nitrous 1. Relating to nitrogen as a trivalent element. 2. Relating to nitrous oxide.

nitrous oxide A colourless gas, chemical symbol N_2O; used to produce temporary general anaesthesia in dentistry and for minor surgical operations.

nociceptive Relating to any pain-producing stimulus, or to pain-receptor nerves.

nocte Latin for *night*; used in prescription writing and abbreviated *noct.*

node A swelling or knob of tissue.
lymph n. One of the many small filtering organs found in clusters along the lymphatic vessels, and through which the lymph is drained.

nodular Relating to a node.

nodule A small node.
enamel n. *Enameloma.
pulp n. *Denticle[2].

nodules, Bohn's *Epstein's pearls.

noma *Cancrum oris.

non- Prefix signifying *not*.

non-carious Not affected with dental caries.

non-infectious Not infectious, not disease-spreading.

non-luetic Not caused by syphilis.

non-malignant Not malignant; benign.

non-metal Any chemical element that is not a metal, such as a gas.

non-occlusion That form of malocclusion in which there is no contact between the opposing teeth; open bite.

non-specific 1. Not produced by only one type of organism. 2. Not indicated for use in the treatment of only one particular disease; as opposed to *specific.*

non-working side The side away from which the mandible is moving during lateral movement.

norm A fixed standard against which other, similar, things may be measured.

norma *In anatomy,* an aspect of the skull from a particular angle and often in outline:
basilaris—the base of the skull, from below (also called *basilis, inferior* or *ventralis*);
facialis—from the front (also called *anterior* or *frontalis*);
lateralis—from the side (also called *temporalis*);
occipitalis—from behind (also called *posterior*);
verticalis—from above (also called *superior*).

normal Relating to the norm; of the regular and ideal standard.

normogenia The chin prominence is in proportion to the rest of the facial skeleton, and to the mandible in particular.

normomandibulism The mandible is in proportion to the rest of the facial skeleton.

normomaxillism The maxilla is in proportion to the rest of the facial skeleton.

Norwegian appliance Myofunctional *appliance.

nose The organ of the sense of smell, and one of the organs of respiration.

nosebleed A haemorrhage from the blood vessels of the nose; epistaxis.

noso- Prefix signifying *disease.*

nosode Any product of a disease that is used in treatment.

nosology The science of the classification of diseases.

nostrate Prevalent in a particular region; endemic.

nostril One of the two external openings of the nose.

notation A set of symbols which may be letters, numbers, or other forms, used to indicate briefly either data or ideas.
dental n. Any form of symbols used to indicate the type and place of a tooth. The ISO designation system consists of two digits for each tooth: the first digit indicates the quadrant; *upper right, upper left, lower left, lower right*, designated 1 to 4 for the permanent dentition and 5 to 8 for the primary dentition; the second digit indicates the actual tooth, numerically designated within each quadrant, distally from the midline—1 to 8 for the permanent teeth, or 1 to 5 for primary teeth.

Notation for permanent teeth:-

right	left
18 17 16 15 14 13 12 11	21 22 23 24 25 26 27 28
48 47 46 45 44 43 42 41	31 32 33 34 35 36 37 38

and for primary teeth:-

right	left
55 54 53 52 51	61 62 63 64 65
85 84 83 82 81	71 72 73 74 75

For example: the lower left lateral permanent incisor would be represented by 32 and the upper right central primary incisor by 51.

Another commonly used notation is:-
for permanent teeth:

right 87654321 | 12345678 left
87654321 | 12345678

and for primary teeth:

right EDCBA | ABCDE left
EDCBA | ABCDE

For example: the lower left lateral permanent incisor would be represented by and the upper right central primary incisor by .

notch A deep depression or indentation, usually in the edge of a bone.

buccal n. The notch found in a denture flange to keep it clear of the buccal frenum.

craniofacial n. A notch in the bony partition between the nasal and orbital cavities; an occasional defect.

digastric n. Mastoid *notch.

ethmoidal n. The space between the orbital plates of the frontal bone which, in an articulated skull, contains the cribriform plate of the ethmoid bone.

frontal n. A notch on the supra-orbital margin of the frontal bone, through which pass the frontal artery and nerve.

hamular n. Pterygomaxillary *notch.

jugular n. of the occipital bone An indentation on the lower edge of the bone, which forms the posterior part of the jugular foramen.

jugular n. of the temporal bone A small depression in the petrous portion of the bone, corresponding to the jugular notch in the occipital bone, with which it forms the jugular foramen.

lacrimal n. A notch on the inner edge of the orbital surface of the maxilla which receives the lacrimal bone.

mandibular n. The crescent-shaped border of the ramus, between the coronoid process and the condyle of the mandible.

mastoid n. A deep groove in the petrous part of the temporal bone, on the mastoid process, providing attachment for the posterior belly of the digastric muscle.

nasal n. A large, uneven notch in the anterior border of the body of the maxilla, forming part of the anterior nasal aperture.

parietal n. The notch that occurs in the angle between the squamous and mastoid processes of the temporal bone.

parotid n. An indentation between the mastoid process of the temporal bone and the ramus of the mandible.

postcondylar n. An indentation on the lower surface of the occipital bone, occurring between the condyle and the foramen magnum.

pterygoid n. The V-shaped notch between the medial and lateral pterygoid plates of the sphenoid bone which is filled by and articulates with the pyramidal process of the palatine bone.

pterygomaxillary n. The notch found at the distal limit of an edentulous alveolar ridge, beyond the maxillary tuberosity; it is formed by the pterygoid process of the sphenoid bone, the pyramidal process of the palatine bone and the hamulus of the medial pterygoid plate.

sigmoid n. Mandibular *notch.

sphenopalatine n. A deep depression that divides the sphenoid and the orbital processes of the palatine bone; when the palatine bone articulates with the body of the sphenoid bone it becomes the sphenopalatine foramen.

supraorbital n. A small notch on the supraorbital margin of the frontal bone, through which pass the supraorbital nerve and vessels. Often converted into the supraorbital foramen.

noxious Poisonous, harmful, pernicious.

nucha, nuche The nape of the neck.

nuchal Relating to the nape of the neck.

nuclear Relating to a nucleus.

nucleated Possessing a nucleus or nuclei.

nucleus (*pl.* nuclei) 1. The spheroidal centre of a cell, separated from the cytoplasm by a membrane, and containing DNA, RNA, lipids and proteins; a nucleus may divide by mitosis or meiosis. 2. A group of nerve cells of similar function within the central nervous system.

Nuhn's gland (A. Nuhn, 1814-89. German anatomist). Anterior lingual *gland.

numbness Partial or total loss of sensation; it may be pathological or deliberately induced, as with a local or surface anaesthetic.

nutrient 1. Nourishing. 2. Any substance that nourishes.

nutriment Any nourishing substance.

nutrition The process by which food is assimilated.

nycterine Occurring at night.

nyctohemeral Relating to or occurring both at night and during the day.

O

O 1. Chemical symbol for oxygen. 2. Occlusal.

OC Occlusocervical.

OG Occlusogingival.

ol. Abbreviation for *oleum*—oil; used in prescription writing.

o.m. Abbreviation for *omni mane*—every morning; used in prescription writing.

omn. bih. Abbreviation for *omni bihora*—every two hours; used in prescription writing.

omn. h. Abbreviation for *omni hora*—every hour; used in prescription writing.

o.n. Abbreviation for *omni nocte*—every night; used in prescription writing.

oz Abbreviation for *ounce*.

obelion The point of juncture of the sagittal suture and a line joining the parietal foramina.

obese Excessively fat, overweight, adipose.

oblique Slanting.

obliquus capitis muscles Aid in lateral movements and extension of the head. *See* Table of Muscles.

obliquus (oculi) muscles Elevate, depress and abduct the eyeball. *See* Table of Muscles.

obliteration Complete removal or closure.

obtundent 1. Able to lessen or relieve pain. 2. Any drug that lessens or relieves pain.

obturator A plate, disc or appliance used to fill or cover a cleft or an orifice; applied particularly to the prosthesis used in the treatment of cleft palate.

buccofacial o. An appliance used to close an opening through the cheek to the mouth.

occipital Relating to the occiput.

occipital artery Supplies neck and scalp muscles. *See* Table of Arteries—occipitalis.

occipital bone The bone forming the posterior part of the skull.

occipital muscle Draws back scalp. *See* Table of Muscles—occipitalis.

occipital nerves Supply skin over scalp. *See* Table of Nerves—occipitalis.

occipital sinus A variable anastomosing venous channel between the transverse and sigmoid sinuses. *See* Table of Veins—sinus occipitalis.

occipito- Prefix signifying *occipital, occiput*.

occipitobasilar Relating to the occiput and the base of the skull.

occipitobregmatic Relating to the occiput and the bregma.

occipitocervical Relating to the occiput and the neck.

occipitofacial Relating to the occiput and the facial bones.

occipitofrontal Relating to the occiput and the frontal bone.

occipitofrontal muscle The scalp muscle. *See* Table of Muscles—occipitofrontalis.

occipitomastoid Relating to the occipital bone and the mastoid process.

occipitomental Relating to the occiput and the chin; used particularly of radiographs, indicating the alignment through these points.

occipitotemporal Relating to the occiput and the temporal bones.

occiput The back part of the skull.

occlude To close or to shut. *In dentistry,* closure of the jaws to bring opposing teeth into contact.

occlusal Relating to the occlusion of the teeth.

occlusion 1. The state or process of being occluded or closed. 2. *In dentistry,* the contact of the upper and lower teeth in any jaw position.
abnormal o. Any occlusal relationship considered to be outside the normal range of variation.
afunctional o. Any occlusal relationship that does not allow normal function.
balanced o. 1. The ideal interdigitation of the teeth, in which there is no cuspal interference in lateral excursions of the mandible. 2. *In prosthetic dentistry,* the simultaneous contact of all occlusal areas to prevent tipping or rotating of the denture base.
centric o. Intercuspal *occlusion.
distal o. A term denoting the position of a tooth which is distal to the normal position in occlusion.
eccentric o. The occlusion of the teeth with the mandible in any position other than that of rest.
hyperfunctional o. Any occlusal relationship placing excessive stress on a tooth or teeth.
intercuspal o. The relationship of the upper and lower dental arches when the teeth are brought into contact from retruded jaw relation.
labial o. A term for the position of an incisor or canine when it is labial to the line of occlusion.
lateral o. The occlusion of the teeth with the mandible moved to one side or the other, not in intercuspal occlusion.
line of o. A term used by Angle to denote the line joining areas of contact of the teeth in normal occlusion.
lingual o. A term for the position of a tooth lying lingual to the line of occlusion.
mesial o. A term to denote the position of a tooth which is mesial of its normal position in occlusion.
pathogenic o. Any occlusal relationship producing pathological changes in the supporting tissues.
posterior o. The occlusion resulting when the mandibular teeth occlude posterior to their normal position in relation to the maxillary teeth.
post-normal o. Distal *occlusion.
protrusive o. The occlusion produced by a protruding mandible.
retrusive o. 1. The occlusion produced by a receding mandible. 2. Distal *occlusion.
traumatic o., traumatogenic o. Any form of malocclusion causing damage to the teeth or to the periodontal tissues.

occlusive Relating to occlusion.

occlusocervical Relating to the occlusal surface and the neck of a tooth.

occlusometer *Gnathodynamometer.

occupational *Of a disease*: caused by the patient's occupation; it may be organic or functional.

oct-, octo- Prefix signifying *eight.*

ocular Relating to the eye.

ocular hypertelorism A craniofacial deformity characterized by enlargement of the sphenoid bone, great breadth across the bridge of the nose, and resulting width between the eyes.

oculo- Prefix signifying *eye.*

oculomotor nerve The third cranial nerve, supplying the muscles of the eye and upper eyelid. *See* Table of Nerves—oculomotorius.

odont-, odonto- Prefix signifying *teeth,* or *tooth.*

odontagra Toothache.

odontalgia Toothache.
phantom o. Toothache felt in the socket from which a tooth has been extracted.

odontalgic Relating to or characterized by toothache.

odontatrophia Atrophy of the teeth.

odontectomy Surgical excision for the removal of retained roots, unerupted or partially erupted teeth.

odonterism Teeth-chattering.

odontexesis Cleaning the teeth, especially by means of a scraping instrument; obsolete term.

odonthaemodia Excessive sensitivity in the teeth.

odontharpaga Toothache.

odonthyalus Tooth enamel; obsolete.

odontia Any dental abnormality.

odontia deformans Any deformity of the teeth.

odontia incrustans Dental *calculus.

odontiasis Eruption of the teeth; dentition.

odontiatria Dental treatment.

odontiatrogenic Resulting from dental treatment.

odontic Relating to the teeth.

odontinoid 1. Resembling a tooth. 2. A tumour containing tooth substance.

odontitis Inflammation of the tooth pulp; pulpitis.

odontium That part of the tooth which consists of enamel, dentine and pulp, but does not include cementum; the word is normally only used with a prefix.

odontoameloblastoma A very rare benign tumour containing dentine, enamel and odontogenic epithelium.

odontoamelosarcoma *Ameloblastosarcoma.

odontoatlantal *Atlantoaxial.

odontoblast 1. One of the germ cells from which dentine is formed. 2. One of the layers of cylindrical cells in the connective tissue surrounding the dental pulp.

odontoblastoma A tumour composed of odontoblasts.

odontobothrion The socket of a tooth; obsolete term.

odontobothritis *Alveolitis; obsolete term.

odontocele An alveolodental cyst.

odontoceramic Relating to porcelain teeth.

odontoceramotechny Dental *ceramics.

odontochalix *Cementum.

odontochirurgical Relating to dental surgery.

odontocia A condition which is characterized by softening of the teeth.

odontoclamis Dental *operculum.

odontoclasia 1. Rampant caries; rapid disintegration of tooth enamel, with dentine decay, occurring in the primary dentition; the remains of the teeth are frequently discoloured, and often black. 2. External tooth *resorption.

odontoclasis 1. Fracture of a tooth. 2. The process of resorption of a tooth.

odontoclast One of the multinuclear cells associated in the process of resorption of the roots of primary teeth. A form of osteoclast, it may also be involved with pathological resorption of the permanent tooth roots.

odontoclastoma Internal tooth *resorption.

odontocnesis An itching sensation of the gums.

odontodynia Toothache.

odontodysplasia A localized disturbance in tooth formation, most commonly involving the maxillary anterior teeth on one side of the midline. Evidence of mineralization may be seen in the pulp; the enamel, however, is thin or absent.

odontogenesis 1. *Odontogeny. 2. *Dentinogenesis.

odontogenesis imperfecta Disturbance in the formation and mineralization of enamel and dentine; it is an hereditary condition.

odontogenic Originating from a tooth or tooth germ.

odontogenic tumour For all the different types of odontogenic tumour *see under* tumour.

odontogenous Originating in or around the teeth, or in a dental condition.

odontogeny The origin and development of the teeth.

odontoglyph A dental scaler.

odontogram The record made by an odontograph.

odontograph An instrument for recording any unevenness of a tooth surface.

odontography 1. The description of tooth anatomy. 2. The use of an odontograph.

odontohyperaesthesia Hypersensitivity of a tooth.

odontoiatria Treatment of the teeth.

odontoid Resembling a tooth.

odontolith Dental *calculus.

odontolithiasis The condition of having deposits on the teeth.

odontologist A scientist engaged in odontology. Often used as synonymous with dentist.

odontology That branch of medical science concerned with the structure and development of the teeth and jaws, and the scientific study of related diseases. Often used as synonymous with dentistry.

odontoloxia Irregularity or slanting of the teeth.

odontolysis The resorption of mineralized tooth substance.

odontoma, odontome A hamartoma derived from or composed of dental tissue.
complex o. A malformation made up of various elements of the tooth germ; individual tissues are mainly well formed but occur as a disordered mixture.
composite o. Complex *odontome or compound *odontome.
compound o. A malformation similar to a complex odontome, but with the dental tissues better ordered, the pulp, dentine and enamel being arranged to form tooth-like structures.
cystic o. A follicular cyst associated with a tumour of odontogenic origin.
dilated o. A type of *dens in dente.
gestant o. *Dens in dente.
invaginated o. *Dens in dente.

odontometry The use of measurement and statistics in the study of the teeth and jaws.

odontonecrosis Gross dental caries.

odontoneuralgia 1. Neuralgia caused by dental disease. 2. Neuralgic pain felt in the teeth.

odontonomy Dental terminology.

odontonosology The study of tooth diseases.

odontoparallaxis Irregularity in the position of the teeth.

odontopathy Any disease of the teeth.

odontoperiosteum *Periodontium.

odontophobia Fear of teeth.

odontoplast *Odontoblast.

odontoplasty 1. *In periodontology*, the modification of tooth contours to aid in maintenance of healthy gingiva. 2. *Orthodontics.

odontoplerosis The operation of filling a tooth cavity.

odontoprisis Grinding the teeth; bruxism.

odontopsis Loss of the teeth.

odontoradiograph A radiograph of the teeth or of a tooth.

odontorrhagia Bleeding after tooth extraction.

odontorthrosis *Orthodontics.

odontosarcoma

ameloblastic o. A very rare malignant tumour, similar in structure to an ameloblastic fibrosarcoma but containing traces of dentine and enamel.

odontoschisis Splitting of a tooth or of teeth.

odontoschism A fissure or cleft in a tooth.

odontoscope 1. A dental mirror. 2. An instrument containing a magnifying lens, used to examine tooth surfaces.

odontoscopy The recording of the occlusion in an individual mouth, used for identification.

odontoseisis Looseness of a tooth or of teeth.

odontosis *Dentition.

odontosteophyte An osseous tumour occurring on a tooth.

odontosteresis Loss of the teeth.

odontosynerismus Teeth-chattering.

odontotechny The practice of dentistry.

odontotheca A tooth follicle.

odontotherapy Treatment of dental diseases.

odontotomy The process of cutting into tooth structure.

prophylactic o. Mechanical modification of the occlusal fissures of teeth and the filling of non-carious pits and fissures in an attempt to prevent dental caries.

odontotripsis Wearing away of the teeth.

odontotrypy The drilling of a tooth in order to drain the pus from the pulp cavity.

odyn- Prefix signifying *pain, ache.*

-odynia Suffix signifying *pain, ache.*

odynolysis The easing or relief of pain.

odynophagia Swallowing which causes pain.

odynophobia Morbid fear of pain.

oedema An abnormal accumulation of fluid in the body tissues, producing swelling.

angioneurotic o. Painless, circumscribed swellings, commonly on the lips, tongue, cheeks or eyelids, due to the rapid escape of fluid following local increased vascular permeability; *also called* Quincke's oedema.

oedematous Relating to or affected by oedema.

oesophagitis Inflammation of the oesophagus.

oesophagus The gullet; the musculomembranous tube extending between the pharynx and the stomach.

-oid Suffix signifying *like.*

oil A liquid which does not mix with, and is generally lighter than, water; oils may be derived from fats, or from chemicals.

ointment A fatty, semisolid substance, used as a base for local medicaments for external application.

oleum Latin for *oil*; used in prescription writing, and abbreviated *ol.*

olfactory Relating to the sense of smell.

olfactory nerve The first cranial nerve, supplying the olfactory mucosa. *See* Table of Nerves—olfactorius.

oligo- Prefix signifying *few, deficient.*

oligodontia *Hypodontia.

oligoptyalism *Hyposalivation.

oligosialia *Hyposalivation.

-ology Suffix signifying *study of, science of.*

-oma Suffix signifying *tumour.*

omnis Latin for *every*; used in prescription writing, and abbreviated *o.* or *omn.*

omnivorous Capable of eating anything; as opposed to *herbivorous, carnivorous*, etc.

omohyoid muscle Depresses hyoid bone and tightens deep cervical fascia in lower part of neck. *See* Table of Muscles—omohyoideus.

onco-, oncho- Prefix signifying *tumour.*

oncocyte One of the individual cells or groups of cells in various glands which, in elderly persons, may change and become larger, with an eosinophilic and granular cytoplasm.

oncocytoma A benign circumscribed and encapsulated adenoma; the term is often used specifically for a tumour of the salivary glands.

oncocytosis The change of acinar and duct-lining cells in the salivary glands into oncocytes, a change which may appear in old age.

oncology The study of neoplasms.

oncosis Any disease characterized by the development of tumours.

oncotic Relating to oncosis.

oncotomy Surgical incision into a tumour or swelling.

Onion's fusible alloy An alloy containing five parts of bismuth to three parts of lead and two parts of tin.

onlay *Overlay.

onychophagia Nail-biting.

opacity The condition of being impervious to light.

opalescent Iridescent, showing various colours.

opalgia Facial neuralgia.

open bite 1. A form of malocclusion in which a group of teeth fail to come into contact when the dental arches are brought into occlusion. 2. *Apertognathia.

anterior o. b. Open bite in which the anterior teeth do not come into contact.

posterior o. b. Open bite in which the posterior teeth on one side (*unilateral*) or both sides (*bilateral*) do not come into contact.

operability The state allowing of operation with a reasonable expectation of recovery.

operable Permitting of an operation; capable of treatment by operation.

operation 1. Anything performed, especially any procedure by a surgeon, either with instruments or by hand. 2. The mode of action of a drug.

For eponymous surgical operations *see* under the personal name by which the operation is known.

operative 1. Relating to an operation. 2. Effective.

operculectomy The surgical removal of the mucosal flap partially or completely covering an unerupted tooth.

operculum A cover or lid, in any form.

dental o. The flap of mucosa which remains over the occlusal surface of an erupting posterior tooth.

ophryon The midpoint of the transverse supra-orbital line; a craniometric landmark.

ophthalmic Relating to the eye.

ophthalmic artery Supplies the eyeball, eye muscles, etc. *See* Table of Arteries—ophthalmica.

ophthalmic nerve Supplies the orbit and eyeball, mucosa of nose, frontal, ethmoidal and sphenoidal air sinuses, skin of forehead. *See* Table of Nerves—ophthalmicus.

ophthalmic veins Veins draining the area supplied by the ophthalmic artery. *See* Table of Veins—ophthalmica.

opisthion The midpoint on the lower edge of the foramen magnum; a craniometric landmark.

opistho- Prefix signifying *back, backwards.*

opisthocranion The point in the mid-line on the occipital bone which marks the maximum antero-posterior skull length, measured from the glabella; a craniometric landmark.

opisthogenia Defective development of the jaws as a result of ankylosis.

opisthognathism Recession of the mandible.

opsialgia Facial neuralgia.

opsigenes A term meaning late born, applied to third molars.

optic nerve The second cranial nerve, supplying the retina. *See* Table of Nerves—opticus.

orad In the direction of the mouth.

oral Pertaining to the mouth.

orale The point on the inner surface of the alveolar process marking the end of the incisive suture; a craniometric landmark.

oralogy The science of the mouth; sometimes used to denote medical and dental co-operation for health.

orbicularis oculi muscle Closes eyelids. *See* Table of Muscles.

orbicularis oris muscle Purses lips and puckers up mouth. *See* Table of Muscles.

orbit The bony eye-socket.

orbital Relating to the orbit.

orbital muscle Vestigial. *See* Table of Muscles—orbitalis.

orbital nerve Supplies the orbit. *See* Table of Nerves—orbitalis.

orbitale The lowest point on the lower border of the orbit; one of a pair of craniometric landmarks on the skull.

order One of the principal divisions of a class in biological classification.

organ Any separate part of the body having a specific function.

absorbent o. Vascular tissue lying between the roots of a primary tooth and its permanent successor during resorption.

dental o. That complex of tissue made up of the tooth, the periodontium and the alveolar bone.

enamel o. A proliferation of the dental lamina enclosing the dental papilla; it determines the shape of the tooth crown and forms the dental enamel.

organic 1. Relating to, having, or characteristic of an organ or organs. 2. Arising from, or relating to substances arising from, living organisms. 3. *In chemistry,* relating to carbon compounds.

organism Any individual plant or animal; an organized body of living cells.

organotrophic *Heterotrophic.

orifice An opening; the mouth or entrance of a body cavity.

orificial Relating to an orifice.

origin The beginning of anything.

origin *of a muscle In anatomy,* the fixed attachment of a muscle, as opposed to its *insertion.*

oro- Prefix signifying *mouth, oral.*

orofacial Relating to the mouth and the face.

orolingual Relating to the mouth and the tongue.

oromandibular Relating to the mouth and the mandible.

oromaxillary Relating to the mouth and the maxilla.

oronasal Relating to the mouth and the nose.

oropharyngeal 1. Relating to both the mouth and the pharynx, as one cavity. 2. Relating to the oropharynx.

oropharynx The continuation of the nasopharynx from below the border of the soft palate to the larynx; the oral portion of the pharynx.

ortho- Prefix signifying *straight, normal.*

orthocephalic Having a vertically straight head, with an index between 70 and 75.

orthodentine Straight-tubed dentine, occurring in mammals.

orthodontia *Orthodontics[1].

orthodontics 1. The study of craniofacial development, especially as related to dentofacial anomalies, malocclusion and irregularities of the teeth, and methods of treatment. 2. The treatment and prevention of malocclusion and irregularities of the teeth.

interceptive o. The alleviation or correction of malocclusion in the mixed dentition, as the occlusion develops.

preventive o. That form of orthodontic treatment designed to maintain a proper occlusion by the prevention of tooth movement.

prophylactic o. Preventive *orthodontics.

surgical o. Treatment of malocclusion by surgical procedures to reposition or reshape the jaws.

orthognathia The study and treatment of conditions causing malposition of the jaws.

orthognathic, orthognathous 1. Relating to orthognathia. 2. Having a straight, unprojecting jaw; having a gnathic index of under 98.

orthopaedics

dental o., dentofacial o. *Orthodontics.

orthopnoea Severely laboured breathing except when in an upright position.

orthopnoeic Relating to or characterized by orthopnoea.

orthostaphyline Having a moderate palatal arch in both height and curvature.

orthosurgical Relating to surgical orthodontics.

os (*pl.* ora) Latin for *mouth* or *opening*; used in anatomical terminology.

os (*pl.* ossa) Latin for *a bone*; used in anatomical terminology.

oscedo 1. The act of yawning. 2. Aphthous *stomatitis.

-osis Suffix signifying 1. *condition* or *process*; 2. *a diseased condition*; 3. *formation* or *development* of a condition.

osphresis The sense of smell.

osphretic Relating to the sense of smell.

osseo-integration The area between an implant and the host site where there is direct contact, with no interposed tissue.

osseous Having the characteristics of bone; bony.

ossicle A small bone.
auditory o's. The stapes, malleus and incus, in the middle ear.

ossification Development of, or conversion into, bone.

ossify To develop or become bone or bone-like.

osteal Bony.

ostectomy The surgical removal of a segment of bone.

osteitis Inflammation of a bone.
dentoalveolar o. *Pyorrhoea alveolaris.
localized alveolar o. An acute inflammatory condition of the walls of a tooth socket following the extraction of a tooth; dry socket.

osteitis deformans A chronic disease of bone, characterized by resorption followed by thickening and distortion; *also called* Paget's disease of bone.

osteitis interna Osteomyelitis of the alveolar process caused by infection from a tooth.

osteo- Prefix signifying *bone.*

osteoblast One of the cells from which bone is developed.

osteocementum Secondary cementum and the tissue of which it is formed.

osteochondral Relating to both bone and cartilage.

osteochondroma A benign tumour containing cells of bone and cartilage.

osteoclasia The destruction of bone tissue by osteoclasts.

osteoclast 1. A bone-consuming multinuclear giant cell. 2. A surgical instrument used to break up bone.

osteoclastoma A giant-cell tumour affecting the bone.

osteodentine 1. Bone-like dentine, found in the teeth of certain fish. 2. A pathological form of dentine found in certain tumours.

osteodentinoma A tumour composed of both bone tissue and dentine.

osteodystrophy Defective bone formation.

osteoectomy *In dentistry,* surgical removal of alveolar bone to correct imperfect bone contour, changing the level of bone on the tooth root.

osteofibroma Ossifying *fibroma.

osteogenesis imperfecta A developmental bone disease in which the bones become abnormally brittle and fracture easily; *also called* fragilitas ossium.

osteogenic Relating to or derived from the tissue from which bone is developed.

osteoid 1. Resembling or having the characteristics of bone. 2. The bone matrix before mineralization.

osteology The study of bone and bones.

osteolysis Absorption of bone, especially demineralization.

osteoma A benign hard tumour composed of bone tissue, and developing on bone or on other structures of the body.

osteomalacia Softening of the bones, caused by vitamin D deficiency in adult life.

osteomyelitis Inflammation of the soft tissues of the bone.
alveolar o. *Pyorrhoea alveolaris.

osteonecrosis Massive bone necrosis.

osteo-odontoma A tumour arising from the odontoblastic processes; an obsolete term.

osteoperiostitis Inflammation of bone and of its periosteum.
alveolodental o. *Periodontitis.

osteopetrosis A familial bone disease, characterized by osteosclerosis, fibrosis of bone marrow, fragility and anaemia; *also called* Albers-Schönberg disease.

osteoplasty Plastic surgery in relation to bone; as, for example, a reshaping of the alveolar process to conform to that required for a healthy periodontium, without loss of support for the tooth roots.

osteoporosis Enlargement of the bone marrow and canals, causing fragility and abnormal porosity of bone.

osteopsathyrosis *Osteogenesis imperfecta.

osteoradionecrosis Necrosis of bone as a result of irradiation.

osteosarcoma A sarcoma composed of osseous tissue; osteogenic sarcoma.

osteosclerosis A condition characterized by abnormal hardness or denseness of bone.

osteosynthesis Internal skeletal *fixation.

osteotomy The surgical operation of cutting through bone.
cortical o. *Corticotomy.

otalgia Ear-ache.

otalgia dentalis Referred pain in the ear caused by dental disease.

otic Relating to the ear.

otitis Inflammation of the ear.

oto- Prefix signifying *ear.*

oul- Prefix signifying *gingiva. See* under ul-

overbite The distance, measured vertically, between the incisal edges of the incisor teeth, with the dental arches in occlusion; vertical overlap.
horizontal o. *Overjet[1].
negative o. Anterior *open bite.

overclosure A form of malocclusion in an edentulous mouth in which the jaws are in abnormally close relationship.

overdenture A form of denture which covers at least one tooth or prepared root.

over-eruption The condition of having the teeth extruded from their sockets more than normal, so that the occluding surfaces are above the normal occlusal plane.

overhang 1. To jut out or project over. 2. *In dentistry,* a filling, especially on an approximal surface, having a projection at the cervical margin of the cavity, causing a shoulder under which food may become lodged.

overjet 1. The distance, measured horizontally, between the labial incisal edges of the incisor teeth, with the dental arches in occlusion. 2. *In prosthetic dentistry,* horizontal *overlap.
reverse o. A relationship of the anterior teeth in which, in centric occlusion, the maxillary incisors are lingual to the mandibular incisors (as in Angle's Class III malocclusion).

overlap
horizontal o. In prosthetic dentistry, the distance, measured horizontally, between the labial incisal edges of the incisor teeth, with the dental arches in occlusion.
vertical o. *Overbite.

overlay 1. A restoration covering the whole of the occlusal surface of a tooth. 2. *In prosthetic dentistry,* an extension of the occlusal rest of a partial denture to fit over the whole of the occlusal surface of a tooth; used as a partial denture support.

overlay appliance A form of overlay, covering the occlusal surfaces of several teeth, used to correct closed bite in prosthetic dentistry, or to splint natural teeth in the treatment of periodontal disease, and in bruxism.

overt *In the medical sciences*, evident or obvious.

ovoid Egg-shaped.

Owen's contour lines (Sir R. Owen, 1804-92. English anatomist). The concentric rings which mark the interglobular spaces in dentine in a transverse section; *also called* Salter's lines.

oxy- Prefix signifying 1. *oxygen*; 2. *sharp*, *pointed*; 3. *acid*.

oxycephaly A condition which is characterized by a pointed and high-domed skull; being both hypsicephalic and acrocephalic.

oxygen A colourless, odourless and tasteless gas, chemical symbol O, which supports combustion and is essential to life in animals and also in many plants. It constitutes one-fifth of the air, and in combination exists in most solids, liquids or gases which are not elements.

oxygeusia The condition of having an especially acute sense of taste.

ozena *Rhinitis sicca.

ozostomia Foul-smelling breath, of oral origin.

P

P 1. Chemical symbol for phosphorus. 2. Abbreviation for *premolar.*

PA Pulpoaxial.

p. ae., part. aeq. Abbreviation for *partes aequales*—equal parts; used in prescription writing.

Pb Chemical symbol for lead.

PBA Pulpobuccoaxial.

p.c. Abbreviation for *post cibum*—after meals; used in prescription writing.

PC Pharmaceutical Codex; used in descriptions of drugs, to indicate the source of the formula in a prescription.

pH Abbreviation for hydrogen ion concentration, based on a scale from 0 (pure acidity) to 14 (pure alkalinity), with neutrality at 7.

pil. Abbreviation for *pilula*—a pill; used in prescription writing.

PL Pulpolingual.

PLa Pulpolabial.

PLA Pulpolinguoaxial.

PM 1. Pulpomesial. 2. Abbreviation for *premolar.*

PMA 1. Pulpomesioaxial.

PMA index An index for measuring gingivitis by scoring the interdental papillae (P), marginal gingiva (M) and attached gingiva (A) for presence (1) or absence (0) of inflammation. The total scores for each arch are then added together to give the index value.

p.p.m. Abbreviation for *parts per million.*

p.r.n. Abbreviation for *pro re nata*—as required; used in prescription writing.

pulv. Abbreviation for *pulvis*—a powder; used in prescription writing.

PUO Abbreviation for *pyrexia of unknown origin.*

PVC Polyvinyl chloride.

pachy- Prefix signifying *thick.*

pachycheilia The condition of having abnormally thick lips.

pachyglossia The condition of having an abnormally thick tongue.

pachygnathous Having a thick, abnormally large jaw.

pack A dressing or blanket, either wet or dry, hot or cold, which is laid on or wrapped round a part or the whole body.

periodontal p. A dressing laid on the gums and about the teeth during treatment of periodontal disease or after gingivectomy.

pad A fleshy cushion or soft tissue mass.

occlusal p. A pad of gingiva covering the occlusal surface of a tooth.

retromolar p. The soft tissue mass at the distal end of the mandibular ridge behind the last molar tooth.

Padgett's operation (E.C. Padgett, 1893-1946. American surgeon). Plastic surgical reconstruction of the lip by tubular grafts from the neck and scalp.

paediadontology Paediatric *dentistry.

paediatrics That branch of medicine which deals with the growth and development, diseases and treatment of children.

paedo- Prefix signifying *child.*

paedodontia, paedodontics Paediatric *dentistry.

Paget's disease of bone (Sir James Paget, 1814-99. English surgeon). *Osteitis deformans.

pain A distressing or unpleasant sensation transmitted by a sensory nerve, usually indicative of injury or of disease.
referred p. Pain felt in a part different from that in which it is caused.

palatal Relating to the palate.

palate The roof of the mouth.
artificial p. An obturator used to close a cleft palate.
bony p. The bony skeleton of the hard palate.
cleft p. Congenital fissure of the palate, due to defective development in embryo; it may be associated with hare-lip. There is a wide range of deformity, from a bifid uvula to complete bilateral cleft of both palate and lip.
gothic p. An abnormally high, pointed palatal arch.
hard p. The bony, front portion of the roof of the mouth, covered by mucosa closely bound to the underlying bone.
primary p. The palate in the embryo, corresponding to the premaxillary region.
primitive p. That part of the median nasal process in the embryo from which the middle portion of the upper lip and the primary palate develop.
secondary p. The palate formed by the joining of the palatal processes of the maxilla in the embryo.
smoker's p. *Leukokeratosis nicotina palati.
soft p. The fleshy rear portion of the roof of the mouth.

palate-hook An instrument used to retract the uvula.

palatiform Shaped like a palate.

palatine Relating to the palatal processes.

palatine arteries Supply hard and soft palates, tonsils and upper portion of pharynx. *See* Table of Arteries—palatina.

palatine bone The bone forming the posterior part of the hard palate and the lateral wall of the nose.

palatine nerves Supply the palatal mucosa and the uvula. *See* Table of Nerves—palatinus.

palatine vein, external The vein draining the palatal region. *See* Table of Veins—palatina externa.

palatitis Inflammation of the palate.

palato- Prefix signifying *palate*.

palatoglossal Relating to the palate and the tongue.

palatoglossal muscle Raises tongue and constricts anterior fauces. *Also called* glossopalatine. *See* Table of Muscles—palatoglossus.

palatognathous Having a congenital cleft palate.

palatograph An instrument for recording movements of the palate during speech.

palatolabial Relating to the palate and the lips.

palatomaxillary Relating to the palate and the maxilla.

palatomyograph An instrument for recording movements of the soft palate.

palatonasal Relating to the palate and the nose.

palatopharyngeal Relating to the palate and the pharynx.

palatopharyngeal muscle Aids in swallowing. *Also called* pharyngopalatine. *See* Table of Muscles—palatopharyngeus.

palatoplasty Plastic surgical repair of the palate.

palatoplegia Palatal paralysis.

palatopterygoid Relating to the palatine bone and the pterygoid processes of the sphenoid bone.

palatorraphy Repair of cleft palate by means of sutures.

palatoschisis Cleft palate; palatal fissure.

palirrhoea. 1. Regurgitation. 2. Recurrence of a mucous discharge.

pallanaesthesia Diminution or complete loss of the sense of vibration.

palliation The act of alleviating or affording relief, without effecting a cure.

palliative 1. Alleviating or relieving without curing. 2. Any medicine that alleviates or relieves.

palpation Examination by touch to determine the position or consistence of an organ or part lying beneath the body surface.

palpebral Relating to the eyelid.

palpebral artery Supplies the conjunctiva, eyelid and lacrimal sac. *See* Table of Arteries—palpebris.

palpebral nerve Supplies the eyelid. *See* Table of Nerves—palpebralis.

palsy *Paralysis.

pantomography Panoramic *tomography.

papilla (*pl.* papillae) Any small nipple-like eminence.
arcuate p. Fungiform *papilla.
circumvallate p. Vallate *papilla.
conical p. Filiform *papilla.
corolliform p. Filiform *papilla.
dental p. The developing tissue that later becomes the dental pulp.
filiform p. One of the minute, conical or cylindrical papillae on the anterior two-thirds of the dorsum of the tongue.
foliate p. One of the three or four short vertical folds on the sides of the tongue at the back; often rudimentary in man.
fungiform p. One of the large, bright red mushroom-like papillae scattered irregularly over the surface of the tongue, particularly at the tip and on the sides.
gingival p. Interdental *papilla.
incisive p. The projection of the palatine mucosa overlying the incisive fossa at the anterior end of the palatine raphe.
interdental p. The gingiva in the spaces between the mesial surface of one tooth and the distal surface of the one adjacent.
lingual p. Any one of the papillae on the dorsum of the tongue.
palatine p. Incisive *papilla.
vallate p. Any one of the large, flat papillae, having a surrounding rim, found in front of the terminal sulcus of the tongue.
villous p. Filiform *papilla.

papillectomy Surgical excision of gingival papillae.

papillitis Inflammation of the optic disc.

papilloma A benign epithelial tumour, having a corrugated surface, with long, finger-like projections.
squamous-cell p. A benign tumour of the squamous epithelium, projecting from the surface.

papillomatosis The development of multiple papillomas.

papillomatous Relating to or characterized by papillomas; having finger-like projections.

Papillon-Lefèvre syndrome (M.M. Papillon and P. Lefèvre, 20th century French dermatologists). An inherited dermatological disease developing in infancy, its oral manifestations include destruction of alveolar bone, inflammatory gingival enlargement and pocket formation; there may also be skin lesions and hyperkeratosis of palmar and plantar surfaces.

papular Relating to or characterized by papules.

papule A circumscribed nodular elevation of the skin.

para- Prefix signifying *by the side of*; sometimes used as synonymous with *peri-*.

paracone The mesiobuccal cusp of a maxillary molar.

paraconid The mesiolingual cusp of a mandibular molar.

paradental Near or next to a tooth; parodontal.

paradenitis Inflammation of the tissues surrounding a gland.

paradentitis *Periodontitis.

paradentosis Any disease affecting the tissues round a tooth.

paraesthesia Perverted sensation; a burning, prickling or crawling sensation of the skin; for example, pins and needles.

parageusia 1. An unpleasant taste in the mouth. 2. Perversion of the sense of taste.

paraglossa Swelling of the tongue.

paraglossia *Paraglossitis.

paraglossitis Inflammation of the tissues and muscles below the tongue.

parakeratosis Any abnormality of the stratum corneum of the epidermis, which may be associated with inflammation of the prickle-cell layer, causing defective formation of keratin and characterized by persistent nuclei; may affect the mucous membrane of the mouth.

paralysis Loss or impairment of muscle function or of sensation due to nerve injury or destruction of neurons.

paralytic Relating to or affected by paralysis.

paramedian, paramesial Near to the median line.

paramolar A small supernumerary tooth which may erupt beside the molar teeth, most commonly in the maxillary arch.

paranasal Near to or in the region of the nose.

paraoral Around, in the region of, the mouth.

parapharyngeal Around, in the area of, the pharynx.

pararhizoclasia Inflammatory ulcerative destruction of the deep layers of tissue and the alveolar process about the root of a tooth.

parasite An organism, plant or animal, living on or within another organism from which it obtains nourishment, to the detriment of the host.

parasitic Relating to parasites.

paratonsillar In the region of a tonsil, around a tonsil.

paratonsillar vein V. palatina externa. *See* Table of Veins.

parenteral Descriptive of methods of drug administration other than by the alimentary canal.

paresis Slight paralysis.

paresthesia *See* paraesthesia.

parietal 1. Relating to the walls of a cavity. 2. Relating to the parietal bone.

parietal bone One of two bones forming the lateral surface of the cranium.

parieto- Prefix signifying *parietal*.

parodontal Near or next to a tooth; sometimes used as synonymous with *periodontal*.

parodontitis *Periodontitis.

parodontium *Periodontium.

parodontopathy Any periodontal disease.

parodontosis *Periodontosis.

parotic, parotid In the region of the ear.

parotid artery Branch of the superficial temporal artery supplying the parotid gland. *See* Table of Arteries—parotidea.

parrot tongue A horny, dry tongue which cannot be protruded, seen in typhus and low fever.

Parrot's ulcer (J.M.J. Parrot, 1839-1883. French physician). Ulceration of the mucous membrane of the mouth and pharynx, seen in thrush.

pars alveolaris The alveolar process, either mandibular or maxillary.

partes aequales Latin for *equal parts*; used in prescription writing, and abbreviated *p.ae.* or *part.aeq.*

partial In part, incomplete.

particle A small piece of a substance.

parulis A subperiosteal abscess; a gumboil.

Passavant's ridge (P.G. Passavant, 1815-93. German surgeon). A bulge, which appears on the posterior wall of the pharynx, caused by the contraction of the superior and middle constrictor pharyngis muscles during speech; occurs generally in a person having a cleft palate. *Also called* P's bar, and P's cushion.

passive Not produced by active efforts, not active or spontaneous.

paste

polishing p. A fine abrasive paste used with special dental instruments in a handpiece to clean and polish the surfaces of teeth and of restorations.

prophylaxis p. Polishing *paste.

patent *In the medical sciences*, open (not closed), unobstructed.

patho- Prefix signifying *disease.*

pathodontia The study of diseases of the teeth; dental pathology.

pathogen Any agent that produces or is able to produce disease.

pathogenesis The development of disease from its inception to the appearance of characteristic symptoms or lesions.

pathognomonic Characteristic of one specific disease or pathological condition as distinct from any others.

pathologic, pathological Relating to pathology.

pathology That branch of medicine which is concerned with the structural and functional changes caused by disease.

patho-occlusion *Malocclusion.

pathosis A disease condition.

-pathy Suffix signifying *disease.*

patrix The male portion of a precision attachment.

pearl, enamel *Enameloma.

pearls, epithelial, Bohn's *Epstein's pearls.

pectinate Comb-like.

pediadontology Paediatric *dentistry.

pediatrics That branch of medicine which deals with the growth and development, diseases and treatment of children.

pediodontia Paediatric *dentistry.

pedo- Prefix signifying *child.*

pedodontia, pedodontics Paediatric *dentistry.

pedodontist A specialist in paediatric dentistry.

peduncle A stem or stalk-like process supporting a part or a tumour.

pedunculated Having a peduncle.

pelican An old form of forceps used in extracting teeth; so called because of its 'beaked' jaws.

pellicle 1. A thin membrane or skin. 2. A scum or film on the surface of a liquid.
acquired p. An acellular film of salivary proteins deposited on the clean tooth surface immediately after eruption.
brown p. A brown or black film on the tooth surface found where there is habitually poor oral hygiene.

pellicular, pelliculous Relating to a pellicle.

pellucid Translucent; not opaque.

pemphigoid 1. Relating to or affected by pemphigus. 2. A chronic skin eruption, with subepidermal bullae; mostly affecting the elderly.
benign mucosal p. A chronic dermatological eruption found primarily on the mucous membranes, especially those of the oral cavity and the eye, characterized by subepithelial vesicles and bullae which break down into ulcers. It is most frequent in middle-aged white women.
cicatricial p. Benign mucosal *pemphigoid.

pemphigus A skin disease characterized by the formation of irregularly distributed bullae which leave pigmented spots, and accompanied by inflammation and itching. It has four main forms: *erythematosus, foliaceus, vegetans* and *vulgaris*. Intra-epithelial bullae in the oral mucosa frequently signal the onset of p. vulgaris.

pendulous Hanging loosely.

penetration 1. The act of piercing or entering beyond the surface. 2. The focal depth of a lens.

penta- Prefix signifying *five*.

penumbra The area surrounding a shadow or *umbra. *In radiography* it denotes the area of blur or fuzziness seen round the edges of an x-ray image.

per- Prefix signifying 1. *through*; 2. *very*.

percolation *Microleakage.

percutaneous Through the skin.

perforate To pierce with a hole or holes.

perforation 1. The process of boring a hole through a part. 2. The hole thus pierced.

peri- Prefix signifying *around, surrounding*.

periadenitis mucosa necrotica recurrens A disease characterized by chronic recurrent ulceration of the buccal and pharyngeal mucosa, extending also to the tongue; now known as major aphthae, sometimes part of Behçet's syndrome. *Also called* Mikulicz's aphthae or Sutton's aphthae.

periapical In the region of the tooth apex.

pericemental Relating to the periodontal *ligament.

pericementitis *Periodontitis.
alveolar p. *Pyorrhoea alveolaris.

pericementoclasia *Periodontitis with chronic pocket formation.

pericementum The periodontal *ligament.

pericision Cutting through the fibres of the periodontal ligament; sometimes used to aid orthodontic treatment.

periclasia *Periodontoclasia.

pericoronal Around, in the region of, a tooth crown.

pericoronitis Inflammation of the gingiva surrounding a partially erupted tooth crown.

peridens A supernumerary tooth found in any position in the mouth other than in the midline.

peridental *Periodontal.

peridentine *Cementum.

peridentitis *Periodontitis.

peridentoclasia *Pyorrheoa alveolaris.

peridontoclasia *Periodontoclasia.

periglossitis Inflammation of the tissues surrounding the tongue.

periglottic Situated near or around the tongue.

periglottis The mucous membrane of the tongue.

perignathic Situated near or around the jaw.

peri-implantitis Any disease process involving the soft tissue surrounding implanted material. It may be exfoliative, resorptive, traumatic or ulcerative.

perikymata The shallow grooves on the surface of the tooth enamel which mark the ends of the striae of Retzius.

perimeter The distance round the outside edge of an object.
dental p. An instrument to measure the circumference of a tooth.

periodontal Pertaining to the gums and the supporting tissues of the teeth.

periodontics, **periodontia** The study, diagnosis and treatment of diseases of the supporting tissues of the teeth and of the gingiva.

periodontitis Inflammation of the periodontal tissues resulting in destruction of the periodontal ligament and the supporting alveolar bone.
acute p. An acute inflammation of the periodontium of (usually) a single tooth, arising as a result of acute trauma to the tooth, or, when localized to the periapical area, as a result of irritation from bacterial toxins, drugs or instruments following pulpal infection and subsequent root canal therapy.
chronic p. A form of periodontitis in which the progress of the condition is slow and usually generalized.
chronic apical p. Apical *granuloma.
juvenile p. A form of periodontitis found in children and adolescents, usually associated with the permanent incisors and the first permanent molars.
marginal p. *Periodontitis.

periodontitis complex A clinical condition thought to be due to chronic periodontitis and periodontosis co-existing in the same mouth.

periodontitis simplex Chronic *periodontitis.

periodontium The tissues that support and surround the teeth: the cementum, the periodontal ligament, the alveolar bone and the gingiva.

periodontoclasia Any destructive or degenerative disease of the periodontium; *also called* Magitot's disease.

periodontology The study of the supporting tissues of the teeth and of the gingiva in health and disease.

periodontolysis The process that produces advanced destruction of the periodontium.

periodontopathy Any disease of the periodontium.

periodontosis Chronic, non-inflammatory destruction of the periodontal ligament and the associated alveolar bone.

perioral Around, in the region of, the mouth.

periosteal Relating to the periosteum.

periosteitis Inflammation of the periosteum.

periosteoma A morbid osseous growth around bone tissue.

periosteum The fibrous membrane covering any bone surface except articulating surfaces.

periosteum alveolaris The periodontal *ligament.

periostitis Inflammation of the periosteum.
alveolar p. *Pyorrhoea alveolaris.

peripheral Relating to the periphery.

periphery The outer edge, farthest from the centre.

periradicular Around a root, especially the root of a tooth.

perirhizoclasia Inflammatory destruction of the periradicular tissues.

peristomal, peristomatous Around, in the region of, the mouth.

perithelioma A telangiectatic sarcoma.

peritonsillar Situated about or near a tonsil.

perlèche Angular *cheilosis.

perlingual Through the tongue; used of drugs administered by resorption through the tongue's surface.

permeability The condition of being permeable; *in physiology,* used of the property in membranes that permits the transit of molecules and ions in solution through fine pores.

permeable Affording passage through; not impassable.

permeation The spreading or extension through tissues or organs, used especially of malignant tumours extending by continuous growth through the lymphatics.

permucosal Through the mucosa; used in implant dentistry.

pernicious Destructive, generally fatal.

peroral Through the mouth; administered by mouth.

pestle An instrument used for rubbing or pounding substances in a mortar.

petechia (*pl.* petechiae) A small red spot or mark on the skin or mucous membrane, caused by an effusion of blood.

petrosa The petrous part of the temporal bone.

petrosal Relating to the petrosa.

petrosal artery Branch of the middle meningeal artery, supplying the tympanic cavity. *See* Table of Arteries—petrosa.

petrosal nerves Supply the palatal mucosa and glands. *See* Table of Nerves—petrosus.

petrosal sinuses Veins draining the cavernous sinus. *See* Table of Veins—sinus petrosus.

petrous Rock-like.

petrous bone The petrous part of the temporal bone.

pharmacal Relating to pharmacy.

pharmaceutic, pharmaceutical Relating to pharmacy.

pharmaceutics 1. The art of *pharmacy[1]. 2. Pharmaceutical *chemistry.

pharmacist A specialist in pharmacy.

pharmaco- Prefix signifying *drug*.

pharmacochemistry Pharmaceutical *chemistry.

pharmacodiagnosis The use of drugs as an aid to diagnosis.

pharmacodynamics The study of drug action.

pharmacognosist A specialist in pharmacognosy.

pharmacognosy That branch of pharmacology which is concerned with crude drugs.

pharmacologist One who studies the composition and action of drugs.

pharmacology The study of drugs, and of drug actions in particular.

pharmacomania Morbid craving to take or administer drugs.

pharmacophobia Morbid fear of drugs.

pharmacopoeia, pharmacopeia A collection of formulae and methods of preparation of drugs; particularly an authoritative book containing recognized standard formulae and methods.

pharmacotherapy The treatment of disease with drugs.

pharmacy 1. The preparation of medicines from prescription. 2. The shop where medicines are made up and sold.

pharyngeal Relating to the pharynx.

pharyngeal artery Supplies pharynx and also membranes of brain, neck muscles and nerves, etc.; two branches: pharyngeal and ascending pharyngeal. *See* Table of Arteries—pharyngea.

pharyngeal nerves Supply the pharyngeal mucosa and the pharyngeal muscles. *See* Table of Nerves—pharyngealis.

pharyngeal plexus The plexus from which arise the pharyngeal veins. *See* Table of Veins—plexus pharyngeus.

pharyngitis Inflammation of the pharynx.
acute lymphonodular p. A virus infection of the soft palate and oropharynx caused by Coxsackie virus A10, characterized by white or yellow papules, sore throat, headache and fever. It is seen mainly in children and young adults.

pharyngo- Prefix signifying *pharynx.*

pharyngoglossal Relating to both the pharynx and the tongue.

pharyngoglossus Muscle fibres extending from the superior constrictor pharyngis to the tongue.

pharyngomaxillary Relating to the pharynx and the maxilla.

pharyngonasal Relating to both the pharynx and the nose.

pharyngo-oral Relating to both the pharynx and the mouth.

pharyngopalatine Relating to both the pharynx and the palate.

pharyngopalatine muscle M. palatopharyngeus. *See* Table of Muscles.

pharyngoplasty A plastic surgery operation performed on the pharynx.

pharynx The musculomembranous canal forming the upper end of the digestive tract, between the mouth and nostrils and the oesophagus.

phatne, phatnoma *Alveolus; an obsolete term.

phatnorrhagia Bleeding from a tooth socket.

philtrum The groove occurring at the median line of the upper lip.

phimosis
labial p. Imperforation of the mouth.
oral p. Labial *phimosis.

phlebo- Prefix signifying *vein.*

phlegm Mucus, especially that secreted by the mucosa of the nose and throat.

phlegmon Acute inflammation of the subcutaneous connective tissue.
p. of the tongue An acute and diffuse form of *glossitis.

phosphonecrosis Jaw necrosis caused by phosphorus poisoning; *also called* phossy jaw.

phosphoric Relating to phosphorus as a quinquevalent element.

phosphorous Relating to phosphorus as a trivalent element.

phosphorus A non-metallic element, chemical symbol P, occurring commonly in two forms: white, or yellow, phosphorus, a semi-transparent solid, which is poisonous and highly inflammable; and red, or amorphous, phosphorus, which is a non-poisonous and non-inflammable red-brown powder.

photo- Prefix signifying *light*.

photomicrograph A photograph of a minute object made with the aid of a microscope, so that the result is visible to the naked eye.

phycomycosis An acute fungal disease of internal organs; one form starts in the nose and later invades the veins and the lymphatics.

phyma (*pl.* phymata) 1. A neoplasm composed of skin or subcutaneous tissue. 2. A circumscribed swelling on the skin caused by exudation, and larger than a tubercle; an obsolete term.

physical 1. Relating to nature. 2. Relating to material substance, or to the body. 3. Relating to physics.

physiologic, physiological Relating to physiology.

physiology The study of the body functions.

physocephaly Emphysematous swelling of the head.

phytosis Any disease produced by bacteria; an obsolete term.

pick *See* toothpick.

Pickerill's lines (H.P. Pickerill, 1879-1956. English surgeon and dentist living in New Zealand). Horizontal imbrication lines on the surface of tooth enamel.

picrogeusia Pathological bitterness of taste.

pier An *abutment; *in prosthetic dentistry*, an intermediate *abutment.

pier band Any band constructed to fit an abutment tooth.

Pierre Robin syndrome (P. Robin, 1867-1950. French histologist and stomatologist). Congenital disease characterized by a small chin, cleft palate, and backward displacement of the tongue; it can cause death by obstruction of breathing.

piezograph *In dentistry*, a plastic shape moulded by pressure from the tongue, lips and cheeks in edentulous areas of the mouth.

pigment 1. Any colouring matter of the body, normal or abnormal. 2. A dye or other colouring agent.

pigmentation 1. The deposit of pigment. 2. The condition resulting from such a deposit.
amalgam p. *Argyria.
bismuth p. Pigmentation of the oral mucous membranes with granules of bismuth sulphide; there may also be a dark line on the gingival margin.
gingival p. Any deposition of colouring matter within the gingival tissues.

pigmented Marked by a deposit of pigment.

pilation A hair-like fracture, found in cranial bones.

pill A small solid mass, either oval or globular, for the internal administration of a medicine.

pillars of fauces Curved muscular folds on either side of the pharyngeal opening, running from the palate to the base of the tongue and the pharynx; they enclose the tonsils. The *anterior* pillars are also known as the palatoglossal arch, and the *posterior* as the palato-pharyngeal arch.

pilula Latin for *a pill*; used in prescription writing and abbreviated *pil.* or *p.*

pin 1. A thin metal rod used to secure the ends of bones in treatment of fractures. 2. A short peg or post used *in dentistry* to attach an artificial crown to a tooth root.

Pindborg's tumour (J.J. Pindborg, b. 1921. Danish oral pathologist). Calcifying epithelial odontogenic *tumour.

piniform Conical.

pink spot Internal tooth *resorption.

pinlay A gold inlay or onlay which is retained by pins, where the tooth surface is too much abraded to permit of a cavity being cut.

pinledge 1. The anchorage for a bridge, held in position by pins extending into the root of the abutment tooth. 2. A form of pinlay retained by pins recessed into small ledges and covering the lingual surface of an anterior tooth.

pinna The external ear.

piriform Pear-shaped.

Pirogoff's triangle (N.I. Pirogoff, 1810-81. Russian surgeon and anatomist). Hypoglossohyoid *triangle.

pit *In dentistry*, a sharp-pointed depression in the enamel of a tooth.
basilar p. A pit on the lingual surface in the crown of a maxillary incisor above the cervix.

pit and fissure sealant Any agent, usually a form of resin, used for pit and fissure sealing.

pit and fissure sealing The filling up of developmental pits and fissures in posterior teeth to prevent the onset of occlusal caries.

pityriasis linguae Geographic *tongue.

pivot 1. *Post. 2. A specific form of post on which something turns or hinges.
occlusal p. An orthodontic device, used in the molar region, providing a raised surface to act as a fulcrum and produce sagittal mandibular rotation.

pivot crown Post *crown.

placebo A medicine having no pharmacological value, given to humour or quieten a patient; it is used also in certain forms of drug trial.

placode A thickened epithelial plate, found in the embryo and forming the anlage of some organ or part.

planagraphy *Tomography.

plane A flat smooth surface, or any imaginary surface tangent to the body or dividing it.
auriculo-infraorbital p. *Frankfort plane.
auriculonasal p. *Camper's plane.
auriculo-orbital p. *Frankfort plane.
axiobuccolingual p. A plane through the buccal and lingual surfaces of a tooth parallel to its axis.
axiolabiolingual p. A plane through the labial and lingual surfaces of a tooth parallel to its axis.
axiomesiodistal p. A plane through the mesial and distal surfaces of a tooth parallel to the axis.
base p. An imaginary plane used to estimate the retention in the construction of artificial dentures.
bite p. 1. Occlusal *plane. 2. Bite *plate[2].
buccolingual p. Any plane passing through both the buccal and lingual surfaces of a tooth.
condylar p. The plane passing through the most posterior points on the condylar head and on the ascending ramus in the region of the angle of the mandible, and perpendicular to the sagittal plane.
coronal p. Frontal *plane.

facial p. The plane passing through the nasion and the pogonion and perpendicular to the sagittal plane.
frontal p. A vertical plane dividing the body into front and back; it is at right angles to the sagittal plane.
horizontal p. A plane passing through the body at right angles to the frontal plane and the sagittal plane; it divides the body into upper and lower parts.
labiolingual p. Axiolabiolingual *plane.
mandibular p. The plane passing through the lowest point on the lower border of the mandible in the region of the angle and through the menton, and perpendicular to the sagittal plane.
maxillary p. In cephalometrics, the plane, perpendicular to the sagittal plane, passing through the anterior and posterior nasal spines as seen on a lateral skull radiograph.
mean foundation p. Base *plane.
median p. The sagittal plane when it passes through the midline of the body, dividing it into right and left halves.
mesiodistal p. Axiomesiodistal *plane.
nasion-postcondylare p. *Bolton plane.
occlusal p. The imaginary plane between the maxillary and mandibular teeth in occlusion; it is used in the construction of artificial dentures.
parasagittal p. *Sagittal plane.
sagittal p. Any plane passing longitudinally through the body from front to back; it divides the body into left and right sides.
S-N p. In cephalometrics, that plane which passes through the centre of the shadow of the sella turcica and the nasion and which is perpendicular to the sagittal plane.
transverse p. Horizontal *plane.
vertical p. Any plane of the body that divides it longitudinally, at right angles to the horizontal plane.

planoconcave Level on one side and concave on the other.

planoconvex Level on one side and convex on the other.

plaque 1. Any patch or flat lesion. 2. Dental *plaque.
bacterial p. Dental *plaque.
dental p. A soft, concentrated mass, consisting of a large variety of bacteria, and their products, together with a certain amount of cellular debris, found adhering to the surfaces of the teeth when oral hygiene is neglected; it cannot be removed by rinsing.
gelatinoid p. Dental *plaque.
mucin p., mucinous p. Acquired *pellicle.

plaque index An index for assessing the amount of plaque in individuals or groups. This may be based on the use of a disclosing rinse or tablets, scoring the plaque revealed on a scale of 0-5, on all teeth other than 3rd molars; the final value is given by dividing the sum of the scores for all teeth by the number of teeth present. Another method of assessment examines the tooth surface at the circumference of the gingival margin on a scale of 0-3, again dividing the total score by the number of teeth present.

plasma The fluid part of blood or lymph, in which cells or corpuscles are suspended.

plasma cell A bone-marrow cell of the lymphocytic series, which makes and secretes antibody.

plasmacytoma A tumour composed of plasma cells.

plasmocytosis A condition characterized by an excess of plasma cells in the blood.

gingival p. Plasma-cell *gingivitis.

plaster of Paris Calcined gypsum, $CaSO_4.H_2O$, which will set hard on drying after being mixed with water. It is used to make dental impressions and casts.

plastic 1. Able to be moulded. 2. Material that can be moulded in processing by pressure or heat. 3. Relating to those processes by which tissue is restored or replaced, and defects rectified, as in *plastic* surgery.

plastics *In dentistry*, those materials used for fillings or prostheses which are soft enough to be moulded while being inserted.

plate 1. Any flat structure, especially a flattened bone process. 2. *In dentistry*, a thin sheet of metal, rubber or plastic, either forming part of an orthodontic appliance or holding teeth in an artificial denture.

base p. 1. Denture *base. 2. *In orthodontics*, an acrylic plate, part of an orthodontic appliance, which is fitted to the mucosa and the necks of the teeth, and may hold the springs or clasps.

bite p. 1. A temporary base plate of rigid material, carrying a rim of wax or plastic (occlusal rim) on which the bite is recorded. 2. An orthodontic appliance designed to correct an abnormal incisor relationship by providing a ledge of metal, vulcanite or acrylic in one arch, against which the opposing incisors strike. Where the ledge is sloped and not flat this appliance is known as a *bite plane*.

bone p's. Perforated metal plates, either flat or L-shaped in cross-section, used in the treatment of fractures, and which can be secured to bone fragments to immobilize them.

cortical p. The superficial outer layer of bone in the alveolar process.

dental p. A plate of metal, acrylic or other material, shaped to fit the roof of the mouth, to which artificial teeth are attached.

die p. A sheet of metal containing dies for forming cusps on a shell crown.

expansion p. An orthodontic appliance consisting of a divided base plate fitted with a screw which will separate the parts and so apply pressure to the teeth.

lingual p. A plate covering part of the lingual surfaces of the crowns of mandibular anterior teeth and the lingual gingiva, used to join and support parts of a partial denture.

mandibular staple bone p. A form of transosseous *implant.

oral p. Buccopharyngeal *membrane.

orbital p. of the frontal bone One of the two processes of the frontal bone which form the vaults of the orbits.

retention p. 1. The foundation for an obturator. 2. Any orthodontic retaining appliance.

simple p. A plate base without teeth attached; generally used for radium or similar therapy.

split p. Expansion *plate.

spring p. A dental plate which is retained by the elasticity of its material pressing against the abutment teeth.

stomodeal p. Buccopharyngeal *membrane.

suction p. A dental plate which is retained in the mouth by suction or atmospheric pressure.

trial p. A temporary dental plate of soft material or wax, used to hold the artificial teeth for fitting in the mouth.

X p. An orthodontic screw-adjusted appliance used to retract protrusive incisors and prevent excessive overbite.

plate culture A bacterial culture grown on a glass plate, or in a Petri dish.

platelet One of the minute circular or oval discs found in the blood of all mammals and concerned in its coagulation mechanism.

platy- Prefix signifying *flat, broad.*

platycephalic Having a broad, flattened skull.

platyglossal Having a flat and broad tongue.

platysma muscle Raises skin from underlying structures, and with M. risorius, retracts angle of the mouth. *See* Table of Muscles.

platystaphyline Having a broad and flat palate.

Plaut's angina (H.K. Plaut, 1858-1928. German physician). Necrotizing ulcerative *gingivostomatitis.

Plaut-Vincent gingivitis (H.K. Plaut, 1858-1928. German physician; J.H. Vincent, 1862-1950. French physician and bacteriologist). Acute ulcerative *gingivitis.

pledget A small compress of cotton wool, lint or gauze.

-plegia Suffix signifying *paralysis.*

pleomorphic Occurring in several distinct shapes.

pleomorphic fibroadenoma *Adenofibroma.

pleurodont Having teeth attached to the side of a bony socket or to the side of the jaw.

plexus 1. A network of nerves. 2. A network of blood or lymphatic vessels.

dental p. A network of nerve fibres about the roots of the teeth; those of the maxilla (*superior dental plexus*) are branches of the maxillary nerve and those of the mandible (*inferior dental plexus*) are branches of the inferior dental nerve.

facial p. A nerve plexus about the facial artery.

lingual p. A nerve plexus about the lingual artery.

maxillary p. One of the nerve plexuses about the external and internal maxillary arteries.

nasopalatine p. A plexus of the nasopalatine nerves in the incisive foramen.

venous p. For venous plexuses *see* Table of Veins—plexus.

plica A pleat or fold. For the anatomical plica of the oral cavity *see under* fold.

plicadentine, plicidentine A form of dentine made up of complex folds, found in the teeth of reptiles and of some fish.

pliers Small pincers, with variously shaped jaws, depending on the purpose for which they are designed, used to hold small objects or to bend or cut metal strips or wire.

plugger *Condenser.

amalgam p. Amalgam *condenser.

Plummer-Vinson syndrome (H.S. Plummer, 1874-1936. American physician; P.P. Vinson, 1890-1959. American surgeon). A syndrome associated with a form of iron-deficiency anaemia; it is characterized by cracks and fissures at the corners of the mouth, a painful, smooth red tongue with atrophy of the lingual papillae and difficulty in swallowing; the skin is pale and lemon-tinted.

plumper
lip p. The labial flange on a denture or obturator built up to hold the cheeks and lip in their normal position.

pneumococcus A single organism of *Streptococcus pneumoniae*.

pocket 1. A pouch, a small bag, or a cavity, into which something may be put. 2. *In dentistry*, an abnormal space developing between the tooth root and the gum.
complex p. A periodontal pocket involving more than one tooth surface but having an outlet on only one surface.
compound p. A periodontal pocket involving more than one tooth surface.
false p. See periodontal pocket.
gingival p. Periodontal *pocket.
infrabony p. Intrabony *pocket.
intrabony p. A form of true periodontal pocket in which the base of the pocket lies below the level of the alveolar bone.
intraoral p. In oral plastic surgery, a pocket created within the mouth, lined with a skin graft, which is used to support a prosthesis in restoration of facial contours caused by the loss or absence of a large portion of the mandible.
periodontal p. An abnormally deep gingival sulcus associated with periodontal disease. A *false* periodontal pocket is one due to the enlargement of the free gingiva in gingivitis; a *true* periodontal pocket is one due to the apical migration of the gingival attachment, associated with periodontitis.
suprabony p. A form of true periodontal pocket in which the base of the pocket lies above the level of the alveolar bone.
true p. See periodontal pocket.

pocket measuring probe, pocket probe A periodontal probe for determining the depth of a periodontal pocket.

pogonion The extreme anterior point on the midline of the mandible; a craniometric landmark.

poikilodentosis Mottled tooth enamel.

point 1. The sharp end of an object, or a small spot. 2. To approach the surface at one place, as of the pus in an abscess.
'A' p. *Subspinale.
alveolar p. *Prosthion.
'B' p. *Supramentale.
contact p. *Contact area.
craniometric p. Any one of the landmarks on the skull used in craniometry.
irritation p. In the testing of vital dental pulp with an electric current, the average reading at which, on application of the current, a tingling sensation is felt, but before pain is produced.
jugal p. *Jugale.
mental p. *Pogonion.
nasal p. *Nasion.
'S' p. *Sella turcica[2].
silver p. A fine cone of silver used to fill a root canal after the removal of the pulp.
supranasal p. *Ophryon.

point angle An angle formed at the junction of three tooth surfaces or cavity walls; point angles are named according to the surfaces or walls that form them.

Poirier's line (P.J. Poirier, 1853-1907. French anatomist). The line joining the lambda to the nasion.

poison Any substance that, when absorbed into the system of a living body, is liable to cause injury and endanger life.

poly- Prefix signifying *many*; *in medicine* it signifies *too many*, or *affecting many parts*.

polycystic Composed of or containing many cysts.

polydontia *Polyodontia.

polylophodont Having teeth with multi-ridged crowns.

polymer The product resulting from the combination of two or more molecules of the same substance, the molecular weight being a whole multiple of the molecular weight of the original substance.
acrylic p. A general term for any of the synthetic polymers or co-polymers derived from acrylic acid; they may be used as synthetic rubbers, adhesives, or plastics.

polymerization The process whereby two or more molecules of the same substance combine to form a polymer.

polyodontia The condition of having supernumerary teeth.

polyostotic Affecting several bones.

polyp, polypus (*pl.* polypi) A pedunculated growth or tumour arising from mucous membrane.
pulp p. Hyperplastic *pulpitis.

polyphyodont Having several successive sets of natural teeth.

polypoid Resembling a polyp.

polyposis A condition characterized by the presence of multiple polyps.

polypous Having the characteristics of a polyp.

polyprotodont Having numerous incisor teeth.

polysialia *Hypersalivation.

polystomatous Having many mouths, or openings.

Pont index The relationship of the width of the four permanent incisors in either the maxillary or the mandibular arch to the distance between the first premolars and the distance between the first permanent molars in the same arch.

pontic A suspended member on a bridge or partial denture, replacing a natural crown.

pontine artery Branch of basilar artery supplying the pons. *See* Table of Arteries—pontis.

porcelain A translucent ceramic product of the fusion of kaolin, feldspar and quartz, with other minerals, used in the making of artificial teeth, inlays, etc.

pore A minute opening on a free surface, especially one of the sweat gland ducts.

porion (*pl.* poria) The median point on the upper margin of the opening of the external auditory canal; one of a pair of craniometric landmarks.

porosity The quality of being porous.

porous Having pores.

porte-polisher A handpiece or carrier used to hold dental polishing instruments.

port-wine stain *Naevus flammeus.

porus A pore or meatus.
p. acusticus externus The opening of the external auditory canal in the tympanic portion of the temporal bone.
p. acusticus internus The opening of the internal auditory canal into the cranial cavity.

posed In position, placed; *in dentistry* it is applied to tooth position.

post *In dentistry*, a peg or pin of metal used to attach an artificial crown to the root of a natural tooth; *also called* a dowel.
screw p. A threaded post, which can be screwed into a prepared root canal.

post cibum Latin for *after a meal*; used in prescription writing, and abbreviated *p.c.*

post crown Any artificial crown attached to the tooth root by means of a post or dowel; *also called* a pivot crown.

post- Prefix signifying *after* or *behind.*

postbuccal Behind the buccal region in the mouth.

postcondylar Behind the condyle.

post-dam A groove along the palatal edge on a model for a denture, which produces a ridge on the finished denture serving as a perfect seal for retention purposes and to prevent food debris from collecting under the plate.

posterior Behind, in the rear.

posterior facial vein V. retromandibularis. *See* Table of Veins.

postero- Prefix signifying *posterior.*

posteroclusion Posterior *occlusion.

postoperative After a surgical operation is completed.

postoral Behind the mouth.

postpalatine Behind the palate, or behind the fauces of the throat.

post-permanent Relating to those teeth that occasionally erupt after the second, permanent dentition.

post-resection filling Retrograde root *filling.

Potts' elevator An instrument similar to *Miller's elevator, but smaller and less strong.

pre- Prefix signifying *before*.

precancerous Relating to any abnormal condition likely to develop into cancer.

precarious *In dentistry*, occurring before or early in the development of caries.

precementum *Cementoid.

predentine The inner, unmineralized layer of dentine formed at the pulp surface.

pregnancy epulis A form of epulis developing during or as a result of pregnancy.

pregnancy gingivitis Gingivitis thought to be caused by the endocrine changes occurring during pregnancy; marked by hypertrophy and haemorrhage of the gums, and occasionally by tumour-like swelling.

premalignant *Precancerous.

premature Occurring early, before the expected time.

premaxilla The frontal bone between the maxillae in the foetus; the intermaxillary bone.

premaxillary 1. Relating to the premaxilla. 2. In front of the maxilla.

premedication The administration of sedatives or other drugs before treatment, to help in patient management especially with nervous patients.

premolar, premolar tooth A bicuspid, found in front of the molar teeth; there are two in each quadrant in the permanent dentition in man.

prenatal Present before birth.

preoperative Before a surgical operation is commenced.

pre-oral In front of the mouth.

prepalatal In front of the palate.

prescribe To write instructions for the preparation, composition and administration of a medicine.

prescription A written instruction on the preparation, composition and administration of a medicine.

presenile Relating to premature old age.

presenility Premature old age.

prevalence The number of cases of a disease at any given time in any given place.

preventive Designed to avert the onset of something.

prickle-cell layer The stratum germinativum of the epidermis or squamous epithelium, excluding the basal cells.

Priestley's mass (J. Priestley, 1733-1804. English scientist). A green or brown stain on the anterior teeth of the young or where reduced enamel epithelium remains over the enamel.

primer *Liner.
cavity p. Cavity *liner.

primitive Original; in its first, simplest form.

primordium The first discernible signs of any organ or part.

prism A solid figure whose sides are parallelograms and which has a triangular or polygonal cross-section.
enamel p. One of the prismatic rods of which tooth enamel is made up.

prismatic Relating to a prism.

prismos Tooth grinding; bruxism.

pro re nata Latin for *as required*; used in prescription writing, and abbreviated *p.r.n.*

pro- Prefix signifying *before, in front of.*

probe A slender, flexible instrument used to explore a cavity or wound.
pocket measuring p., pocket p. A periodontal probe for determining the depth of a periodontal pocket.

procelous Concave at the front.

procerus muscle Wrinkles skin over nose. *See* Table of Muscles.

process *In anatomy*, a slender projection of bone, or a tissue protuberance.
alveolar p. The bony ridge on the maxilla or the mandible containing the tooth sockets.
ameloblastic p's. Projections of cytoplasm from an enamel cell, about which mineralization occurs; *also called* Tomes' processes.
anterior clinoid p. A process projecting backwards at the medial end of the posterior border of the lesser wing of the sphenoid bone.
condyloid p. One of the two mandibular condyles.
coronoid p. A thin and flattened projection of bone from the anterior upper border of the ascending ramus of the mandible into which the temporal muscle is inserted.
dental p. Alveolar process of the maxilla.
ethmoid p., ethmoidal p. A projection from the upper border of the inferior nasal concha.
frontal p. of the maxilla A projection of the maxilla articulating with the frontal bone and forming part of the side of the nasal cavity and of the margin of the orbit.
frontal p. of the zygomatic bone A thick ascending serrated process of the zygomatic bone articulating with the frontal bone and the great wing of the sphenoid.
frontonasal p. The front portion of bone in the head of an embryo which develops into the forehead and the bridge of the nose.
frontosphenoidal p. Frontal *process of the zygomatic bone.
globular p. One of the bulbous expansions at either angle of the nose in the embryo, later fusing to form the philtrum.
hamular p. Pterygoid *hamulus.
infrajugular p. of the occipital bone A bony spike in the jugular notch of the occipital bone; together with the intrajugular process of the temporal bone it divides the jugular foramen.

infrajugular p. of the temporal bone A small ridge on the margin of the petrous part of the temporal bone, within the jugular notch; together with the intrajugular process of the occipital bone it divides the jugular foramen.
jugular p. An irregular plate on the internal aspect of the condyle of the occipital bone, projecting laterally from the foramen magnum; it articulates with the petrous part of the temporal bone.
lacrimal p. A vertical extension on the superior border of the inferior nasal concha, forming part of the medial wall of the nasolacrimal canal.
mandibular p. That part of the mandibular arch in the embryo from which the mandible develops.
mastoid p. A conical bony projection behind the external auditory meatus, on the surface of the temporal bone, giving attachment to the longissimus capitis, splenius capitis and sternocleidomastoid muscles.
maxillary p. in the embryo A protuberance from the mandibular arch in the embryo from which the maxilla, the zygomatic bone and the upper cheek and lip region develop.
maxillary p. of the inferior nasal concha A thin, triangular plate from the ethmoid process, forming part of the medial wall of the maxillary sinus.
maxillary p. of the palatine bone A thin plate projecting forward from the anterior border of the palatine bone, closing the lower posterior end of the opening of the maxillary sinus.
maxillary p. of the zygomatic bone A blunt descending process of the zygomatic bone articulating with the maxilla.
nasal p. of the maxilla Frontal *process of the maxilla.
odontoblast p's. The branching processes of the odontoblasts which occur in the dentinal canals; *also called* Tomes' fibres.
orbital p. of the palatine bone A bone process from the palate bone, pointing upwards and outwards.
palatine p. of the maxilla The flat plate of bone on the maxilla which forms the front portion of the roof of the mouth and articulates with the palatine bone.
posterior clinoid p. One of the tubercles at the angle on either side of the dorsum sellae on the body of the sphenoid bone.
pterygoid p. One of two descending processes from the junction of the body of the sphenoid bone with the greater wings.
pterygospinous p. The sharp projecting spine on the posterior edge of the lateral pterygoid plate of the sphenoid bone, providing attachment for the pterygospinous ligament.
retromandibular p. The narrow part of the parotid gland found in the fossa behind the mandible.
sphenoidal p. of the palatine bone A thin bony plate running upwards and inwards from the palatine bone and articulating with the sphenoid bone and the vomer.
styloid p. of the temporal bone A sharp spine projecting downwards from the lower surface of the petrous portion of the temporal bone.
temporal p. The posterior angle of the zygomatic bone which articulates with the zygomatic process of the temporal bone.
vaginal p. A bony plate extending down from the base of the medial pterygoid plate of the sphenoid bone to the vomer.

zygomatic p. of the frontal bone A thick, strong lateral projection of the frontal bone which articulates with the zygomatic bone.
zygomatic p. of the maxilla A rough triangular eminence articulating with the maxillary process of the zygomatic bone.
zygomatic p. of the temporal bone A long process from the lower squamous portion of the temporal bone, articulating with the zygomatic bone.

processes, Tomes' Ameloblastic *processes.

procheilia The condition in which one lip protrudes forward of its normal position.

procheilon The central prominence on the upper border of the upper lip.

procynodontos A canine tooth, especially one that is protruded; obsolete term.

profunda linguae artery Supplies the lower surface of the tongue. *Also called* ranine artery. *See* Table of Arteries.

progenia *Prognathism.

proglossis The tip of the tongue.

prognathic Having a projecting jaw.

prognathism Protrusion of the jaw.

prognathometer An instrument for measuring the degree of prognathism.

prognathous Having a gnathic index of over 103; having a protruding jaw.

prognosis A forecast, from the symptoms, of the probable course of an attack of a disease and the prospects for recovery.

progonoma
melanotic p. Melanotic neuroectodermal *tumour of infancy.

prolabium 1. The red outer part of the lip. 2. *Procheilon.

proliferation Reproduction or multiplication.

prominent Projecting, standing out.

prop
dental p. Jaw *prop.
jaw p. An appliance for holding the jaws open during an operation performed under general anaesthesia.
mouth p. Jaw *prop.

prophylactic Relating to prophylaxis; a preventive remedy.

prophylactodontia, prophylactodontics Preventive *dentistry.

prophylactodontist One who specializes in preventive dentistry.

prophylaxis The use of mechanical or medical means to prevent the occurrence of disease.
dental p. 1. Preventive treatment for diseases of the teeth. 2. Scaling, cleaning and polishing the teeth.
oral p. Preventive treatment for diseases of the oral cavity.

prophylaxis paste Polishing *paste.

propriodentium The tooth tissues.

prosencephalon The anterior brain vesicle in the embryo, from which develop the cerebral hemispheres, the olfactory lobes and corpora striata; the forebrain.

prosopalgia Facial pain; facial neuralgia.

prosopanoschisis A congenital oblique facial cleft.

prosopo- Prefix signifying *face*.

prosopodiplegia Paralysis of both sides of the face.

prosopodynia Facial neuralgia.

prosoponeuralgia Facial neuralgia.

prosopoplegia Facial paralysis.

prosoposchisis Congenital facial cleft or fissure.

prosopospasm Spasm of the facial muscles; risus sardonicus.

prosopus varus Congenital hemiatrophy of the cranium and the facial bones, resulting in an oblique facies.

prosthesis A manufactured appliance to take the place of a natural part or to correct a congenital abnormality.
combined p. A removable dental prosthesis which is combined with some fixed elements.
dental p. Partial or full dentures, crown or bridge, or any appliance to correct cleft palate.
fixed p. A non-removable dental prosthesis firmly attached to implants, roots or abutment teeth.
fixed/removable p. A form of dental prosthesis in which some parts are fixed and others may be removed and inserted only by the dental practitioner.
maxillofacial p. An artificial substitute for some facial structure which has been too severely damaged to be repaired by surgery.
removable p. Any dental prosthesis designed to be inserted or removed by the patient.
tissue-borne p. A removable dental prosthesis in which the load-bearing is provided entirely by the mucosa and underlying tissue.
tooth-borne p. A dental prosthesis in which the attachments are provided entirely by the teeth or implants.

prosthetic Relating to a prosthesis.

prosthetics The design, construction and fitting of prostheses.

prosthion The mid-point, between the central incisors, on the maxillary alveolar arch; a craniometric landmark.

prosthodontia, prosthodontics Prosthetic dentistry; the design and construction of artificial dentures, and crown- and bridge-work.
implant p. That branch of restorative dentistry which follows the placement of an implant or implants.

prosthodontist A specialist in prosthetic dentistry.

protein
enamel p's. Those proteins synthesized by the ameloblasts during amelogenesis and forming part of the enamel matrix. Those newly secreted are termed *young* enamel proteins, and those remaining in the fully developed enamel are termed *mature* enamel proteins.

proteolysis The process of digestion of protein and its conversion by enzymes into peptones, proteoses, etc.

proteolytic 1. Relating to or effecting proteolysis. 2. Any agent effecting proteolysis.

Proteus A genus of Gram-negative, motile, rod-shaped micro-organisms of the Enterobacteriaceae family, capable of the rapid decomposition of carbohydrates and of proteins.

proto- Prefix signifying *first.*

protocone The mesiolingual cusp on a maxillary molar.

protoconid The mesiobuccal cusp on a mandibular molar.

protomere *In dentistry*, the buccal half of the enamel organ of a tooth.

protraction *of the jaws* The condition in which the jaw is forward of its normal position in relation to the orbital plane; it may be *mandibular* or *maxillary.*

protrusion 1. A forward thrust, especially a forward movement of the mandible. 2. The forward thrust of teeth, usually the incisors.

bimaxillary p. The forward projection of both upper and lower jaws, beyond the normal limits.
jaw p. 1. *Prognathism. 2. Mandibular *protraction of the jaws.
maxillary p. Abnormal projection of the maxilla.
palatine p. *Torus palatinus.

protuberance A swelling, eminence or knob of tissue.
maxillary p. One of the eminences marking the embryonic rudiments of the jaws.
mental p. The prominence on the body of the mandible in the midline of the face.

proximal *Approximal.

proximobuccal Relating to both the approximal and buccal surfaces of a posterior tooth.

proximo-incisal Relating to both the approximal surface and the incisal edge of an anterior tooth.

proximolabial Relating to both the approximal and labial surfaces of an anterior tooth.

proximolingual Relating to both the approximal and lingual surfaces of a tooth.

proximo-occlusal Relating to both the approximal and occlusal surfaces of a posterior tooth.

pseudarthrosis, pseudo-arthrosis A false joint, the site of a poorly united fracture.

pseudo- Prefix signifying *false* or *seemingly*.

pseudo-alveolar Simulating an alveolus, or alveolar tissue.

pseudo-anodontia A condition in which the teeth, although developed, are all unerupted.

pseudo-arthrosis *See* pseudarthrosis.

pseudocolloid *of the lips* *Fordyce's spots.

pseudo-exposure A dental condition in which caries has progressed through the dentine but has not quite exposed the pulp.

pseudomembrane A false membrane; a skin-like layer formed by a fibrinous exudate containing leukocytes and bacteria.

Pseudomonadaceae A family of Gram-negative, aerobic, rod-shaped micro-organisms.

pseudopocket A false periodontal *pocket.

psilosis *Sprue[1].

psoriasis buccalis *Leukoplakia (*buccalis*).

psoriasis linguae *Leukoplakia (*linguae*).

psychosomatic Relating to the mind and the body; *in medicine* particularly relating to the interdependence of mental processes and bodily function.

pterion The point of articulation of the great wing of the sphenoid bone, at the junction of the frontal, parietal and temporal bones.

pterygoid In the shape of a wing.

pterygoid artery Branch of the posterior temporal artery to the pterygoid muscles. *See* Table of Arteries—pterygoidea.

pterygoid canal, artery of Supplies levator and tensor veli palatini muscles, pharyngotympanic tube and upper portion of pharynx. *See* Table of Arteries—canalis pterygoidei.

pterygoid canal, nerve of Supplies the lacrimal glands and the glands of the nose and palate. *See* Table of Nerves—canalis pterygoidei.

pterygoid muscles Muscles involved in the closing of the mouth. *See* Table of Muscles—pterygoideus.

pterygoid plexus, pterygoid venous plexus A venous plexus accompanying the maxillary artery through the pterygoid muscles. *See* Table of Veins—plexus pterygoideus.

pterygomandibular Relating to the pterygoid process and the mandible.

pterygomaxillary Relating to the pterygoid process and the maxilla.

pterygomeningeal artery Branch of the maxillary artery supplying the trigeminal ganglion. *Also called* accessory meningeal. *See* Table of Arteries—pterygomeningea.

pterygopalatine Relating to the pterygoid process and the palatine bone.

pterygopalatine canal 1. Greater palatine *canal. 2. Palatovaginal *canal.

pterygopalatine nerve Supplies the mucosa of the hard palate and the nose. *See* Table of Nerves—pterygopalatinus.

pterygopharyngeal muscle Part of constrictor pharyngis superior. *See* Table of Muscles—pterygopharyngeus.

ptosis Drooping of the eyelid.

ptyalism *Hypersalivation.

ptyalith A salivary *calculus[1].

ptyalo- Prefix signifying *saliva*.

ptyalocele A cyst or cystic tumour containing saliva.
sublingual p. *Ranula.

ptyalogogue *Sialogogue.

ptyalolith A salivary *calculus[1].

ptyalolithiasis The condition of having multiple salivary calculi.

ptyalorrhoea *Hypersalivation.

ptyalosis *Salivation.

ptychodont An animal in which the crowns of the molar teeth are formed in folds.

ptysma Saliva.

Puente's disease *Cheilitis glandularis.

pulmonary Relating to the lungs.

pulmonary artery The artery that conveys deoxygenated blood from the heart to the lungs.

pulmonary vein One of the short, thick blood vessels conveying oxygenated blood from the lungs to the heart.

pulp Any soft and juicy tissue.
coronal p. That part of the dental pulp found within the crown of the tooth.
dental p. The vascular and connective tissue, highly innervated, found at the core of a tooth.
enamel p. The stellate *reticulum.
necrotic p. Dental pulp which, for any reason, has lost its nerve and blood supply, and is no longer vital.
putrescent p. Necrotic pulp which has become putrefied and gives off a foul smell.
radicular p. That part of the dental pulp found within the root of the tooth.

pulp abscess, pulpal abscess Acute or chronic inflammation of the dental pulp associated with an area of necrotic tissue and pus; it may occur in the early stage of acute pulpitis.

pulp amputation *Pulpotomy.

pulp atrophy A degenerative process seen in old age and characterized by a shrinking of the dental pulp and a decrease in the number of cells.

pulp calcification Deposition of calcium salts in the tissues of the dental pulp, leading to hardening, mineralization and progressive narrowing of the pulp chamber; it may be caused by old age, caries or trauma.

diffuse p.c. Calcification of the dental pulp with deposits in columns or strands throughout the tissue.

pulp canal Root *canal.

pulp capping The application of a protective covering to the dental pulp; it may be *direct*, onto exposed vital pulp, or *indirect,* onto sound or carious dentine to promote dentine formation over the pulp.

pulp cavity The cavity at the core of a tooth, comprising the pulp chamber and the root canal.

pulp chamber The cavity at the core of a tooth crown, surrounded by dentine and containing dental pulp.

pulp devitalization Any procedure that destroys the vitality of the dental pulp.

pulp horn One of the horn-like projections of the pulp chamber into the crown of a tooth.

pulp nodule *Denticle[2].

pulp polyp Hyperplastic *pulpitis.

pulp protection The act of inserting intermediate linings in a cavity to prevent conduction of heat or cold to the pulp from the filling material.

pulpal Relating to the dental pulp.

pulpalgia Pain affecting the dental pulp.

pulpectomy Complete removal of the pulp of a tooth.

pulpitis Inflammation of the dental pulp; where the pulp is sufficiently exposed for any exudate to drain out it is known as *open* pulpitis; where no such drainage is possible it is called *closed* pulpitis.

chronic hyperplastic p. Hyperplastic *pulpitis.

hyperplastic p. A chronic inflammation of the dental pulp, usually associated with gross caries, and most frequently seen in children and adolescents; there is a characteristic proliferation of pulp tissue producing a pedunculated fleshy mass in the exposed pulp cavity.

suppurative p. Pulpitis caused by the extension of a carious lesion into the dental pulp.

pulpless Having no pulp.

pulpo-axial Relating to the pulpal and axial walls in the step portion of a proximo-incisal cavity.

p. angle The angle formed at the junction of these walls; a *line* angle.

pulpobucco-axial Relating to the pulpal, buccal and axial walls in the step portion of a proximo-occlusal cavity in a molar or premolar.

p. angle The angle formed at the junction of these walls; a *point* angle.

pulpodistal Relating to the pulpal and distal walls in the step portion of a proximo-incisal cavity.

p. angle The angle formed at the junction of these walls; a *line* angle.

pulpodontics That branch of endodontics concerned with the pulp of the tooth.

pulpolabial Relating to the pulpal and labial walls in the step portion of a proximo-incisal cavity.

p. angle The angle formed at the junction of these walls; a *line* angle.

pulpolingual Relating to the pulpal and lingual walls in the step portion of a proximo-occlusal cavity.

p. angle The angle formed at the junction of these walls; a *line* angle.

pulpolinguo-axial Relating to the pulpal, lingual and axial walls in the step portion of a proximo-occlusal cavity in a molar or premolar.

p. angle The angle formed at the junction of these walls; a *point* angle.

pulpomesial Relating to the pulpal and mesial walls of a cavity.
p. angle The angle formed at the junction of these walls; a *line* angle.

pulpotomy The removal of vital pulp from the crown of a tooth in order to preserve the pulp in the tooth root.

pulpstone A deposit of calcareous matter within the dental pulp, associated with degenerative changes; *also called* a denticle.

pulsation A rhythmic throb or beating, as that of the heart.

pulse The expansion and contraction of an artery due to increased tension of its walls following contraction of the heart and subsequent relaxation. It is usually felt at the wrist, but may be felt over any palpable artery.

pulvis Latin for *a powder*; used in prescription writing, and abbreviated *pulv.*

pumice A hard, abrasive substance of volcanic origin, used in dentistry as a polishing agent.

punch 1. Any instrument used to pierce or indent. 2. An instrument used to extract a tooth root.
rubber-dam p. An instrument used to punch holes of various sizes in a rubber dam; *also called* Ainsworth's punch.

puromucous Mucopurulent; containing both pus and mucus.

purpura A disease characterized by the presence on the skin and mucous membranes of purple patches, caused by subcutaneous haemorrhage.

purpuric Relating to or affected with purpura.

purulence The condition of containing pus.

purulent Relating to or forming pus.

pus A yellowish fluid containing leukocytes, necrotic tissue, bacteria, cell debris and tissue fluid, produced as a result of inflammation.

pustular Relating to or characterized by pustules.

pustule A small circumscribed elevation of the skin containing pus or lymph.

putrefaction The decomposition of organic matter through the action of micro-organisms, resulting in the production of various solid and liquid compounds and gases, giving off a foul odour.

putrescent In the process of rotting; undergoing putrefaction.

putrid Rotten, in a state of putrefaction.

pyaemia Generalized septicaemia caused by pyogenic micro-organisms in the blood stream, and marked by the formation of multiple abscesses.

pyemia *See* pyaemia.

pyic Relating to pus.

pyo- Prefix signifying *pus*.

pyogenic Pus-producing.

pyorrhea *See* pyorrhoea.

pyorrhoea 1. A discharge of pus. 2. *In dentistry*, a lay term used to denote any form of periodontal disease.
paradental p. Periodontitis with deep pocketing and discharge of pus, even after the removal of local irritants.

pyorrhoea alveolaris Usually applied to advanced forms of chronic periodontitis where pus can be expressed from the associated periodontal pockets; it is now a fairly rare condition. *Also called*

Fauchard's disease, Jourdain's disease or Riggs' disease.

pyosis *Suppuration.

pyostomatitis Inflammation and suppuration in the mouth.

pyostomatitis vegetans An oral condition characterized by numerous small and closely grouped papillary projections on a broad base, with chronic inflammation, which later develops tiny pustules on the papillomata.

pyrexia Fever.

pyrexial Relating to or affected by fever.

pyriform *See* piriform.

pyro- Prefix signifying *burning, fire*.

pyroglossia A burning sensation affecting the tongue.

Q

q. Abbreviation for *quaque—each, every;* used in prescription writing.

q.d. Abbreviation for *quaque die*—every day; used in prescription writing.

q.h. Abbreviation for *quaque hora*—every hour; used in prescription writing. q.2h., *quaque secunda hora*—every two hours; q.3h., *quaque tertia hora*—every three hours, etc.

q.i.d. Abbreviation for *quater in die*—four times a day; used in prescription writing.

q.l. Abbreviation for *quantum libet*—as much as desired; used in prescription writing.

q.p. Abbreviation for *quantum placeat*—as much as desired; used in prescription writing.

q.q.h. Abbreviation for *quaque quarta hora*—every four hours; used in prescription writing.

q.s. Abbreviation for *quantum satis*—a sufficient amount; used in prescription writing.

q.suff. Abbreviation for *quantum sufficit*—as much as needed; used in prescription writing.

quadrangle *Of an instrument*: having four angles in the shank; a term introduced by G.V. Black.

quadrant *In dentistry*, one half of each arch, the dividing line being the mid-point of the arch; in ISO nomenclature the quadrants are called *upper right, upper left, lower left, lower right* and designated 10, 20, 30, 40.

quadrate bone The upper jaw in non-mammalian vertebrates.

quadratus labii inferioris muscle M. depressor labii inferioris. *See* Table of Muscles.

quadratus labii superioris muscle M. levator labii superioris. *See* Table of Muscles.

quadratus menti M. depressor labii inferioris. *See* Table of Muscles.

quadri- Prefix signifying *four*.

quadricuspid Having four cusps.

quadritubercular Having four tubercles.

quantum libet Latin for *as much as desired*; used in prescription writing, and abbreviated *q.l.*

quantum placeat Latin for *as much as desired*; used in prescription writing, and abbreviated *q.p.*

quantum satis Latin for *a sufficient amount*; used in prescription writing, and abbreviated *q.s.*

quantum sufficit Latin for *as much as is needed*; used in prescription writing, and abbreviated *q.suff.*

quaque Latin for *each, every*; used in prescription writing, and abbreviated *q.*

quaque die Latin for *every day*; used in prescription writing and abbreviated *q.d.*

quaque hora Latin for *every hour*; used in prescription writing, and abbreviated *q.h.*

quaque quarta hora Latin for *every four hours*; used in prescription writing, and abbreviated *q.q.h.*

quasi- Prefix signifying *resembling* (but not being), or *seeming* (but not being).

quater in die Latin for *four in a day*; used in prescription writing, and abbreviated *q.i.d.* or *q.d.*

Quatrefages' angle (J.L.A. Quatrefages de Bréau, 1810-92. French anthropologist). Parietal *angle.

queen's metal An alloy composed of tin and antimony.

Queyrat's erythroplasia (L.A. Queyrat, 1856-1933. French dermatologist). Frequently used as a synonym for *erythroplakia.

quicksilver *Mercury.

quin-, quinqu- Prefix signifying *five*.

Quincke's oedema (H.I. Quincke, 1842-1922. German physician). Angioneurotic *oedema.

quinquecuspid Having five cusps.

quinquetubercular Having five tubercles.

quinsy Peritonsillar *abscess.

quotidian Recurring daily.

R

Symbol for *recipe*—take; used in prescription writing.

rad. Abbreviation for Latin *radix*—root.

rep. Abbreviation for *repetatur*—let it be repeated; used in prescription writing.

radectomy Root *amputation.

radiability The condition of being easily penetrated by x-rays.

radiation mucositis Characteristic diffuse inflammatory change in the mucosa produced by radiation therapy.

radiciform In the shape of a root, especially a tooth root.

radicular Relating to a root.

radiectomy Root *amputation.

radiodontia, radiodontics Dental *radiology.

radiograph A film negative produced by the use of radiography.
bitewing r. An intraoral radiograph showing the crowns of the teeth and the interdental areas in both the maxilla and mandible, taken on a special individual x-ray film held in place in the mouth by a central wing or *tab* on which the teeth can close.
cephalometric r. A radiograph taken in a standardized position for the purposes of cephalometric analysis; used in orthodontics and oral surgery.
oral r. Any radiograph of the teeth, jaws and related structures. It may be taken with the film in the mouth (*intraoral*) or placed outside (*extraoral*).
panoramic r. A type of radiograph giving an uninterrupted view of the whole dental arch, or of both arches; it may be obtained either by wide-angle beam techniques, by slit-beam methods or by tomography.

radiography Photography by means of x-rays. *In dentistry* it may be intraoral or extraoral.
body-section r. *Tomography.
layer r. *Tomography.
slit-beam r. A technique for obtaining panoramic radiographs using a narrow x-ray beam which moves round while the film and the object remain stationary.
wide-beam r. A method of producing panoramic radiographs using divergent x-ray beams with a technique similar to conventional intraoral radiography; the x-ray source may be intraoral or extraoral.

radiology The science of radiant energy; more particularly the application of radiant energy to medical diagnosis and treatment.
dental r. The radiography and interpretation of x-ray films of the teeth and surrounding structures.

radiolucent Offering little resistance to x-rays in radiography; almost transparent.

radionecrosis Tissue destruction or ulceration caused by radiation.

radio-opaque Resistant to the passage of x-rays in photography and appearing opaque on a radiograph.

radiotherapy Treatment, usually of malignant neoplasms, with ionizing radiation.

radisectomy Root *amputation.

radula Any scraping instrument such as a scaler, used to remove dental calculus from the teeth.

rake teeth Descriptive of widely separated teeth.

Ramfjord index (S.P. Ramfjord, contemporary American dentist). Periodontal *index.

rampart A broad encircling ridge.
maxillary r. A ridge of epithelial cells found in the embryo in that part of the jaw which will develop into the alveolar border.

ramus 1. A branch or process projecting from a bone, as the *ramus* of the mandible. 2. A branch, especially of a blood vessel or nerve.

ranine 1. Relating to a ranula. 2. Relating to the under surface of the tongue.

ranine artery A. profunda linguae. *See* Table of Arteries.

Ranke's angle (J. Ranke, 1836-1916. German physician and anthropologist). The angle made by a line through the centre of the nasofrontal suture and the centre of the maxillary alveolar process with the horizontal plane of the skull.

ranula A retention cyst of the sublingual or submandibular glands, occurring under the tongue.

ranular Relating to a ranula.

raphe A suture, ridge or crease marking the line of union between two symmetrical halves.
buccal r. The line marking the union of those parts of the cheek derived from the maxillary process with those derived from the mandibular process.
lingual r. The furrow along the midline of the dorsal surface of the tongue, corresponding to the fibrous septum which divides the tongue in two.
palatine r. The narrow mucosal ridge on the midline of the hard palate.
pterygomandibular r. A sinewy ligament dividing the buccinator muscle from the constrictor pharyngis superior.

rarefaction The lessening in density but not in volume of any substance.

Raschkow's plexus (I. Raschkow, 1811-72). A fine nerve plexus below the odontoblasts in the dental papilla, found during the formation of dentine.

rash A temporary cutaneous eruption.
gum r. *Strophulus.
tooth r. *Strophulus.
wandering r. Geographic *tongue.

Rathke's pouch (M.H. Rathke, 1793-1860. German anatomist). A dorsal diverticulum from the embryonic buccal cavity which develops into the anterior lobe of the pituitary body.

ratio A quantitative or numerical relationship between two substances or between groups, expressed in its lowest terms.

re- Prefix signifying *again, back*.

reaction Response to a stimulus.

reamer A thin corkscrew-like instrument, used either by hand or with a dental engine, for enlarging root canals.

reattachment 1. The re-uniting of separated parts. 2. *In dentistry*, the process whereby a loosened or a replanted tooth becomes attached again to the alveolus. 3. *In restorative dentistry,* the process of replacing a loosened artificial tooth crown or a bridge. 4. *In periodontics*, the process whereby fibres of the periodontium become reattached to the cementum and/or alveolar bone following therapy to reduce pocket depth.

rebase The process of fitting a new denture base without altering the occlusal relations of the teeth.

recession The drawing back or falling away.
gingival r. The gradual shrinking back of the gums leaving the tooth cervix, and part of the root, exposed.

recipe Latin for *take*; used in prescription writing, and abbreviated

Recklinghausen's disease (F.D. von Recklinghausen, 1833-1910. German pathologist). *Neurofibromatosis.

record 1. An account or representation in a permanent form, which may be referred to in future. 2. To make such an account or representation.
check r. An impression taken in hard wax or in modelling compound to record the various occlusal positions of the teeth in the mouth, and used to check these positions in artificial dentures in an articulator.

recrudescence The return of symptoms or the recurrence of disease after a temporary remission.

rectus capitis muscles Muscles involved in movements of the head. *See* Table of Muscles.

rectus (oculi) muscles Muscles involved in the movement of the eyeball. *See* Table of Muscles.

recumbent Lying down.

recurrence The return of symptoms or of a disease, after a period of remission, or of a malignant tumour after surgical removal or other therapy.

recurrent 1. Returning at intervals. 2. Turning back on itself or on its course.

recurrent nerve N. laryngeus recurrens. *See* Table of Nerves.

reduction *of a fracture* The replacing of the displaced bone ends or fragments to the correct position; if the fracture is corrected without surgery it is known as a *closed* reduction; if surgery is necessary it is called an *open* reduction.

reflect Turn back on itself; transmit, as with light rays, back in the direction of origin.

reflection 1. A turning or bending back upon itself. 2. The image that may be produced, as in a mirror.

reflex 1. Reflected. 2. An involuntary invariable reaction to certain stimuli.
chin r. Closure of the mouth produced by stroking the chin.
conditioned r. A reflex that is not normal and instinctive but is developed as a result of repeated association.
delayed r. A conditioned reflex occurring some time after the application of stimuli.
faucial r. Vomiting or gagging caused by irritation of the fauces.
flexor r., flexion r. Nociceptive *reflex.
gag r. Pharyngeal *reflex.
jaw clonus r. Jaw jerk *reflex.
jaw jerk r. Clonic contraction of the muscles of mastication and upward jerking of the mandible, produced by a downward blow on the relaxed and open jaw. Observed in sclerosis of the lateral columns of the spine.
laryngeal r. Coughing caused by irritation of the larynx and fauces.
mandibular r. Jaw jerk *reflex.
nasal r. *Bekhterev's reflex.
nasomental r. Contraction of the mentalis muscle causing elevation of the lower lip, as a result of a tap on the side of the nose with a percussion hammer.
nociceptive r. Any reflex produced by a painful stimulus.
oesophagosalivary r. Stimulation of the oesophagus producing salivation; *also called* Roger's reflex.

palatal r. Swallowing caused by stimulation of the palate.
palm-chin r. Palmomental *reflex.
palmomental r. Irritation of the thenar eminence on one hand producing contraction of the facial muscles on the same side.
pathologic r. Any reflex that is the result of a pathological condition, and not normal; a diagnostic sign.
pharyngeal r. Contraction of the constrictor pharyngis muscles produced by stimulation of the posterior pharyngeal wall.
zygomatic r. Lateral movement of the mandible to the percussed side in response to a tap over the zygomatic bone with a percussion hammer.

reflex, Bekhterev's *See* Bekhterev's reflex.

reflex, Roger's Oesophagosalivary *reflex.

regainer A device used to recover something which has been lost.
space r. A form of space maintainer used to restore the space between teeth which may have been lost after tooth extraction.

registration *In dentistry,* the record of jaw relations in certain desired positions.

regression 1. A going or turning back; a return to an earlier state. 2. Subsidence of fever or of a disease.

regressive Relating to or characterized by regression.

regurgitation The return of undigested or partially digested food from the stomach or oesophagus to the mouth, or of fluid or semifluid to the nose.

rehabilitation Restoration of health, form and function after damage or disease.
oral r. Comprehensive treatment designed to restore health, function and appearance to the mouth and the teeth.

Reid's base line (R.W. Reid, 1851-1939. Scottish anatomist). An imaginary line from the infraorbital ridge through the external auditory meatus to the midline of the skull.

reimplantation *Replantation.

Reiter's syndrome (H.C.J. Reiter, 1881-1969. German physician). A disease characterized by arthritis, conjunctivitis and urethritis, frequently with oral lesions which are painless, red raised areas on the tongue and oral mucosa.

rejection An immune response resulting in the failure of the body to accept grafted tissue.

relation The position or association of one object to another.
acentric r. Eccentric jaw *relation.
centric r. Retruded jaw *relation.
eccentric jaw r. Any jaw relation of the mandible to the maxilla which is protruded or lateral to retruded jaw relation.
jaw r. Any relationship of the mandible to the maxilla.
maxillomandibular r. Jaw *relation.
retruded jaw r. The relation of the jaws that obtains when the condyles are in the most retruded unstrained position in the glenoid fossa from which lateral excursions of the jaw can be made. In an edentulous mouth it is applied to the position of the alveolar processes with the jaws at rest.

relief 1. The easing of pain or anxiety. 2. The outline of ridges and hollows within the mouth which are reproduced in a denture.

relief chamber A recess in the surface of a denture base to reduce pressure on a specific area in the mouth.

reline *In dentistry*: 1. To resurface or rebase a denture for a more accurate fit. 2. To apply a new lining to the inside of a prepared cavity.

remedy Any cure or preventive measure.

remission 1. The abatement of disease symptoms. 2. The period of such an abatement.

repetatur Latin for *let it be repeated*; used in prescription writing, and abbreviated *rep.*

replantation Replacement of a tooth into the socket from which it has been removed.

resection The cutting away of part of an organ, used especially of the ends of bones which form a joint.
root r. *Apicectomy.

residual Left behind; relating to a residue.

residue That which is left after some part has been removed; a remainder.

resin An amorphous, inflammable vegetable substance, exuded from plants and trees; it is transparent or translucent, insoluble in water but readily soluble in ether, alcohol or volatile oils, and readily fusible.
acrylic r. Acrylic *polymer.
bonding r. An unfilled resin used to help the bonding of a resin cement to etched enamel.
composite r. A synthetic resin containing a high proportion of inorganic filling material.
epoxy r. A synthetic form of resin containing a hardening agent; it is used in dies and for coating, and for adhesive purposes, and is resistant to heat and chemicals.
filled r. A type of resin-based material that contains a proportion of inorganic material such as quartz; the set material is translucent.
glazing r. A form of resin that can be used to coat the surface of filled resin.
quick-cure r. Self-curing *resin.
self-curing r. One that can be hardened without heat, using a chemical catalyst and an activator.
synthetic r. Any synthetic form of resin used in the manufacture of dentures, etc.
thermosetting r. One that hardens and solidifies with the application of heat.

resinous Relating to resin.

resistance form *of a cavity* The shape of a cavity designed to withstand the stress to which the restoration is subjected during mastication.

resorbable Capable of being reabsorbed; used of materials which can be resorbed into the body.

resorption Physiological reabsorption of tissues or secreted matter. *In dentistry,* applied to absorption of the roots of primary teeth, and of the alveolar process after tooth extraction.
external tooth r. Resorption of a tooth root from the outer surface or the apex; it may be a normal process, or have some pathological cause.
internal tooth r. A form of tooth resorption thought to be initiated by trauma or associated with inflammatory pulp hyperplasia; the tooth crown becomes a pinkish colour as the vascular pulp expands into the resorbed area. *Also called* 'pink spot'.

resorption lacuna One of the absorption spaces under the periosteum, semilunar hollows which are, or have been, occupied by osteoclasts.

respiration The act of drawing air into the lungs and the process of the body tissues taking in oxygen and expelling carbon dioxide.

rest 1. Repose after activity. 2. Embryonic *rest. 3. *In dentistry*, an extension on a partial denture or orthodontic appliance to assist in its support or stabilization.
embryonic r. The remnants of embryonic tissue retained within a fully developed organism.
epithelial cell r's. The remains of the epithelial root sheath (Hertwig's sheath) found in the periodontal ligament, and contributing to the formation of dental cysts; *also called* rests of Malassez.
epithelial r. Embryonic *rest.
foetal r. Embryonic *rest.
incisal r. An extension or projection on a partial denture which rests on or engages with the incisal edge of an anterior tooth.
lingual r. An extension or projection on a partial denture which rests on or engages with the lingual surface of an anterior tooth.
occlusal r. A cast metal projection on a partial denture, extending over and resting upon the occlusal or other prepared surface of a natural tooth, and acting as an indirect retainer.

restbite The relationship of the dental arches with the jaws at rest.

restoration 1. Replacement of missing or removed substance or tissue, as in the filling of teeth, or in prosthetic work in the mouth. 2. A dental filling.

rests of Malassez Epithelial cell *rests.

retainer, retaining appliance 1. *In prosthetic dentistry*, any form of attachment by which a restoration is fastened to an abutment tooth. 2. *In orthodontics*, any appliance that holds in position teeth that have been moved.
continuous bar r. A metal bar along the lingual surfaces of the teeth, used in prosthetic dentistry to stabilize them and to act as an indirect retainer for a bridge or partial denture; *also called* Kennedy bar.
direct r. An attachment or clasp on a partial denture which connects with the abutment tooth.
indirect r. Part of a partial denture which acts indirectly on the opposite side of the fulcrum line from the direct retainers, to prevent displacement in free-end dentures.
secondary r. Indirect *retainer.
space r. Space *maintainer.

retainer, Hawley's *See* Hawley retainer.

retardation Delay or slowness of development, or hindrance of function.

retention 1. Keeping in place permanently, as of dentures in the mouth. 2. Keeping within the body matter normally excreted, as of urine in the bladder.

retention cyst One caused by the retention of glandular secretion.

retention form The shape of a cavity, designed to prevent displacement of the restoration by lifting or tipping stress.

retention index An index for assessing the potential of the tooth surfaces in an individual to retain food debris, etc. Each tooth is scored round the gingival margin, in four areas, on a scale of 0-3, based on the presence of calculus and carious cavities and on the state of the margins of any restorations; each score is divided by 4 and the sum of all the scores is divided by the number of teeth present.

retention plate 1. The foundation for an obturator. 2. Any orthodontic retaining appliance.

reticular Relating to a net or net-like structure.

reticulo-endothelial system The system of specialized reticular and endothelial cells concentrated in the bone marrow, liver, spleen and lymph glands; they are concerned in the formation and destruction of blood cells, and in iron metabolism, and are part of the defensive mechanisms in inflammation and immunity.

reticulo-endothelium The tissue that forms the reticulo-endothelial system.

reticulum Fibrous net-like tissue. *stellate r.* The tissue between the outer and inner dental epithelium of the enamel organ before amelogenesis.

retina The light-sensitive innermost coat of the eye.

retina, central artery of the *See* Table of Arteries—centralis retinae.

retraction *of the jaws* 1. The condition in which the mandible is drawn back from its normal position in relation to the orbital plane. 2. The process of drawing back the mandible in this way.

retractor A surgical instrument for drawing back the edges of a wound to allow access to deeper structures, or holding back other tissues or organs.

retro- Prefix signifying *behind, backward.*

retro-alveolism A condition in which the alveolar process is positioned posterior to the base of the jaw; it may be *maxillary* or *mandibular.*

retrobuccal Relating to the region of the mouth behind the cheeks.

retrocheilia The condition in which one lip is farther back than normal.

retrofilling Retrograde root *filling.

retrogenia A condition in which the chin is set back in relation to the rest of the facial skeleton.

retrognathia, retrognathism 1. The condition of having a retruded lower jaw. 2. Underdevelopment of the mandible or of the maxilla, or of both.

retrolingual Behind the tongue.

retromandibular Relating to the region of the mouth behind the mandible.

retromandibular vein Joins common facial vein and drains into the external jugular. *See* Table of Veins—retromandibularis.

retromandibulism A condition in which the body of the mandible is positioned posteriorly.

retromaxillary Behind the maxilla, relating to that region of the mouth situated behind the maxilla.

retromaxillism A condition in which the maxilla is positioned posteriorly.

retromolar Situated behind the molar teeth.

retronasal Behind the nose.

retropharyngeal Behind the pharynx.

retroposed Displaced backwards.

retrusion *of the jaws* *Retraction of the jaws.

retrusion *of the teeth* Malposition of teeth behind the line of the normal arch.

Retzius' lines (M.G. Retzius, 1842-1919. Swedish anatomist). *Enamel striae of Retzius.

rhabdo- Prefix signifying *rod* or *rod-shaped.*

rhabdomyoblastoma *Rhabdomyosarcoma.

rhabdomyoma A rare benign tumour made up of striated muscle cells.

rhabdomyosarcoma A malignant connective tissue tumour in which some cells appear as abnormal striated muscle.

rhabdosarcoma *Rhabdomyosarcoma.

rhagades Chaps or excoriations of the skin; often syphilitic lesions, appearing on the lips and round the mouth.

rhaphe *See* Raphe.

rhinion The lower end of the internasal suture.

rhinitis Inflammation of the nasal mucosa.

rhinitis sicca Inflammation and wasting of the mucous membranes of the nose, with no secretion. Part of the syndrome complex known as *Sjögren's syndrome*.

rhino- Prefix signifying *nose*.

rhinocheiloplasty Plastic surgery of both the nose and the upper lip.

rhinolalia A nasal intonation, caused by defect or disease in the nasal passages.

rhinolith A calculus or concretion occurring in the nose.

rhinopharyngitis mutilans *Gangosa.

rhinorrhagia Nosebleed.

rhinorrhoea Any discharge of fluid from the nose.

rhinoschisis Congenital nasal cleft.

rhinoscopy Examination of the nasal passages by means of a speculum.

rhizagra An old instrument used to extract the roots of teeth.

rhizo- Prefix signifying *root*.

rhizodontropy The attachment of an artificial crown to the tooth root by means of a pivot.

rhizodontrypy Surgical perforation of a tooth root to allow for the discharge of fluid.

rhizoid Resembling a root, root-like.

rhizotomy Surgical division of either a tooth root or a nerve root.

rhodo- Prefix signifying *red*.

rhyparia *Materia alba; an old term.

ribbon arch An orthodontic appliance of flattened wire conforming to the dental arch, used for anchorage in the movement of teeth; a type of expansion arch.

riboflavin Vitamin B_{12}, occurring in milk, liver, cheese, eggs and malt, and in other foods; used therapeutically in deficiency states.

Richmond crown (C.M. Richmond, 1835-1902. American dentist). A porcelain-veneer faced gold crown attached by means of a post to the tooth root.

rickets Defective skeletal mineralization in childhood associated with vitamin D deficiency; oral defects may include retarded mandibular development, delayed eruption and malposition of teeth.

Rickettsia (H.T. Ricketts, 1871-1910. American pathologist). A genus of the tribe Rickettsieae; seen as short, non-motile rods, Gram-negative and aerobic; parasitic agents of typhus and spotted fever.

Rickettsieae (H.T. Ricketts, 1871-1910. American pathologist). The first tribe of the Rickettsiaceae family, small pleomorphic intracellular parasitic organisms, pathogenic or related to species that are pathogenic to humans and some other vertebrates.

rictal Relating to a rictus or fissure.

rictus 1. A fissure or cleft. 2. Any gaping condition.

rictus lupinus Cleft *palate.

ridge A projecting or raised edge.
alveolar r. The crest remaining in an edentulous mouth after the resorption of the alveolar process.
basal r. *Cingulum².
buccocervical r. A ridge on the buccal surface of a primary molar near to the cervix of the tooth.

buccogingival r. Buccocervical *ridge.
dental r. Any elevation on a tooth, forming a cusp or tooth margin.
edentulous r. Alveolar *ridge.
external oblique r. A smooth ridge on the buccal surface of the body of the mandible, extending from the anterior border of the ramus to the region of the mental foramen.
linguocervical r. A ridge on the lingual surface of an anterior tooth near to the cervix.
linguogingival r. Linguocervical *ridge.
marginal r. Any one of the ridges forming the outer margins on the occlusal surface of a molar or premolar, or the lingual surface of an incisor or canine.
maxillary r. Dental *lamina.
mylohyoid r. The ridge on the internal surface of the mandible to which the mylohyoid muscle is attached.
oblique r. A ridge running obliquely across the occlusal surface of a maxillary molar.
palatine r's. The median raphe and the lateral mucosal corrugations on the hard palate.
residual r., residual alveolar r. The remaining alveolar bone once the tooth has been removed; particularly an alveolar ridge that has undergone resorption.
sublingual r. 1. Sublingual *fold. 2. *Frenulum linguae.
supplemental r. Any abnormal or extra ridge on a tooth surface.

ridge lap That area of the surface of an artificial tooth adapted to fit over the alveolar ridge.

Riga's aphthae (A. Riga, 1832-1919. Italian physician). Cachectic aphthae of the tongue, mucous membranes of the mouth and gastrointestinal tract.

Riga's disease (A. Riga, 1832-1919. Italian physician). 1. *Fede's disease; *also called* Riga-Fede's disease. 2. *Riga's aphthae.

Riggs' disease (J.M. Riggs, 1810-85. American dentist). *Pyorrhoea alveolaris.

rim A narrow edging or well-defined edge.
bite r. Occlusal *rim.
occlusal r. A rim of wax mounted on a denture base; it is used in the recording of the relationships of the jaws.

rima glottidis The *glottis.

rima oris The mouth opening.

ring
infancy r. A line marking the arrested mineralization of tooth enamel, formed at about 12 months.
neonatal r. Neonatal *line.

Ringer's solution (S. Ringer, 1835-1910. English physiologist). A solution of sodium chloride, calcium chloride and potassium chloride used, *in dentistry*, as a vehicle in anaesthetic injection.

risorius muscle Draws angle of mouth sideways. *See* Table of Muscles.

risus sardonicus A grinning distortion of the face produced by spasm of the facial muscles; seen in tetanus.

Rivalta's disease (S. Rivalta, 1852-1893. Italian veterinary surgeon). *Actinomycosis.

Rivet's angle The angle basion-prosthion-nasion.

Rivinus' gland (A.Q. Rivinus, 1652-1723. German anatomist). The sublingual *gland.

Roach's attachment (F.E. Roach, 1868-1960. American dentist). A form of attachment for removable partial dentures, consisting of a ball and socket joint, the socket being in a prepared crown or inlay.

Rochette bridge A bridge in which the abutments are bonded to the acid-etched surfaces of the supporting teeth. Although the teeth undergo little preparation, the metal abutments are perforated to improve the mechanical retention of the bonding agent.

rod

enamel r. Enamel *prism.

rodent ulcer A basal-cell carcinoma of superficial origin, arising in the epidermis, and occurring generally on the face or neck.

roentgenogram (W.K. von Roentgen, 1845-1923. German physician). A photograph taken using roentgen rays or x-rays.

roentgenography (W.K. von Roentgen, 1845-1923. German physician). *Radiography.

body-section r. *Tomography.

roentgenology (W.K. von Roentgen, 1845-1923. German physician). The science of the diagnostic and therapeutic uses of roentgen rays or x-rays.

Roger-Anderson extraoral splint (R. Anderson, 1891-1971. American orthopaedic surgeon). A type of splint using threaded steel pins and rod connectors to stabilize complex mandibular fractures.

Roger's reflex (G.H. Roger, 1860-1946. French physiologist). Oesophagosalivary *reflex.

roll

cotton-wool r. A small and tightly packed roll of cotton wool used in the mouth to absorb saliva and assist in keeping the operative field dry.

rongeurs Bone-cutting forceps.

root *In dentistry*, that part of the tooth in the gums, covered by cementum.

accessory r. A supplemental tooth root, differing in size, shape and direction from the main root or roots.

anatomical r. That portion of a tooth which is covered by cementum.

clinical r. That portion of a tooth which is attached by the periodontal ligament to the alveolar bone.

lingual r. That root of a multirooted mandibular tooth which is situated nearest to the tongue.

palatal r. That root of a multirooted maxillary tooth which is situated nearest to the palate.

physiological r. Clinical *root.

retained r. A tooth root, or part of a root, left in the bone or soft tissue after extraction, as a result of severe caries, or to prevent alveolar resorption.

root *of the tongue* The pharyngeal, fixed portion of the tongue.

root abscess An apical *granuloma.

root amputation Surgical excision of the apical portion of a tooth root.

root canal The canal, containing dental pulp, running through the root of the tooth to the pulp chamber.

root dehiscence A pathological condition in which the vestibular surface of a tooth root is exposed to the oral cavity over some or all of the apical two-thirds of its length.

root diaphragm That part of the epithelial root sheath which angles beneath the dental papilla early in dental development.

root filling 1. The process of inserting material into a root canal to fill it up and seal it. 2. Any material used for this purpose.

retrograde r. f. The placing of a root filling in the apex of a tooth, which is surgically exposed, to seal the end of the root canal after apicectomy; the material is inserted through the apex, rather than through the pulp chamber.

reverse r. f. Retrograde *root filling.

root planing Smoothing of the roughened root surfaces of a tooth after subgingival scaling.

root sheath Epithelial root *sheath.

root trunk That portion of a multi-rooted tooth between the cervical line and the branching of the roots.

rostral 1. Relating to a rostrum or beak. 2. Relating to the front end of a body, as opposed to *caudal.*

rostrum A beak or beak-like appendage.

rotation *In dentistry,* the turning of a tooth about its central axis, either correcting a malposed tooth, or the gradual twisting of a normal one to malposition.

Rothia (named after G.D. Roth, 20th century American bacteriologist, who first isolated it). A genus of bacteria of the order *Actinomycetales,* Gram-positive, aerobic and non-sporing.

R. dentocariosa A species found in the oral cavity and on the teeth of primates, especially in carious material, plaque and calculus. *Also called Actinomyces dentocariosus.*

rouge Powdered iron oxide, used *in dentistry* to polish gold restorations.

-rrhagia Suffix signifying *excessive discharge.*

-rrhaphy Suffix signifying *suturing.*

rubber dam A thin sheet of rubber, pierced to fit over the teeth leaving their crowns exposed, used to exclude moisture from the field of operation during cavity preparation and other dental procedures.

rubber-dam clamp A form of spring clip which holds the rubber dam round the neck of an exposed tooth.

rubber-dam clamp forceps Specially designed forceps for placing rubber-dam clamps on the teeth.

rubber-dam holder A strap device for holding a rubber dam in position over the mouth, and for keeping the edges back clear of the field of operation.

rubber-dam punch An instrument used to punch holes of various sizes in a rubber dam.

rubefacient 1. Causing a reddening of the skin. 2. Any agent that causes redness or erythema of the skin; applied to substances used as counter-irritants.

rudiment An organ or part either imperfectly developed or at an early stage in its development.

rudimentary Only partially, or imperfectly, developed.

ruga (*pl.* rugae) A ridge, fold or wrinkle.

ruga palatinae Palatine *fold.

Russell index (A.L. Russell, contemporary American dentist). Periodontal disease *index.

S

'S' point *Sella turcica[2].

sig. Abbreviation for *signatur*—let it be labelled; used in prescription writing.

sing. Abbreviation for *singulorum*—of each; used in prescription writing.

Sn Chemical symbol for tin.

SNA *In cephalometrics,* the angle between the S-N plane and the line joining the nasion to the subspinale (point 'A').

SNB *In cephalometrics,* the angle between the S-N plane and the line joining the nasion to the supramentale (point 'B').

S-N plane *In cephalometrics,* that plane which passes through the centre of the shadow of the sella turcica and the nasion and which is perpendicular to the sagittal plane.

saburra A foul condition of the mouth and teeth or of the stomach due to food debris.

sac A pouch or bag-like covering.
dental s. The vascular tissue enclosing the enamel organ.

saccular nerve Supplies filaments for the macula sacculi. *See* Table of Nerves—saccularis.

sacro- Prefix signifying *flesh*.

saddle *In prosthetic dentistry,* that part of a partial denture which is supported by and in contact with the underlying alveolar tissue.
bounded s. One limited by the presence of a natural tooth at each end.
free-end s. One having no natural tooth distally.

sagittal 1. Shaped like an arrow. 2. *In anatomy,* running antero-posteriorly.

sagittal sinus *inferior*: A venous sinus joining the great cerebral vein to form the straight sinus. *See* Table of Veins—sinus sagittalis inferior.
superior: A venous sinus draining into the transverse sinus. *See* Table of Veins—sinus sagittalis superior.

Saint Apollonia's disease Toothache.

saline Salty; relating to a salt.

saliva Clear, slightly alkaline fluid secreted by the salivary glands, assisting in the mastication and digestion of food.

saliva ejector An apparatus used to suck saliva from the mouth during operative dentistry, thus keeping the field of operation free from moisture.

salivant Producing a flow of saliva.

salivary Relating to saliva.

salivation Production and secretion of saliva.

salivatory Causing or promoting salivation.

salivolithiasis The condition of having a salivary *calculus[1].

Salmonella (D.E. Salmon, 1850-1914. American bacteriologist). A genus of the Enterobacteriaceae family of bacteria; non-spore forming, motile rods, facultatively anaerobic, Gram-negative, found primarily as intestinal parasites, pathogenic for man and many animal species.

salpingopalatal, salpingopalatine Relating to the pharyngotympanic tube and the palate.

salpingopharyngeal muscle Part of M. palatopharyngeus. *See* Table of Muscles.

Salter's lines (Sir Samuel J.A. Salter, 1825-97. English dentist). *Owen's contour lines.

sandarac varnish A solution of transparent resin in alcohol, used *in dentistry* as a separating fluid and protective coating for plaster casts.

Sandwith's bald tongue (F.M. Sandwith, 1853-1918. English physician). The smooth tongue surface seen in the later stages of pellagra.

sanguine 1. Bloody. 2. Hopeful, optimistic.

sanguineous Relating to blood; bloody.

sapid Of agreeable flavour.

sapro- Prefix signifying *rotten, decaying*.

saprodontia Dental *caries.

saprophyte A plant living on decaying or putrefying matter.

Sarcina A genus of Gram-positive cocci, non-motile and relatively aerotolerant, in which cell division occurs in three planes.

sarcoidosis A benign generalized granulomatous disease with lesions most commonly seen in the lungs, the liver, the spleen, the lymph nodes, lymphoid tissue and the skin; the salivary glands, particularly the parotid gland, may be involved, and lesions may also occur in the soft palate, the floor of the mouth, gingiva and cheek, presenting as submucosal nodules.

sarcoma A malignant tumour arising from any non-epithelial embryonic tissue.
ameloblastic s. Ameloblastic *fibrosarcoma.
endothelial s. *Ewing's sarcoma.
granulocytic s. *Chloroma.
osteogenic s. *Osteosarcoma.

sarcomatous Relating to a sarcoma.

saucerization The wide and shallow depression occurring about a wound or bone cavity, as in osteomyelitis.
pericervical s. A circular area of bone loss occurring about the necks of endosteal implants.

saucerize To shape a wound or bone cavity to a wide and shallow depression.

sausarism 1. Lingual paralysis. 2. A dry condition of the tongue.

saw An instrument having a thin blade with a sharp, serrated edge, used for cutting bone or other hard tissue.

scaler A hand instrument used for the removal of calculus and other deposits from the tooth surface.
ultrasonic s. Electromechanical device with a handpiece and interchangeable tips which are vibrated at a very high frequency; it is used to dislodge dental calculus from tooth surfaces.

scaling The removal of calculus and other accretions from the surfaces of the teeth with specially designed instruments.

scalpel A small, straight surgical knife.

scalpriform In the shape of a chisel.

scapho- Prefix signifying *boat-shaped*.

scaphocephalic, scaphocephalous Having a ridged, keel-shaped skull.

scar The mark left in tissue after the healing of a wound or sore.

Scarpa's foramen (A. Scarpa, 1747-1832. Italian anatomist and surgeon). A foramen occasionally present in the midline fossa in the hard palate.

Scarpa's nerve (A. Scarpa, 1747-1832. Italian anatomist and surgeon). The *nasopalatine nerve.

schindylesis A type of fibrous joint in which one bone fits into the other.

-schisis Suffix signifying *fissure* or *cleft*.

schisto-, schizo- Prefix signifying *fissure* or *cleft*.

schistoglossia A tongue fissure.

schistoprosopia Congenital facial cleft.

schizo- Prefix signifying *division*.

schizodontia *Gemination[2].

schizognathism Jaw cleft.

schizoprosopia Any congenital fissure of the face.

schmutz pyorrhoea Old term for a chronic form of periodontitis, caused by persistently poor dental hygiene.

Schour-Massler index (I. Schour, 1900-64. American oral histologist; M. Massler, b. 1912. American paedodontist). PMA *index.

Schreger's lines (C.H.T. Schreger, 1768-1833. German anatomist). *In dentine*: concentric rings which appear in transverse section parallel to the amelodentinal junction and mark the coincidence of the primary curvatures of dentinal tubules. *In enamel*: a series of lines or bands in the enamel, visible, in a longitudinal section of a human tooth, by reflected light.

schwannoma (T. Schwann, 1810-82. German anatomist). 1. *Neurilemmoma. 2. The name formerly given to a rare malignant tumour of the nerve-sheath tissue, found in the mandible and histologically similar to the fibrosarcoma.

Schwarz activator, Schwarz appliance (A.M. Schwarz, b. 1887. American orthodontist). Bow *activator.

scion tooth A tooth used for transplantation, to replace one extracted.

scirrhous Hard; especially relating to a hard carcinoma or scirrhus.

scirrhus A hard carcinoma containing dense connective tissue.

sclero- Prefix signifying *hard*.

scleroderma A systemic disease affecting the fibrous connective tissue and characterized by progressive hardening and thickening of patches of the skin and mucous membranes; it may also involve the periodontal ligament.

scleroid Hard; of a hard texture.

sclerosis Hardening of a vessel or part; applied particularly to arteries, and to proliferation of connective tissue in the nervous system as a result of degeneration.
dentinal s. Mineralization of the dentinal tubules producing translucent areas and tissue changes in the tooth.

sclerotic Relating to or affected by sclerosis.

scobinate Having a rough or roughened surface.

scoliodontic Having a tooth that has twisted in its socket.

-scopy Suffix signifying *examination*.

scorbutic Relating to or affected with scurvy.

scorbutus *Scurvy.

screen
oral s. A thin plastic plate used in orthodontic treatment and constructed so that it is in contact with the tips of protruding maxillary incisors whilst appearing to cover the labial surfaces of all the maxillary teeth; lip pressure tips the incisors lingually. It is also used as an inhibitor of mouth-breathing and thumb-sucking.
vestibular s. Oral *screen.

screw A threaded pin, post or peg, used for attachment.
adjustable s. A very accurately threaded type of orthodontic screw, which enables exact adjustments to be made to appliances.
cover s. A thin covering designed to fit the implant abutment and connect it to the prosthesis or superstructure.

jack s. See jackscrew.
orthodontic s. A type of screw used in certain orthodontic appliances to separate or to approximate the parts during treatment.
traction s. A screw used in orthodontics to produce a pulling force sufficient to move malposed teeth.

screw elevator An instrument that can be screwed into a retained root in order to draw it out.

screw post A threaded post, which can be screwed into a prepared root canal, and by which a denture may be attached.

scurvy A disease produced by vitamin C deficiency and characterized by general weakness and anaemia, swollen gums and mucocutaneous haemorrhage; it used to be common amongst sailors, but is now chiefly seen amongst the elderly.

sealant
pit and fissure s. Any agent, usually a form of resin, used for pit and fissure sealing.

sealing
pit and fissure s. The filling up of developmental pits and fissures in posterior teeth to prevent the onset of occlusal caries.

seat
basal s. The tissue area on which the denture base rests.

seat *of a cavity* In simple cavities, the floor of the cavity; in proximo-occlusal or proximo-incisal cavities, the gingival wall.

sebaceous Relating to sebum.

sebaceous gland One of the glands that secrete sebum.

Sebileau's hollow (P. Sebileau, 1860-1953. French surgeon). The depression beneath the tongue between the sublingual glands.

sebum A semi-fluid substance containing fat, keratin and epithelial debris secreted by the sebaceous glands.

secodont Having cutting edges on the tubercles of the molar teeth.

secretion 1. The production and ejection of a specific fluid material by a gland. 2. Any substance thus produced and ejected.

sectorial Cutting.

sedation 1. A condition of decreased functional activity. 2. The production of calm, or lessened excitement.

sedative 1. Relating to sedation. 2. Any agent that produces sedation.

segment When applied to the dentition this refers to a group of teeth within a single arch. In the ISO nomenclature a segment is called a 'sextant'.
anterior s. Term used in ISO nomenclature for the labial *segment.
buccal s. The molar and premolar teeth; there are two buccal segments in each dental arch—left and right; in ISO nomenclature these are called *upper right, upper left, lower left, lower right* and are designated 03, 05, 06, 08.
labial s. The incisor and canine teeth as a single group within one arch; in the ISO nomenclature the labial segments are called *upper anterior* and *lower anterior* and designated 04 and 07.

selenodont Having teeth with longitudinal crescentic ridges, as, for example, the molar teeth in herbivores.

sella turcica 1. The depression on the inner surface of the sphenoid bone, forming the pituitary fossa. 2. A cephalometric landmark, 'S', in the centre of the shadow of the sella turcica on a lateral skull radiograph.

semi- Prefix signifying *half.*

semicohesive Only partially cohesive.

semispinalis muscles Muscles involved in extending the head and vertebral column. *See* Table of Muscles.

senescence Ageing.
dental s. The changes occurring in the mouth and in the teeth as a result of ageing.

senile Relating to old age.

senility Old age.

separator Anything used to effect a separation. *In dentistry,* a device for forcing apart adjoining teeth.

sepsis Poisoning as a result of the absorption of putrefactive products.
focal s. A local source of infection which may spread to cause systemic disease.
oral s. A septic condition in the mouth producing excessive bacterial activity which may affect the general health.

septal Relating to a septum.

septal artery Supplies the nasal mucous membrane. *See* Table of Arteries—septalis posterior.

septal bone Interalveolar *septum.

septic Relating to or caused by sepsis.

septicaemia A systemic condition due to the presence of bacteria and their poisons in the blood.

septicaemic Relating to or affected with septicaemia.

septicemia *See* septicaemia.

septum A thin partition between two masses of soft tissue or two cavities.
alveolar s. Interalveolar *septum.
enamel s. Enamel *cord.
gingival s. That part of the gingiva lying between two teeth.
gum s. Gingival *septum.
interalveolar s. That portion of the alveolar process between adjoining tooth sockets.
interdental s. Interalveolar *septum.
interradicular s. The bony partition between the roots of a multirooted tooth.
intra-alveolar s. A bony partition within the tooth socket.
lingual s. The median, vertical fibrous partition of the tongue, providing attachment for the intrinsic muscles.

sequela (*pl.* sequelae) Any condition following on a disease, of which it is the direct or indirect result.

sequential 1. In sequence. 2. Relating to sequelae.

sequestrectomy The removal of a bone sequestrum by surgery.

sequestrum A piece of necrotic bone that has become detached from the sound bone.

sero- Prefix signifying *serum.*

serous 1. Relating to a serum. 2. Serum-producing.

serpiginous Creeping.

serrated Having a toothed edge, like a saw.

serration 1. The condition of being toothed or having a saw-like edge. 2. A notch, as between two teeth on a saw edge, or a row of such notches.

Serres' glands (A.E.R.A. Serres, 1786-1868. French physiologist). Gingival *glands.

serum 1. The clear, amber-coloured fluid obtained by the separating out of the solid elements in blood by clotting. 2. Blood serum obtained from immune animals or humans and used in the prevention and treatment of disease.

serum hepatitis A form of hepatitis caused by hepatitis B virus and spread by blood transfusion or contaminated instruments, especially syringes; it is very similar to acute infective hepatitis, but may be fatal in the acute stage.

sesqui- Prefix signifying *one-and-one-half; in the ratio of two to three.*

sesquihora An hour and a half.

sessile Having a broad base; as opposed to *pedunculated.*

setiform Bristle-shaped.

set-up Trial *denture.

sextant Term used in ISO nomenclature for *segment.

shaft *of an instrument.* The handle.

shank *of an instrument.* The slender portion joining the handle to the blade or nib.

Sharpey's fibres (W. Sharpey, 1802-80. English anatomist). 1. The collagen fibres of connective tissue between bone and periosteum. 2. *In dentistry*, those parts of the collagen fibres of the periodontal ligament which are embedded in the alveolar bone or in the cementum of the tooth.

Shea-Anthony antral balloon *Sinus balloon.

sheath A covering or sac; applied to the outer envelope of nerves and arteries.

carotid s. The envelope containing the common carotid artery, the internal jugular vein, and the vagus nerve.

dentinal s. *Neumann's sheath.

epithelial root s. A continuation of the internal and external enamel epithelium at the lower rim of the enamel organ, which provides the inductive stimulus for root dentine formation and determines root morphology; *also called* Hertwig's sheath.

root s. Epithelial root *sheath.

sheath of Hertwig Epithelial root *sheath.

shell crown A crown consisting of a metal shell, contoured to fit over the crown of an existing natural tooth; *also called* a cap crown.

shingles *Herpes zoster.

shock Acute circulatory failure, marked by a fall in blood pressure, rapid and feeble pulse, pallor and clamminess of the skin, shallow respiration, and similar symptoms.

shoulder crown An artificial crown shaped at the base to sit on a prepared root without a metal collar.

siagonagra Pain of the jaw-bone.

siagonantritis Inflammation of the maxillary antrum.

sial-, sialo- Prefix signifying *saliva.*

sialadenitis Inflammation of a salivary gland.

sialadenoncus Any salivary gland tumour.

sialagogue *Sialogogue.

sialaporia Deficiency in the amount of saliva secreted.

sialectasia, sialectasis *Sialoangiectasis.

sialic Relating to or characteristic of saliva.

sialitis *Sialadenitis.

sialo-adenitis *Sialadenitis.

sialo-angiectasis Distention of the salivary ducts.

sialocele A tumour or cyst of the salivary glands.

sialodochitis *Sialoductitis.

sialoductitis Inflammation of the salivary ducts.

sialogenous Saliva-producing.

sialogogue 1. Saliva-producing. 2. An agent that promotes the flow of saliva.

sialography Radiography of the salivary glands and ducts.

sialoid 1. Relating to saliva. 2. Saliva-like.

sialolith A salivary *calculus[1].

sialolithiasis The process of formation of salivary *calculi[1].

sialoma A salivary tumour.

sialometaplasia
necrotizing s. An ulcerous condition of the hard and soft palates with necrosis of the mucous cells of the salivary glands, some of which may be replaced by squamous epithelium.

sialoncus A tumour of the sublingual gland caused by obstruction of the duct.

sialorrhoea *Hypersalivation.

sialoschesis Suppression of the secretion of the salivary glands.

sialosemeiology Diagnosis by chemical examination and analysis of saliva.

sialosis 1. Recurrent, non-inflammatory bilateral swelling of the parotid glands, which may eventually develop as lipomatosis; it has been seen in cases of malnutrition, hormonal disturbance, chronic alcoholism and cirrhosis of the liver. 2. *Hypersalivation.

sialotic Relating to or characterized by saliva.

sialozemia Uncontrolled flow of saliva, often with dribbling.

sigmoid sinus A venous sinus, continuous with the transverse sinus and draining into the internal jugular vein. *See* Table of Veins—sinus sigmoideus.

signatur Latin for *let it be labelled*; used in prescription writing, and abbreviated *sig.*

signature That part of a prescription written on the label of the medicine, with the directions for administration.

silicone A plastic material based on silicon. *In dentistry* it is used as an impression compound.

silver A soft, white, malleable and ductile metal, chemical symbol Ag; soluble in dilute nitric acid, hot concentrated sulphuric acid, and solutions of alkali cyanides.

silver cone Silver *point.

silver point A fine cone of silver used to fill a root canal after the removal of the pulp.

sinciput The top of the head.

singulorum Latin for *of each*; used in prescription writing, and abbreviated *sing.*

sino-, sinu- Prefix signifying *sinus.*

sinus 1. A hollow or cavity. 2. A channel for venous blood, especially in the cranium. 3. An air cavity, especially one communicating with the nose. 4. A tract lined with granulations and leading from a suppurating cavity to the body surface.
air s. *Sinus[3].
ethmoidal s. One of the many small intercommunicating cavities forming the labyrinth of the ethmoid bone, opening into the nasal cavity.
frontal s. One of two cavities in the frontal bone, varying in size in different skulls, and found above the root of the nose.
maxillary s. A large air sinus in the maxilla communicating with the middle meatus of the nose; *also called* the maxillary antrum or the antrum of Highmore.
oral s. *Stomodeum.
palatine s. A variable cavity in the orbital process of the palatine bone, opening into the sphenoidal or a posterior ethmoidal sinus.

paranasal s. One of the air cavities in the skull bones of the face, communicating with the nasal cavity; they are named after the bones in which they occur.

sphenoidal s. A cavity, of variable size, in the body of the sphenoid bone, above the nasopharynx and the nasal cavity; it is divided by a bone septum into a right and left sinus.

venous s. *Sinus^2. For venous sinuses *see* Table of Veins—sinus.

sinus balloon A plastic or rubber device, like a balloon, which can be expanded either with air or with liquid, and which is used to support depressed fractures of the zygomaxillary process. *Also called* Shea-Anthony antral balloon.

sinusal Relating to a sinus.

sinusitis Inflammation of the mucosal lining of an air sinus, most commonly that of the maxillary sinus.

skeletal Relating to a skeleton.

skeletal classification of malocclusion *See under* malocclusion.

skeletal fixation, external *In surgery*, a method of immobilizing the ends of a fractured bone by external metal pins or screw appliances, used especially for an edentulous mouth.

skeletal fixation, internal *In surgery*, the immobilization of fractured bone by direct wiring, by the use of bone plates or by fixation by medullary pins.

skeleton The bony framework of an animal body.

skeleton denture A form of partial denture which is mainly tooth-borne, and which has connectors of the smallest size consistent with adequate strength, leaving the mucous membrane and the gingival margins exposed.

skiagram A radiograph or roentgenogram.

skin The outer covering of the body, consisting of the epidermis and the dermis.

Skinner classification (C.N. Skinner, contemporary American dentist). A classification of removable partial dentures, very similar to the *Kennedy classification.

Class I: Partial dentures with abutment teeth both anterior and posterior to the denture base; unilateral or bilateral, maxillary or mandibular.

Class II: All remaining teeth are posterior to the denture base; unilateral or bilateral, maxillary or mandibular.

Class III: All abutment teeth are anterior to the denture base; unilateral or bilateral, maxillary or mandibular.

Class IV: The denture base is both anterior and posterior to the abutment teeth, which may be central or between the sections of the base.

Class V: All abutment teeth are unilateral to the denture base.

skull The bony framework of the head.

slough The necrotizing tissue that scales or peels off in ulcerative conditions.

smoker's palate *Leukokeratosis nicotina palati.

smoker's tongue *Leukoplakia (*linguae*).

Snawdon's operation An operation to treat large maxillary cysts by opening the cyst into the nasal cavity and removing the partition between the cyst and the maxillary sinus.

socket The cavity or depression into which a corresponding part fits.

dry s. An acute inflammatory condition of the walls of a tooth socket following extraction of a tooth; localized alveolar osteitis.
tooth s. An *alveolus.

sodium A silver-white alkaline metallic element, chemical symbol Na, which oxidizes rapidly on exposure to air.

sodium fluoride A white powder form of fluoride, chemical formula NaF, used to adjust the concentration of fluoride ion in a water supply to an optimum level of 1 p.p.m. in water fluoridation, in tablet form for administration where the water supply is not so adjusted and in solution as a topical application for the prevention of dental caries.

sol A colloidal solution, in which the disperse medium is a liquid.

solder 1. A fusible alloy used to join two metal surfaces or edges. 2. The process of joining a metal in this way.

solubility The degree to which any substance is soluble.

soluble Capable of dissolving in a liquid to make a solution.

solution
disclosing s. A staining agent applied to the tooth surface in a mouthwash, which attaches to the plaque and other surface deposits and shows them up in some distinct colour against the normal clean enamel.
saline s. A solution of sodium chloride.

somato- Prefix signifying *body.*

sophronistae dentes Old term for a third molar tooth.

soporific Sleep-producing.

sorbifacient 1. Causing or promoting absorption. 2. Any agent that causes or promotes absorption.

sordes 1. Dirt; particularly the dark brown crust which forms on the teeth and lips in continued low fever. 2. *In dentistry,* food *debris.

sore 1. Painful. 2. Any lesion of the skin or mucous membrane.
cold s. *Herpes labialis.
hard s. *Chancre.

space
apical s. The area between the bony wall of the tooth socket and the apex of the tooth root; the site of an apical abscess.
buccal s., buccinator s. The space between the buccinator muscle and the masseter muscle.
denture s. The potential space available in an edentulous mouth within which a denture should lie.
freeway s. Interocclusal *clearance.
interdental s. The triangular space between two adjacent teeth, opening out into the embrasure.
interglobular s's. Large spaces found in dentine close to the amelo-dentinal junction, caused by incomplete mineralization.
interocclusal s. Interocclusal *clearance.
interproximal s. Interdental *space.
interradicular s. The space between the roots of a multirooted tooth.
leeway s. See Nance's leeway space.
periodontal s. A radiological term for the radiolucent area between the cementum and the alveolar bone seen on a radiograph.
proximal s., proximate s. Interdental *space.
retromylohyoid s. The space within the alveolingual sulcus along the lingual surface of the mandible behind the attachment of the mylohyoid muscle.
septal s. That area of the interdental space below the tooth contact point.
subgingival s. Gingival *sulcus.

submandibular s. The space formed by the division of the deep cervical fascia about the submandibular salivary gland.
submasseteric s. The space between the masseter muscle and the ascending ramus of the mandible.
submaxillary s. Submandibular *triangle of the neck.

space of Donders (F.C. Donders, 1818-89. Dutch physician and ophthalmologist). The space between the tongue and the palate with the mandible at rest.

space maintainer A passive orthodontic appliance used to prevent overcrowding of teeth or closure of a space into which a tooth is expected to erupt; it may be *fixed, removable* or *fixed-removable* (that is, removable only by the dentist).

span bridge Fixed *bridge.

spasm A sudden, involuntary and violent muscular contraction.

spasmodic 1. Relating to or characterized by spasm. 2. Intermittent, irregular.

spatula A flexible, blunt knife-shaped instrument used for mixing or spreading plaster or ointment.

spatulator A mechanical apparatus for mixing cements or amalgams.

species A group of organisms having certain characteristics distinguishing them from similar organisms within the same genus.

specific 1. Relating to a species. 2. Produced by one type of organism. 3. A medicine indicated for use in the treatment of a particular disease.

Spee, curve of (F. Graf von Spee, 1855-1937. German embryologist). *See* curve of Spee.

spheno- Prefix signifying *sphenoid bone*.

sphenoid Shaped like a wedge.

sphenoid bone The wedge-shaped bone at the base of the skull.

sphenoid fissure Superior orbital *fissure.

sphenoidal Relating to the sphenoid bone.

sphenomandibular Relating to the sphenoid bone and the mandible.

sphenomaxillary Relating to the sphenoid bone and the maxilla.

sphenopalatine Relating to the sphenoid bone and the palate.

sphenopalatine artery Supplies the lateral nasal wall and septum; *also called* A. nasopalatina. *See* Table of Arteries—sphenopalatina.

sphenopalatine nerve N. pterygopalatinus.
long s.n. N. nasopalatinus.
short s.n. N. nasalis posterior superior lateralis.
See Table of Nerves.

sphenoparietal sinus A venous sinus draining the dura mater and terminating in the cavernous sinus. *See* Table of Veins—sinus sphenoparietalis.

spheroid In the shape of a sphere.

spheroiding The tendency of amalgam to become round as a result of excess mercury in the mass.

sphincter muscle One that surrounds and closes a natural opening.

spillway *Embrasure.

spinal Relating to a spine.

spinalis muscles Muscles involved in extending the head and vertebral column. *See* Table of Muscles.

spindle A rod-like structure, tapered at both ends.
enamel s's. Short extensions into the enamel, across the amelodentinal junction, of dentinal tubules.

spine 1. A thorn-like, slender bone process. 2. The vertebral column of the body.
anterior nasal s. A median spine of bone projecting from the maxillae and supporting the septal cartilage of the nose.
mental s. Mental *tubercle.
posterior nasal s. The spine at the lower, posterior end of the nasal crest of the palatine bone.

spinous Relating to a spine.

Spirillum A genus of bacteria seen as rigid spiral rods, Gram-negative, motile, and generally aerobic.

Spirochaetaceae A family of slender spiral micro-organisms of the order Spirochaetales, Gram-negative, anaerobic and motile.

Spirochaetales An order of spiral micro-organisms, unicellular and motile.

Spironema **Treponema*.

Spix's spine (J.B. Spix, 1781-1826. German anatomist). The bony spine on the median border of the inferior dental foramen, to which is attached the sphenomandibular ligament.

splanchnology The study of the viscera of the body.

splenius muscles Muscles involved in extending the head and spinal column. *See* Table of Muscles.

splint 1. An appliance, which may be rigid or flexible, used to immobilize the ends of fractured bones or to restrict the movement of joints. 2. To immobilize by the use of such an appliance. *In dentistry*, to immobilize loose teeth with a fixed appliance, or to immobilize fractured jaws.
acrylic s. A plastic splint or stent used in dental surgery to immobilize fractures of the mandible or the maxilla, or to support bone grafts of the jaw.
anchor s. A type of splint used in fractures of the jaw, in which wire loops are passed over the teeth and anchor them to a rod to immobilize the broken bone.
cap s. 1. A cast metal dental splint fitting accurately over the crowns and occlusal surfaces of the teeth and cemented into place; used to assist in immobilizing jaw fractures. 2. An acrylic splint covering the crowns of the teeth, and used as a provisional fixation for fractured teeth or those loosened as a result of periodontal disease.
dental s. Any form of appliance or device used to fasten and immobilize the teeth.
extraoral s. *Roger-Anderson extraoral splint.
fenestrated s. Open-cap *splint.
flange s. A metal splint used in fracture of the mandible; it is cemented to several of the posterior mandibular teeth and has a high flange which rests on the buccal surfaces of the opposing maxillary teeth.
interdental s. A type of splint used in fracture of the jaw, held in place by wires passed round the teeth.
open-cap s. A form of cap splint in which the occlusal surfaces of the teeth are left exposed.

splinter 1. A small, sharp-pointed fragment. 2. To break up into small fragments.

splinting The process of applying a splint or splints.

sponge
absorbable gelatin s. A sponge-like absorbable material inserted into a wound to act as a haemostatic; it may be impregnated with anti-septic.

sponge gold Cohesive gold in the form of spongy crystals.

spongiosa *Substantia spongiosa.

spoon denture A form of upper partial denture for the replacement of one or more anterior teeth, the teeth being attached to a plastic base plate which extends over the whole of the hard palate, but does not cover the gingival margins of the natural teeth.

spoon excavator A type of excavator having a spoon-shaped head.

sporotrichosis A chronic fungal infection caused by *Sporotrichum (Sporothrix) schenckii*, in which there may be ulceration of the oral, nasal and pharyngeal mucosa, and lymphadenitis.

spot grinding The correction of occlusion by grinding down high areas on the teeth, fillings, or prosthetic appliances, disclosed by articulating paper.

spots, Filatov's *Koplik's spots.

sprew *See* sprue.

spring A coil of fine wire which possesses the property of elasticity.

spring plate A dental plate retained by the elasticity of its material pressing against the abutment teeth.

sprue 1. A chronic disease affecting the intestines, characterized by diarrhoea, blood changes, wasting, and a raw mouth and tongue. 2. *In dentistry*, the hole through which molten metal is poured into a closed mould; also the small sprig of waste metal which is left in this hole, or on the casting.

sprue former A small pin used to remove a wax pattern from a cavity.

spur *In dentistry*, a small metal projection on an appliance or partial denture.

sputum Matter expelled from the mouth by spitting; it may be saliva alone, or mixed with mucous secretions from the respiratory tract.

squama A scale, or scale-like matter.

squamomandibular Relating to the squamous portion of the temporal bone, or of the occipital bone, and the mandible.

squamous Scale-like; scaly.

squash bite A bite taken to register the relationship of the cusps of the upper and lower teeth, but not to give any clear reproduction of the teeth.

stab culture A culture made by inoculating the medium by means of a needle thrust deeply into it.

Stafne's cavity, Stafne's cyst (E.C. Stafne, b. 1894. American oral pathologist). A developmental fold within the mandible filled by salivary gland tissue.

stagnation 1. The cessation of flow of any circulating fluid in the body. 2. *In dentistry*, the accumulation of debris on a tooth.

stain 1. Any mark discolouring a surface. 2. The process of colouring tissue for microscopical examination. 3. Any colouring agent used for this process.
port-wine s. *Naevus flammeus.

stannous fluoride A form of fluoride, chemical formula SnF_2, used in toothpaste and for topical application for the prevention of dental caries.

stapedius muscle Retracts stapes. *See* Table of Muscles.

stapedius nerve A motor nerve to the stapedius muscle. *See* Table of Nerves.

staphyle The palatine *uvula.

staphyline Relating to the palatine *uvula; also used to refer to the palate as a whole.

staphylion The point in the midline on the posterior edge of the hard palate; a craniometric landmark.

staphylitis *Uvulitis.

staphylococcal Relating to or caused by staphylococci.

Staphylococcus A genus of the Micrococcaceae family of bacteria, non-motile, aerobic or facultatively anaerobic and Gram-positive cocci, seen as irregular clusters of cells, or as short chains; species of this genus are found in suppurative lesions, boils, inflammatory conditions, etc.

staphylococcus A type of *coccus arranged in clusters.

staphyloptosis *Uvuloptosis.

staphylorraphy Surgical repair of a cleft soft palate, or cleft uvula and soft palate.

staphyloschisis Cleft uvula, or cleft of the uvula and the soft palate.

staphylotomy *Uvulotomy.

statoacusticus nerve N. vestibulocochlearis. *See* Table of Nerves.

staurion The point at which the transverse palatine suture intersects the median suture; a craniometric point.

steel A metal formed by the combination of iron and a small quantity of carbon; it is tough and elastic.
stainless s. A form of steel containing some nickel or chromium, or both; it does not easily tarnish.

stelengis Grinding of the teeth.

stellate Star-shaped.

stenion One of two craniometric points on the sphenosquamous suture, located nearest to the midline on each side, being at each end of the smallest transverse diameter of the temporal region.

stenocephalic Having an abnormally narrow skull.

stenocompressor An instrument used in oral and dental surgery to close the parotid duct.

stenodont Having abnormally narrow teeth.

stenosis Constriction or narrowing of an aperture, canal or duct.

stenostenosis Constriction of Stensen's (parotid) duct.

stenostomia Constricture of the mouth.

Stensen's duct (N. Stensen, 1638-86. Danish anatomist). Parotid *duct.

stent 1. A mould of plastic compound (Stent's compound) used to immobilize certain forms of skin graft. 2. An impression of the oral cavity in Stent's compound.
acrylic s. A plastic splint or stent used in dental surgery to immobilize fractures of the mandible or maxilla, or to support bone grafts of the jaws.
occlusal s. A form of bite plate used in treatment of temporomandibular joint dysfunction.
paedodontic s. An acrylic stent used to prevent premature closure and assist in the eruption of surgically exposed unerupted teeth.
periodontal s. One designed to hold dressings in place after periodontal surgery.
trismus s. A form of Kingsley's splint designed to assist in opening and closing the mouth, or to exercise the temporomandibular joint.

Stent's compound or mass (C.R. Stent, 19th century English dentist). A resinous, thermoplastic material, which sets very hard, used in dentistry as an impression compound and in plastic surgery for moulds to immobilize skin grafts.

step *of a cavity* The auxiliary part of a compound mortise form, in complex cavities, consisting of the pulpal and axial walls.

stephanial Relating to the stephanion.

stephanion The junction of the coronal suture and the temporal line of the frontal bone.

stereo- Prefix signifying *three-dimensional.*

stereograph An instrument used to reproduce mandibular movements as a series of carved or moulded three-dimensional records.

sterile 1. Aseptic, germ-free. 2. Infertile.

sterilization 1. The process of rendering germ-free or aseptic. 2. The process of rendering incapable of reproduction.

sterilizer An apparatus used for sterilization.

sternocleidomastoid artery Two branches, from the occipital and the superior thyroid arteries, supplying the sternocleidomastoid muscle. *See* Table of Arteries—sternocleidomastoidea.

sternocleidomastoid muscle Flexes head and turns it to the opposite side; *also called* M. sternomastoideus. *See* Table of Muscles—sternocleidomastoideus.

sternohyoid muscle Depresses hyoid bone. *See* Table of Muscles—sternohyoideus.

sternomastoid muscle M. sternocleidomastoideus. *See* Table of Muscles.

sternothyroid muscle Depresses thyroid cartilage and larynx. *See* Table of Muscles—sternothyroideus.

Stevens-Johnson syndrome (A.M. Stevens, 1884-1945. American paediatrician; F.C. Johnson, 1894-1934. American paediatrician). Erythema multiforme with involvement of the conjunctiva and the oral tissues; dermatostomatitis.

Stillman's cleft (P.R. Stillman, 1871-1945. American periodontologist). A fissure in the gum margin, seen in periodontal disease.

stimulus Any agent or impulse that excites or promotes a functional reaction.

stippled Having a mottled or spotted appearance with light and dark patches.

stoma (*pl.* stomata) A mouth, orifice or opening.

stomacace Acute ulcerative *stomatitis.

stomadeum *Stomodeum.

stomatal Relating to a stoma.

stomatalgia Pain in the mouth.

stomatic Relating to the mouth; oral.

stomatitis Inflammation of the soft tissues of the mouth.

acute ulcerative s., acute necrotizing s. A severe form of stomatitis, characterized by painful shallow ulcers on the tongue, lips and buccal mucosa, and necrosis of the oral tissues; *also called* Vincent's stomatitis.

angular s. Angular *cheilitis.

aphthous s. A form of stomatitis, often recurring, characterized by painful aphthae affecting the oral mucous membranes.

fusospirochaetal s. Acute ulcerative *stomatitis.

gangrenous s. *Cancrum oris.

herpetic s. Herpetic *gingivostomatitis.

membranous s. Any form of stomatitis in which there is pseudomembrane formation.

mycotic s. *Thrush.
nicotinic s. *Leukokeratosis nicotina palati.
ulceromembranous s. Acute ulcerative *stomatitis.
vesicular s. with exanthem Caused by a Coxsackie virus, which produces painless vesicles, most often seen on the buccal mucosa, and also on the mucosa of the lips, palate, gingiva and tongue; *also called* 'hand-foot-mouth' disease.

stomatitis areata migrans Lesions similar to those seen in geographic tongue, found on the buccal and oral mucosa, appearing as red patches with white raised rims, the patterns changing continuously.

stomatitis herpetiformis An uncommon form of stomatitis, characterized by multiple ulcers, possibly viral in origin and simulating herpes simplex infection.

stomatitis scarlatina An oral manifestation of scarlet fever, characterized by congested palatal mucosa and fiery red throat; a white coated tongue with red fungiform papillae (strawberry tongue) is followed by a deep red, smooth and glistening tongue surface (raspberry tongue); there may also be ulceration of the buccal mucous membrane and palate.

stomato- Prefix signifying *mouth*.

stomatocace Acute ulcerative *stomatitis.

Stomatococcus A genus of the Micrococcaceae family of bacteria, seen as spherical cells, grouped in clusters, Gram-positive, non-motile and facultatively anaerobic.

stomatodeum *Stomodeum.

stomatodynia Pain in the mouth; stomatalgia.

stomatodysodia *Halitosis.

stomatogastric Relating to the mouth and the stomach.

stomatoglossitis Inflammation of the mucosa of the oral cavity and the tongue, seen most commonly in nutritional deficiency disorders.

stomatognathic Relating to the mouth and the jaws.

stomatognathic system Masticatory *apparatus.

stomatolalia Speaking through the mouth with the nostrils obstructed.

stomatologic, stomatological Relating to stomatology.

stomatologist A dentist, especially one concerned principally with oral diseases.

stomatology The medical specialty concerned with the mouth and its diseases; sometimes used as synonymous with dentistry.

stomatomalacia Pathological softening of the mouth structures.

stomatomenia Bleeding of the oral mucosa occurring at the time of menstruation.

stomatomycosis Any fungal disease of the mouth.

stomatonecrosis *Cancrum oris.

stomatonoma *Cancrum oris.

stomatopanus Inflammation of the oral lymph glands.

stomatopathy Any disease or disorder of the mouth.

stomatophylaxis Prevention of diseases of the mouth and teeth; oral prophylaxis.

stomatophyma Any circumscribed swelling.

stomatoplasty Plastic surgery of the mouth.

stomatorrhagia Oral haemorrhage.

stomatoschisis *Hare-lip.

stomatoscope A type of torch for illuminating the oral cavity for examination.

stomatosis *Stomatopathy.

stomenorrhagia Vicarious menstruation occurring in the mouth.

stomion Soft-tissue cephalometric landmark; the most anterior point on the line of contact between the upper and lower lips, in the midline.

stomodeum The primitive oral cavity in the embryo; an invagination of the embryonic ectoderm which later develops into the mouth and the upper pharynx.

stomoschisis Mouth fissure.

stone 1. A hard mineral concretion. 2. *In prosthetic dentistry*, a hard form of plaster of Paris, which sets like cement, and is used to make casts. 3. *In conservative dentistry*, a rotary abrasive head, mounted for use in a handpiece and used for grinding and smoothing.

pulp s. A deposit of calcareous matter within the tooth pulp, associated with degenerative changes; *also called* a denticle.

salivary s. Salivary *calculus[1].

straight sinus A venous sinus formed by the union of the inferior sagittal sinus and the great cerebral vein. *See* Tables of Veins—sinus rectus.

strap

cervical s. *Neckstrap.

stream

cutting s. The jet of abrasive particles used with an airbrasive to cut tooth cavities.

Streptococcus A genus of the Micrococcaceae family of bacteria, seen as spherical to ovoid cells forming clusters; Gram-positive, facultatively anaerobic, non-motile and non-sporing. They are found in the upper respiratory tract and mouth in vertebrates; some species are highly pathogenic.

S. mitior A species of *Streptococcus* seen as spherical or ovoid cells occurring singly, in pairs or chains; found in human saliva, dental plaque and sputum. *Also called Streptococcus sanguis type II.*

S. mutans A species of *Streptococcus* similar to *S. salivarius*, Gram-positive cocci in pairs or chains, non-motile. It colonizes the tooth surface and aids the adhesion of dental plaque; it also produces organic acids which are thought to be involved in the initiation of dental caries.

S. pneumoniae A species of *Streptococcus*, one of the most common causes of pneumonia and of a variety of other infectious diseases; it has spherical or ovoid cells occurring in pairs or short chains, is non-motile and Gram-positive. *Also called Diplococcus pneumoniae, Micrococcus pneumoniae* or pneumococcus.

S. salivarius A non-haemolytic species of *Streptococcus*, the most common found in the mouth, with spherical or ovoid cells occurring in chains of varying length; associated in particular with the tongue and saliva.

S. sanguis A species of *Streptococcus* found in dental plaque and in the mouth; only established in infants after the eruption of the first primary teeth. *Streptococcus sanguis type II* is known as **Streptococcus mitior.*

streptococcus A type of *coccus which is found as chains.

Streptothrix A suggested name for a group of micro-organisms including *Actinomyces*, *Streptomyces* and *Nocardia*.

stress 1. Force exerted by some mechanical means; pressure. 2. *In dentistry*, the pressure or force exerted by the mandibular teeth on the maxillary teeth during mastication.

stress breaker A device in a partial denture designed to take some of the load from abutment teeth.

striae of Retzius (M.G. Retzius, 1842-1919. Swedish anatomist). *See* enamel striae of Retzius.

striate, striated Striped or streaked.

striation 1. A stripe or streak, or a series of stripes or streaks. 2. The condition of being striped.

stricture Abnormal contraction of any aperture or vessel.

stridor A harsh whistling sound produced by the respiratory system.

stridor decutum The noise made by the grinding of teeth.

stridor dentium Grinding the teeth.

strip 1. A thin and narrow piece of material. 2. To peel off, in layers, so revealing the surface below.
abrasive s. A strip of linen coated on one side with an abrasive, used in dentistry for contouring and polishing.
separating s. A strip of metal, having one side coated with a coarse abrasive, used to increase the space between adjacent teeth.

stroma The tissue forming the matrix or the framework of an organ.

strophulus A papular eruption sometimes seen on the gums of infants who are cutting teeth.

struma *Goitre.

struma *of the tongue* A tumour developing from aberrant thyroid tissue in the tongue.

stump *Of a tooth:* that part of the tooth which remains after the destruction or removal of the crown.

styloglossal Relating to the styloid process of the temporal bone and the tongue.

styloglossal muscle Raises tongue. *See* Table of Muscles—styloglossus.

stylohyoid muscle Raises tongue and hyoid bone, and draws them back. *See* Table of Muscles—stylohyoideus.

styloid Long and pointed; like a stylus.

stylomandibular Relating to both the styloid process and the mandible.

stylomastoid Relating to both the styloid process and the mastoid process.

stylomastoid artery Supplies the middle ear. *See* Table of Arteries—stylomastoidea.

stylomaxillary Relating to both the styloid process and the maxilla.

stylomyloid Relating to the styloid process and the molar teeth.

stylopharyngeal muscle Raises and opens pharynx. *See* Table of Muscles—stylopharyngeus.

stylostaphyline Relating to the styloid process of the temporal bone and the soft palate.

styptic An astringent haemostatic agent.

sub- Prefix signifying *below, underneath*.

subacute Less severe than acute; the stage between chronic and acute illness.

subapical Below the apex.

subclavian artery *Right* from the brachiocephalic trunk, and *left* from the aortic arch, supplying the upper limb, spinal cord, brain, etc. *See* Table of Arteries—subclavia.

subclinical Relating to a mild form of infection, with no clinical symptoms or manifestations.

subcranial Below the cranium.

subcutaneous Beneath the skin.

subdental Below a tooth or teeth.

subgingival Below or beneath the gums.

subglossal Below the tongue.

subglossitis Inflammation of the sublingual tissues, or of the under side of the tongue.

subjugal Beneath the zygomatic bone.

sublingual Under the tongue.

sublingual artery Supplies the lower jaw muscles, sublingual glands, etc. *See* Table of Arteries—sublingualis.

sublingual nerve A sensory nerve supplying the area about the sublingual gland. *See* Table of Nerves—sublingualis.

sublinguitis Inflammation of the sublingual salivary glands.

subluxation A partial dislocation or sprain.

submandibular Below the mandible.

submandibular gland One of a pair of salivary glands lying on the inner edge of the mandible, in the region of the angle.

submasseteric Beneath the masseter muscle.

submaxilla *Mandible.

submaxillaritis Adenitis occurring in one of the submandibular (submaxillary) glands.

submaxillary Below the mandible or lower maxilla; submandibular.

submental Beneath the chin.

submental artery Branch of facial artery, supplying the tissues below the jaw. *See* Table of Arteries—submentalis.

submucosa The layer of tissue beneath the mucous membrane.

subnasale The point at which the nasal septum forms an angle with the philtrum; a cephalometric soft-tissue landmark.

subnasion The lowest point on the mid-sagittal plane of the lower anterior margin of the nasal aperture.

suboccipital nerve A motor nerve from the first cervical, supplying the semispinalis capitis muscle and the muscles of the occipital triangle. *See* Table of Nerves—suboccipitalis.

suboccipital plexus *See* suboccipital venous plexus.

suboccipital venous plexus A plexus of veins found in the posterior portion of the scalp, draining into the vertebral vein. *See* Table of Veins—plexus venosus suboccipitalis.

suborbital Below the orbit.

subperiosteal Below or beneath the periosteum.

subpulpal Beneath the tooth pulp.
s. wall. The base of the pulp chamber in a cavity where the pulp has been removed and the pulp wall, therefore, does not exist.

subscription That part of a prescription containing directions for the preparation and compounding of the ingredients of a medicine.

subspinale The deepest point on the midline of the premaxilla, between the anterior nasal spine and the lower border of the alveolus; a subsurface landmark.

substantia adamantina Tooth enamel.

substantia spongiosa Cancellous bone.

substructure 1. *In dentistry,* that part of an implant denture which is covered by the tissues. 2. *Of an implant:* *Infrastructure.

succedaneous Succeeding and replacing.

suction chamber Air *chamber.

suction disc A flexible disc attached to the fitting surface of an upper denture in an attempt to improve its retention. This method is no longer used.

suction plate A dental plate retained in the mouth by suction or atmospheric pressure.

sulcoplasty *Vestibuloplasty.

sulcular Relating to a sulcus.

sulcus 1. A long groove or depression. 2. *In dentistry*, a long groove or depression in a tooth surface, the sides meeting at an angle.
alveolabial s. The sulcus between the lips and the alveolar process.
alveolingual s. The sulcus between the tongue and the alveolar process and teeth.
gingival s. The space lying between the inner aspect of the free gingiva and the tooth enamel or cementum, depending on the level of the epithelial attachment.
greater palatine s. of the maxilla The groove on the nasal surface of the body of the maxilla which, with the corresponding groove on the perpendicular plate of the palatine bone, forms the channel for N. palatinus major.
greater palatine s. of the palatine bone The groove on the perpendicular plate of the palatine bone which, with the corresponding groove on the nasal surface of the body of the maxilla, forms the channel for N. palatinus major.
infraorbital s. A groove on the body of the maxilla which runs a short distance backwards from the orbital surface into the infraorbital canal; in it lie the infraorbital nerve and vessels.
labiodental s. Vestibular *lamina.
lacrimal s. of the maxilla A deep groove on the nasal surface of the body of the maxilla, just in front of the maxillary sinus and forming part of the wall of the nasolacrimal canal.
median lingual s. A narrow and shallow groove on the dorsum of the tongue in the midline.
mylohyoid s. A groove on the medial surface of the ramus of the mandible, extending obliquely forward from the mandibular foramen to a point on the body of the mandible just below the end of the mylohyoid line; the mylohyoid nerve and vessels run in this sulcus.
nasolacrimal s. Lacrimal *sulcus of the maxilla.
palatine s. of the maxilla One of the longitudinal furrows on the lower surface of the palatine process of the maxilla, between the palatine spines; they carry the greater palatine nerves and vessels.
pterygopalatine s. Greater palatine *sulcus of the palatine bone.
terminal s. A shallow groove on the posterior portion of the dorsum of the tongue, dividing it from the root of the tongue.

sulcus of the nasal process of the maxilla Lacrimal *sulcus of the maxilla.

sulfonamide *See* sulphonamide.

sulphonamide Any one of the compounds derived from sulphanilamide, and used in the treatment of bacterial infections.

super- Prefix signifying *above*, or *excessive*.

superficial Immediately below the surface; as opposed to *deep*.

superior Above; higher of two parts.

superior sagittal sinus A venous sinus draining into the transverse sinus. *See* Table of Veins—sinus sagittalis superior.

supermaxilla *Maxilla.

supernumerary More than the usual number.

supernumerary tooth An extra tooth, above the normal number occurring in the mouth.

superscription The symbol —*recipe*; used at the beginning of a prescription.

superstructure *Of an implant:* a metal framework fitted to an implant abutment or abutments which provides retention for a prosthesis.

supplemental tooth A supernumerary tooth which is identical in form to the normal teeth in that area of the mouth in which it occurs.

suppuration The formation and discharge of pus.

suppurative Relating to or characterized by suppuration; pus-producing.

supra- Prefix signifying *over, above, upon.*

suprabuccal Above, or in the upper part of, the cheek region.

suprabulge That part of the tooth crown which converges on the occlusal surface.

supraclusion *Over-eruption.

supracondylism Deviation of the mandibular condyles in an upward direction.

supragingival Above the gingival margin.

suprahyoid artery Supplies muscles above the hyoid bone. *See* Table of Arteries—suprahyoidea.

supralabial Above the area of the lips.

supramandibular Above the mandible.

supramaxilla *Maxilla.

supramaxillary 1. Relating to the maxilla. 2. Above the maxilla.

supramental Above the chin.

supramentale The deepest point on the midline of the mandible between the pogonion and the upper border of the alveolus; a subsurface landmark.

supraocclusion *Over-eruption.

supraorbital Above the orbit.

supraorbital artery Supplies the supraorbital muscles. *See* Table of Arteries—supraorbitalis.

supraorbital nerve Supplies skin of forehead and upper eyelid. *See* Table of Nerves—supraorbitalis.

supratrochlear artery Supplies the anteromedial part of the forehead. *See* Table of Arteries—supratrochlearis.

supratrochlear nerve Supplies skin of forehead, bridge of nose and upper eyelid. *See* Table of Nerves—supratrochlearis.

supraversion *Close-bite.

surface *of a tooth* Any specifically designated area on a tooth crown or root.

approximal s. One of the surfaces of a tooth which adjoin each other in the same dental arch; it may be either a *mesial* or a *distal* surface.

axial s. A cavity surface parallel with the long axis of the tooth.

buccal s. That surface on the crown of a molar or premolar tooth facing the cheek; ISO designation: V.

contact s. Approximal *surface.

distal s. That surface on the crown of a tooth farthest away from the midline of the dental arch; ISO designation: D.

facial s's of the teeth Vestibular *surfaces of the teeth.

interproximal s. Approximal *surface.

interstitial s. Approximal *surface.

labial s. That surface on the crown of a canine or incisor tooth facing the lip; ISO designation: V.

lingual s. That surface on the crown of a tooth facing the tongue; ISO designation: L.

masticatory s. Occlusal *surface.

mesial s. That surface on the crown of a tooth nearest to the midline of the dental arch; ISO designation: M.

occlusal s. The grinding surface of a posterior tooth, which comes into contact with a corresponding surface of another tooth in the opposing jaw in occlusion; ISO designation: O.

palatal s. The lingual surface of a maxillary tooth; ISO designation: L.

proximal s. Approximal *surface.

pulpal s. A cavity surface that lies over the tooth pulp.

radicular s. The surface of the root of a tooth; ISO designation: G.

vestibular s's of the teeth The buccal and labial surfaces collectively; ISO designation: V.

surface anaesthesia, surface analgesia Topical *anaesthesia.

surgery That branch of medical science which is concerned with the manual or operative treatment of disease or injury.

dental s. That branch of dentistry which is concerned with the operative or manual treatment of the teeth; generally used as synonymous with dentistry.

maxillofacial s. That branch of surgery which is concerned with operative treatment of the jaws and facial bones.

oral s. That branch of dentistry which is concerned with the diagnosis and surgical treatment of diseases, defects and injuries of the jaws and their associated structures.

plastic s. That branch of surgery concerned with the correction or reconstruction of parts that are deformed or injured.

reconstructive s. Plastic *surgery.

surgical Relating to surgery.

Sutton's aphthae (R.L. Sutton, 1878-1952. American dermatologist). *Periadenitis mucosa necrotica recurrens.

sutural Relating to a suture.

suture 1. The line of junction between bones of the skull. 2. A surgical stitch.

coronal s. The transverse suture at the junction of the parietal bones with the frontal bone.

false s. A line of junction between two bone surfaces without any real interosseous union.

frontoparietal s. Coronal *suture.

incisive s. An indistinct line on the palatine process of the maxilla, extending from the incisive fossa to the space between the canine and the lateral incisor, marking the junction of the premaxilla and the maxilla.

intermandibular s. *Symphysis menti.

interparietal s. Sagittal *suture.

jugal s. Sagittal *suture.

lambdoid s. The suture at the junction of the parietal bones with the occipital bone; the name derives from its resemblance to the Greek letter lambda.

limbous s. A type of serrated squamous suture in which there is bevelling of the interdigitating surfaces.

longitudinal s. Sagittal *suture.

metopic s. The suture joining the two halves of the frontal bone; the frontal suture when it persists in the adult skull.

occipital s. Lambdoid *suture.

occipitoparietal s. Lambdoid *suture.

parietal s. Sagittal *suture.

premaxillary s. Incisive *suture.

sagittal s. The suture between the two parietal bones, which lies in the midline of the skull.

scaly s. Squamous *suture.

serrated s. One in which the borders of the bones are finely serrated and interdigitate at the junction.

simple s. One in which the borders of the bones are smooth or nearly smooth along the joining edge.
squamous s. One in which the borders of the bones are bevelled so that one overlaps the other at the junction.
squamous s. of the cranium The articulation between the squamous part of the parietal bone and the squamous part of the temporal bone.
temporal s. Squamous *suture of the cranium.
true s. One in which the united bones are interlocked and cannot move at the junction; an obsolete term.
The sutures between the facial bones are named after the bones they join.

suture needle A sharp-pointed and generally curved needle with an eye for thread, used for surgical suturing.

suture shears A pair of scissors having short blades, the upper one straight and the lower with a half-moon notch at the end, used for cutting ligatures or sutures.

Suzanne's gland (J.G. Suzanne, b. 1859. French physician). An oral mucous gland found in the alveolingual sulcus near the midline.

swage 1. The contouring of metal using dies and counterdies. 2. A tool used in this work.

symbiosis 1. An intimate association of two organisms of different species; it includes parasitism and commensalism. 2. More specifically it is used of an association which is to the mutual advantage of both partners.

symbiotic Relating to symbiosis.

symmetrical Relating to symmetry.

symmetry The correspondence or balance of parts about a common axis, or their regular distribution and relationship within a plane.

symphysion The midpoint of the anterior border of the mandibular alveolar process; a craniometric point.

symphysis A joint with limited movement, the bony surfaces being covered with cartilage but separated by fibrous tissue.

symphysis mandibulae *Symphysis menti.

symphysis menti The centre line of the chin, where the two halves of the mandible fused at birth; *also called* symphysis mandibulae, intermandibular suture.

symptom Any indication of the presence or course of a disease, either by functional or other change occurring in the patient.

symptomatic Relating to a symptom or set of symptoms.

syn- Prefix signifying *with, in association with.*

synalgia Pain in one part caused by injury or a lesion in another, distant, part; referred pain.

synarthrosis Fibrous *joint.

syncheilia Congenital imperforation of the mouth opening.

synchondrosis Cartilaginous *joint.

synchronous Occurring together, at the same time.

syncleisis Old term for *occlusion[2].

syncope Fainting; temporary unconsciousness caused by cerebral hypoxia or changes in cerebral blood flow.

syndesmosis The joining of two bone surfaces by the interposition of connective tissue which forms an interosseous membrane.

syndesmotome A surgical instrument used to cut the periodontal ligament fibres.

syndesmotomy The cutting of the periodontal ligament fibres before tooth extraction.

syndrome A complex of symptoms, occurring together, which characterize one disease or lesion.
acquired immune deficiency s. AIDS. A viral disease, often sexually transmitted, in which changes in infected lymphocytes lead to immune deficiency that predisposes to severe, usually fatal, secondary infections; oral manifestations include candidosis, 'hairy' leukoplakia and Kaposi's sarcoma.
aglossia-adactylia s. A congenital absence or hypoplasia of the tongue, with hypoplasia of the mandibular alveolar process and missing teeth, regression of the mandible, and absence of some or all fingers and toes.
first arch s. A congenital abnormality syndrome, which includes cleft lip and palate, mandibulofacial dysostosis, hypertelorism, and deformities of the ear, all stemming from developmental deficiency in the first branchial arch.
hypoglossia-hypodactyly s. Aglossia-adactylia *syndrome.
For eponymous syndromes *see* under the name of the person first describing or exhibiting the syndrome.

synergist 1. A muscle or other organ that acts together with another. 2. A drug or chemical that aids the action of another.

synodontia *Fusion^3.

synostosis Osseous fusion of parts of a single bone or of adjacent bones.

synovial Relating to or secreting synovial fluid (synovium).

synovial fluid, synovium A viscid, transparent alkaline and albumen-like fluid contained in joint cavities and tendon sheaths, secreted by the synovial membranes.

synovium Synovial *fluid.

syphilis A contagious venereal disease, manifesting oral and facial lesions.

syringe An instrument for injecting liquid or gas into the tissues or into a vessel or cavity.
air s. A syringe used in dental surgery, by means of which compressed air may be blown into a cavity or root canal to dry it or to remove loose debris.
aspirating s. One used for removing fluid from a cavity or vessel.
cartridge s. A syringe in which the solution to be injected is delivered from a pre-packed cartridge in the form of a glass phial.
chip s. A type of air syringe consisting of a metal nozzle and a rubber bulb, used to remove loose debris during operative procedures, or for drying the area.
combination s. One designed to deliver either water or compressed air, or an air/water spray.

systematic 1. Relating to a system. 2. Methodical.

systemic 1. Relating to or affecting the whole body. 2. *Systematic^1.

systole The contraction period in each heart beat.

systolic Relating to the systole.

T

t.d.s. Abbreviation for *ter die sumendus*—to be taken three times a day; used in prescription writing.

t.i.d. Abbreviation for *ter in die*—three a day; used in prescription writing.

tab. Abbreviation for *tablet*; used in prescription writing.

tinct. Abbreviation for *tinctura*—a tincture; used in prescription writing.

TPA Transpalatal *arch.

table
occlusal t. 1. The total occlusal surface of the molars and premolars. 2. The total occlusal surface of a complete or partial denture.

tablet A small solid disc containing one dose of a drug.
disclosing t. A staining agent applied to the tooth surface as a tablet to be chewed, which attaches to plaque and other surface deposits and shows them up in some distinct colour against the normal clean enamel.

tachy- Prefix signifying *fast, swift.*

tactile Relating to touch.

talon A low distal cusp on an upper molar; an extension of the trigon.

talonid A low distal cusp on a lower molar; an extension of the trigonid.

tapinocephalic Having a low, flattened top to the cranium.

tapir mouth A condition characterized by loose, thickened lips, and caused by atrophy of the orbicularis oris muscle.

tartar Lay word for dental *calculus.

taste The perception of flavour, a sensation produced by stimulation of the gustatory nerve endings in the tongue with a soluble substance.

taste buds The end organs of the gustatory nerve, situated at the base of the filiform and vallate papillae on the tongue.

tattoo
amalgam t. An area of pigmentation on the oral tissues as a result of the implantation of amalgam restorative materials; it may be black or brown in colour.

taurodontism Vertical deepening of the pulp cavity in molar teeth, at the expense of the roots.

tectocephalic Having a roof-shaped cranium.

tectonic Relating to plastic surgery or plastic restoration.

teeth Plural of tooth.
accessorial t. Those permanent teeth that do not have deciduous predecessors.
anterior t. The incisors and canines, those teeth found in the front of the mouth.
ciliiform t. Very fine, closely-set teeth, as found in certain fish.
cross-pin t. Artificial teeth which are attached by pins running at right angles to the long axis of the tooth.
deciduous t. Primary *teeth.
fused t. Teeth, especially incisors, that have become joined together during development, and erupt as one large tooth.
milk t. Primary *teeth.
permanent t. Those teeth in the second dentition in man; teeth that will not be replaced as a matter of course.
posterior t. The premolars and molars, collectively.
primary t. The first teeth to erupt in the mouth in man, later shed and replaced by the permanent teeth.

rake t. Descriptive of widely separated teeth.
scalpriform t. The chisel-like incisors of a rodent, used for cutting or gnawing.
sectorial t. The cutting teeth of Carnivora.
setiform t. Ciliiform *teeth.
succedaneous t. Those teeth in the permanent dentition that replace primary teeth.

teething The process of eruption of the primary teeth in infants.

telalgia Referred pain.

telangiectasia, telangiectasis Dilatation of the capillaries and small arteries, forming types of angioma.

telangiectatic Relating to telangiectasis.

telescope crown A double metal crown, composed of two tubular or conical crowns, placed one over the other.

temper To render a metal hard and elastic by successive heating and cooling.

temperature The degree of intensity of heat or cold.

template A mould or pattern.

temple The flattened part of the head above the zygomatic arch and in front of the ear.

temporal 1. Relating to time. 2. *In anatomy*, relating to a temple.

temporal artery Supplies the temporal fascia and zygomatic bone, etc.; three branches: deep, middle, superficial. *See* Table of Arteries—temporalis.

temporal bone The bone of the temple, at the side and base of the skull.

temporal muscle Retracts protruded mandible and closes mouth. *See* Table of Muscles—temporalis.

temporalis profundi nerve Supplies the temporal muscles. *See* Table of Nerves.

temporo- Prefix signifying *temple.*

temporofacial Relating to the temporal bones and the facial bones.

temporomandibular Relating to the temple and the mandible.

temporomaxillary Relating to the temporal bone or region and the maxilla.

temporoparietal muscle Tightens the scalp. *See* Table of Muscles—temporoparietalis.

tender Sensitive; abnormally susceptible to pressure; sore.

tendinous Relating to, having the characteristics of, a tendon.

tendon The fibrous connective tissue that attaches muscle fibres to bone or to some other structure.

teno- Prefix signifying *tendon.*

tenon 1. Any projection fitting into a slot or mortise to make a joint. 2. *In dentistry*, the pin or post used to attach an artificial crown to a tooth root.

tensor muscles Muscles that tense or tighten. *See* Table of Muscles.

tensorius nerve Supplies the meninges. *See* Table of Nerves.

ter die sumendus Latin for *to be taken three times a day*; used in prescription writing, and abbreviated *t.d.s.*

ter in die Latin for *three a day*; used in prescription writing, and abbreviated *t.i.d.*

teratoma A tumour, sometimes found on the palate, derived from more than one germ layer and containing hair, teeth, etc., in places where these would not normally occur; it is most commonly seen in childhood. In a *benign* tumour the tissues are well differentiated; in a *malignant* tumour they may be immature or undifferentiated.

teratomatous Relating to or characteristic of a teratoma.

terminal nerve Supplies the nasal septum. *See* Table of Nerves—terminalis.

terminal vein V. thalamostriata superior. *See* Table of Veins.

tetanus An acute infectious disease, caused by the toxin of *Clostridium tetani*; it is characterized by tonic spasm of the voluntary muscles, and is generally fatal. *Also called* lockjaw.

tetany A syndrome caused by abnormal calcium metabolism, and characterized by muscle spasm, cramp, and, occasionally, stridor.

tetarcone *Tetartocone.

tetartocone The distolingual cusp on a maxillary molar or premolar.

tetartoconid The distolingual cusp on a mandibular molar or premolar.

tetra- Prefix signifying *four.*

tetracoccus A form of coccus in which cell division occurs in two planes, and the cells form into groups of four.

thalamostriate vein, superior With the choroid veins forms the internal cerebral vein; *also called* terminal vein. *See* Table of Veins—thalamostriata superior.

thecodont Having teeth contained in bony sockets or alveoli.

therapeutic Relating to treatment.

therapist

dental t. A person trained to carry out simple operative procedures on children's teeth, together with those performed by a dental *hygienist, under the direction of a dentist. Formerly known as a *dental auxiliary.*

therapy The treatment of disease. *See* treatment.

thermal Relating to or characterized by heat.

thermocautery The use of heated points for cauterization.

thermohardening material A plastic material which undergoes a chemical change during processing, so that the material of the finished product is different from the original material; *e.g.* vulcanite.

thermoplastic material A plastic material in which the material of the finished product is chemically identical with the original, having undergone no change, except of shape, during processing; *e.g.* celluloid.

thick-necked Descriptive of a tooth in which the mesiodistal diameter of the cervix is almost as great as that of the crown.

thimble *Coping[1].

thirst A desire for water or any other form of drink.

throat The gullet; the pharynx and the fauces; the anterior part of the neck.

thrombus A blood clot, formed and remaining in a blood vessel or in the heart, which may cause serious obstruction to the circulation.

thrush A type of candidiasis caused by infection with *Candida albicans*, and occurring generally in children and old people; it is characterized by the formation of whitish spots on the tongue and mucous membrane.

thyro- Prefix signifying *thyroid gland.*

thyroarytenoid muscle Closes larynx and relaxes vocal cords. *See* Table of Muscles—thyroarytenoideus.

thyrocele *Goitre.

thyroepiglottic muscle Closes larynx. *See* Table of Muscles—thyro-epiglotticus.

thyroglossal Relating to the thyroid gland and the tongue.

thyrohyoid Relating to both the thyroid gland and the hyoid bone.

thyrohyoid muscle Depresses hyoid bone or raises larynx. *See* Table of Muscles—thyrohyoideus.

thyroid, thyroid gland A large ductless endocrine gland situated in front of the trachea, and consisting of two lateral lobes joined by an isthmus. It is made up of follicles lined with epithelium and secretes a colloid material.
lingual t. A tumour of thyroid tissue at the upper end of the original thyroglossal duct, on the dorsum of the tongue; it is caused by the failure of an embryonic thyroid gland to descend. *Also called* lingual goitre.

thyroid artery Supplies the thyroid gland, and the muscles of the neck, the oesophagus and the larynx; two branches: inferior and superior. *See* Table of Arteries—thyroidea.

thyroid veins The veins draining the thyroid gland. *See* Table of Veins—thyroidea.

thyroidea ima artery An inconstant branch of the brachiocephalic trunk, supplying the thyroid gland. *See* Table of Arteries.

thyropharyngeal muscle Part of constrictor pharyngis inferior. *See* Table of Muscles—thyropharyngeus.

tic A spasmodic twitching, particularly of the facial muscles; a habit spasm.

tic douloureux Trigeminal *neuralgia.

tin A silver-white metallic element, chemical symbol Sn; used especially in metal alloys.

tinctura Latin for *tincture*; used in prescription writing, and abbreviated *tinct.*

tincture A solution of a medicinal substance in alcohol.

tinnitus A ringing noise in the ears.

tissue A mass of similar cells performing a specialized function.

tissue-borne *In prosthetic dentistry*, descriptive of a partial denture in which the masticatory loads are transmitted to the soft tissues rather than the teeth, as opposed to *tooth-borne*.

Tomes' fibres (Sir John Tomes, 1815-95. English dentist). Odontoblast *processes.

Tomes' granular layer (Sir John Tomes, 1815-95. English dentist). The outer layer of interglobular dentine near to the cemento-enamel junction.

Tomes' processes (Sir Charles Tomes, 1847-1928. English dentist). Ameloblastic *processes.

tomography A radiographic technique used to produce a detailed and distinct image of structures in a predetermined tissue plane by moving the film and the x-ray source simultaneously in opposite directions about the object while retaining the focus.
panoramic t. A technique for producing a panoramic radiograph using a combination of slit-beam radiography and rotational tomography.
rotational t. A method of tomography in which the movement of the film and the x-ray source follows a circular or elliptical path; there may be only a single centre of rotation, multiple centres, or continuously moving centres.

-tomy Suffix signifying *cutting*, in surgery.

tone 1. The state of slight tension maintained in healthy muscle tissue. 2. The quality of a sound.

tongue 1. A muscular body situated in the floor of the mouth, attached to it by the lingual frenum, and to the hyoid bone, the epiglottis and the soft palate by muscles and membranes; the organ of taste, and also an important adjunct in speech, mastication and deglutition. 2. Any structure having a similar shape.
adherent t. A tongue attached to both the floor and the sides of the mouth by folds of mucous membrane.
bald t. A clean, smooth tongue having no prominent papillae on its surface, seen in conditions such as vitamin B deficiency.
bifid t. A tongue split into two down the midline from its tip.
black t. Black patches of pigmentation on the tongue, composed of hypertrophied filiform papillae and micro-organisms.
burning t. *Glossodynia.
cardinal t. A tongue that has a bright red appearance, being denuded of epithelium.
cleft t. Bifid *tongue.
coated t. A whitish covering of the tongue surface containing food particles, epithelial debris and bacteria.
cobblestone t. Hypertrophy of the lingual papillae and a whitish coating, associated with leukoplakia and glossitis.
crocodile t. Fissured *tongue.
ectopic geographic t. *Stomatitis areata migrans.
fissured t. One having numerous furrows on the upper surface, possibly radiating from the midline.
frog t. *Ranula.
furred t. A tongue having the papillae coated, thus giving the mucous membrane a whitish, furry appearance.
geographic t. A tongue having scaly patches with no filiform papillae, and resembling maps, on the dorsal surface; these heal in a short time, to be replaced by others of different shape, in a different area, giving the impression of migrating. *Also called* benign migratory glossitis or erythema migrans linguae.
hairy t. A tongue having hair-like papillae.
hobnail t. Cobblestone *tongue.
magenta t. Glossitis associated with ariboflavinosis, giving the tongue a magenta-coloured appearance.
mappy t. Geographic *tongue.
parrot t. A horny, dry tongue seen in typhus and low fever, which cannot be protruded.
raspberry t. The deep red, smooth and glistening tongue surface associated with the later stages of scarlet fever, and developing from strawberry tongue.
scrotal t. Fissured *tongue.
smoker's t. *Leukoplakia (*linguae*).
strawberry t. A tongue having prominent red fungiform papillae, seen in the early stages of scarlet fever.
struma of the t. A tumour developing from aberrant thyroid tissue in the tongue.
wooden t. One affected by actinomycosis.

tongue-tie *Ankyloglossia.

tonsil One of the two almond-shaped bodies situated one on each side of the fauces, between the pillars.
faucial t. *Tonsil.
lingual t. The collective term for the nodules, produced by the lingual follicles, and found on the pharyngeal portion of the dorsum of the tongue.
palatine t. *Tonsil.

tonsillar Relating to a tonsil.

tonsillar artery Branch of the facial artery supplying the faucial tonsil and the base of the tongue. *See* Table of Arteries—tonsillaris.

tonsillectomy Surgical excision of the tonsils.

tonsillith *Tonsillolith.

tonsillitis Inflammation of the faucial tonsils.
acute ulcerative t. An acute ulceration of the tonsils in which the predominant infection is fuso-spirochaetal; *also called* Vincent's angina.

tonsillolith A calculus occurring in tonsillar tissue.

tonus *Tone[1].

tooth (*pl.* teeth) One of the mineralized structures in the maxillary and mandibular alveolar processes in the mouth, retained in its socket by means of a root or roots. The tooth body consists of a central cavity, containing the dental pulp and surrounded by dentine; the exposed portion or crown is covered by enamel, and the root or roots by cementum. *See also* dentition; teeth.
abutment t. A natural tooth used to support a bridge or partial denture.
anatomical t. In prosthetic dentistry, an artificial tooth whose crown is designed to look as like that of a natural tooth as possible.
artificial t. A prefabricated element designed for use on a dental prosthesis to represent a natural crown.
axle t., azzle t. An obsolete term for a molar *tooth.
canine t. A single-cusped tooth, resembling a dog's, found between the lateral incisor and the first molar or premolar. There is one in each quadrant in both the primary and the permanent dentition in man.
deciduous t. Primary *tooth.
eye t. A maxillary canine *tooth.
impacted t. One so placed in the jaw that it cannot erupt.
incisor t. A cutting tooth in the centre of the dental arch. There are two incisors in each quadrant in both the primary and the permanent dentition in man, one *central* and one *lateral.*
malacotic t. A poorly formed tooth with a high susceptibility to dental caries.
molar t. One of the back, grinding teeth. There are two in each quadrant in the primary dentition and three in each quadrant in the permanent dentition in man. The *third* molar is *also called* wisdom tooth.
neonatal t. A primary tooth present in the mouth at birth or erupting within a few days of birth.
non-anatomical t. An artificial tooth having the occlusal surface designed functionally rather than carved to reproduce the anatomic form.
permanent t. A tooth in the second, permanent, dentition in man.
premolar t. A bicuspid, found in front of the molar teeth; there are two in each quadrant in the permanent dentition in man.
primary t. One of the first teeth to erupt in the mouth in man; later shed and replaced by permanent successors.
scion t. A tooth used for transplantation, to replace one extracted.
straight-pin t. A porcelain tooth facing having vertical pin attachments.
supernumerary t. An extra tooth, above the normal number occurring in the mouth.
supplemental t. A supernumerary tooth that is identical in form to the normal teeth in that area of the mouth in which it occurs.

tube t. An artificial tooth having a cylindrical hollow running from the occlusal surface to the cervix.
wall t. A molar *tooth.
wisdom t. A third molar *tooth.

tooth angle The angle formed by the surfaces of the tooth, named according to the surfaces that form it.

tooth germ The enamel organ, dental papilla and sac; the rudiments of the developing tooth.

tooth hood Dental *operculum.

tooth pick A small pointed implement, of wood or metal, used to remove surplus food from the interdental spaces.

tooth rash *Strophulus.

tooth socket An *alveolus.

toothache Any pain associated with a tooth.

tooth-borne *In prosthetic dentistry,* descriptive of a prosthesis in which the masticatory loads are transmitted to the supporting abutment teeth rather than the soft tissue underlying the denture; as opposed to *tissue-borne.*

toothbrush A small brush head on a long handle, designed for cleaning the teeth and applying stimulation to the gingival tissues.

toothpaste Paste form of *dentifrice.

tophus Dental *calculus; an obsolete term.

topical Relating to or affecting only a specific surface area; local.

Topinard's line (P. Topinard, 1830-1912. French anthropologist). The line joining the mental point to the glabella.

torque *In dentistry,* the rotation of a tooth about its long axis.

torsiversion *Rotation.

torso-occlusion *Rotation.

torulosis *Cryptococcosis.

torus A rounded projection or swelling; a bony tumour.

torus mandibularis An exostosis occurring on the lingual aspect of the mandible, between the canines and the molars.

torus palatinus An exostosis occurring at the junction of the hard palate and the intermaxillary bone.

toxaemia Generalized blood poisoning caused by the absorption of toxins from a local focus of infection into the blood stream.

toxic Relating to a poison; poisonous.

toxicoid Resembling a toxin or poison.

toxicosis Any pathological condition due to poisoning.

toxin A poisonous substance produced by animal or vegetable cells, more particularly by bacteria; if injected into animals or man it causes the formation of specific antibodies or antitoxins.

toxoid A detoxified toxin which still retains its antigenic properties.

trabecula (*pl.* trabeculae) 1. A septum extending from the outer capsule or envelope into an organ. 2. One of the bony lamellae or spicules found in cancellous bone.

tracer *In dentistry,* a mechanical device used to record the pattern of mandibular movement.

trachea The windpipe; a cartilaginous tube which extends from the lower end of the larynx to the bronchi.

tracheal Relating to the trachea.

tracheal artery Branch of the inferior thyroid artery, supplying the trachea. *See* Table of Arteries—trachealis.

trachelomastoid muscle M. longissimus capitis. *See* Table of Muscles.

tracing 1. The process of copying by following and reproducing the lines of a drawing through transparent paper. 2. The copy so made. 3. The record produced by a tracer.
cephalometric t. An outline of facial bones and craniometric landmarks taken directly from a radiograph.

tract
dead t's. Areas of dentine tubules beneath a carious lesion in which the odontoblast processes have died and the pulpal ends have been blocked by calcific matter.

traction The act of moving by pulling or drawing.

traction screw A screw used in orthodontics to produce a pulling force sufficient to move malposed teeth.

tragale The most distal point on the tragus; a cephalometric soft-tissue landmark.

tragion The most forward point in the supratragal notch, above and in front of the porion; a cephalometric landmark.

tragus The small cartilaginous prominence over the external auditory meatus.

trans- Prefix signifying *through* or *across*.

transillumination The illumination of the interior of an object by means of a strong light shining through the walls.

translucent Capable of partial transmission of light rays, but not of a visual image.

transmucosal component Implant *abutment.

transparent Clear; affording transmission of light rays, and able to be seen through.

transplantation The transfer of tissue, either from another donor or from one site to another.

transplantation *of the teeth* The operation of removing teeth from one site and inserting them into empty sockets, either in the same mouth or in another mouth.

transposition *of the teeth* The interchange in position of two adjacent teeth.

transversa colli artery A. transversa cervicis. *See* Table of Arteries.

transverse cervical artery Supplies the root of the neck and the muscles of the scapula; *also called* A. transversa colli. *See* Table of Arteries—transversa cervicis.

transverse facial artery Supplies the masseter muscle, the parotid gland and the facial skin. *See* Table of Arteries—transversa faciei.

transverse muscle of the tongue M. transversus linguae. *See* Table of Muscles.

transverse sinus A venous sinus, found in the groove on the occipital bone and the posterior inferior angle of the parietal bone, into which drain the superior sagittal or the straight sinus, the cerebral and cerebellar veins and the superior petrosal sinus. *See* Table of Veins—sinus transversus.

transversion *Transposition of the teeth.

transversus colli muscle M. longissimus cervicis. *See* Table of Muscles.

transversus colli nerve Supplies the skin of the anterior triangle of the neck. *See* Table of Nerves.

transversus linguae muscle Changes the shape of the tongue. *Also called* lingualis transversus. *See* Table of Muscles.

transversus menti muscle Superficial fibres of M. depressor anguli oris. *See* Table of Muscles.

trapezius muscle Raises shoulder and draws back scapula. *See* Table of Muscles.

trauma Any injury or wound.

traumatic Relating to or produced by trauma.

traumatism A condition resulting from a trauma.
periodontal t. Degenerative changes occurring in the periodontium as a result of excessive stress transmitted through the teeth over a prolonged period of time.

traumatogenic Capable of producing trauma.

tray
impression t. A metal receptacle, usually shaped like the dental arch, in which wax or plastic impression material is placed when taking mouth impressions.

Treacher Collins syndrome (E. Treacher Collins, 1862-1919. English ophthalmologist). Mandibulofacial *dysostosis.

treatment 1. The means used to combat or cure a disease. 2. The care and management of a sick patient.

trench mouth Acute ulcerative *gingivitis.

trephination
dental t. *Apicostomy.

trephine bur A type of dental bur having either a hollow cylindrical or truncated cone head; it is primarily an end-cutting bur.

Treponema A genus of the Spirochaetaceae family of bacteria, a thread-like, spiral micro-organism, anaerobic, Gram-negative and motile, found in the oral cavity; some species are pathogenic to man.

tri- Prefix signifying *three*.

triangle Any three-sided figure.
cephalic t. Formed by lines from the chin to the forehead and occiput, and a line joining occiput to forehead.
cervical t's. *Triangles of the neck.
facial t. Formed by lines joining the alveolar and nasal points and the basion.
hypoglossohyoid t. The triangular space bounded by the posterior border of the mylohyoid muscle, the intermediate tendon of the digastric muscle, and the hypoglossal nerve; it lies within the submandibular triangle. *Also called* Pirogoff's triangle.
palatal t. Formed by a line across the greatest transverse diameter of the palate, and lines from either end of this base to the alveolar point.
retromandibular t., retromolar t. A shallow fossa on the mandible behind the third molar.
For eponymous triangles *see* under the personal name by which the triangle is known.

triangle of the neck
anterior Formed by anterior margin of sternocleidomastoid muscle, anterior median line of neck, base of mandible, continued to the mastoid process; apex at the sternum.
carotid Formed by sternocleidomastoid, superior belly of omohyoid, styloid, and posterior belly of digastric muscles.
digastric *See* submandibular.
muscular Formed by anterior margin of sternocleidomastoid muscle, median line of neck from sternum to hyoid bone, and superior belly of omohyoid muscle.
occipital Formed by sternocleidomastoid, trapezius and omohyoid, splenius capitis, levator scapulae, and scalenus medius et posterior muscles.

posterior Formed by sternomastoid and anterior margin of trapezius muscles, and middle third of clavicle.
subclavian See supraclavicular.
submandibular or *submaxillary* Formed by base of mandible, continued to mastoid process, posterior belly of digastric and styloid, and anterior belly of digastric muscles.
submental or *suprahyoid* Formed by anterior belly of digastric muscle, hyoid bone, and mylohyoid muscles; apex at mandible.
supraclavicular Formed by inferior belly of omohyoid muscle, clavicle and lower part of posterior border of sternocleidomastoid muscle.

triangular muscle M. depressor anguli oris. *See* Table of Muscles.

tribe An intermediate division in biological classification, coming between the family and the genus.

trichoglossia Hairy *tongue.

Trichomonas A genus of flagellate protozoa of the class Mastigophora and having a pear-shaped body and several flagella.
T. buccalis, T. elongata **Trichomonas tenax*.
T. tenax A form of *Trichomonas* found in the mouth.

triconodont A tooth having three cusps in a line.

tricuspal, tricuspid Having three cusps.

trifurcate Divided into three branches or roots.

trigeminal nerve The fifth cranial nerve, which divides into N. ophthalmicus, N. maxillaris and N. mandibularis. *See* Table of Nerves—trigeminus.

trigon, trigone The three main cusps, in a group, of a trituberculate maxillary molar.

trigonid The first three cusps on a mandibular molar.

trigonodont A tooth having three cusps in the form of a triangle.

trilobate Having three lobes.

trimmer Any instrument used to trim or shape.
gingival margin t. A type of chisel designed for bevelling gingival enamel margins.

triple-angle *Of an instrument*: having three angles in the shank.

trismus 1. Inability to open the mouth because of tonic spasm of the jaw muscles. 2. Lockjaw, caused by muscle spasm, associated with tetanus.

trismus stent A form of Kingsley's splint designed to assist in opening and closing the mouth, or to exercise the temporomandibular joint.

tritocone The distobuccal cusp on a maxillary premolar; not found in man.

tritoconid The distobuccal cusp on a mandibular premolar; not found in man.

tritubercular Having three cusps or tubercles.

triturate 1. To rub to a fine powder. 2. *Trituration[2].

trituration 1. The reduction of a solid substance to a powder by rubbing. 2. A substance so reduced.

trochlear nerve The fourth cranial nerve, supplying the obliquus superior muscle of the eyeball. *See* Table of Nerves—trochlearis.

trunk 1. The main part of the body, excluding the limbs and the head and neck. 2. A major part of a nerve or of a blood or lymphatic vessel, usually short and unbranched.
brachiocephalic t. The blood supply for the right upper limb, and the right side of the head and neck.

Also called the innominate artery. *See* Table of Arteries—truncus brachiocephalicus.
costocervical t. The blood supply for the deep muscles of the neck and back, 1st and 2nd intercostal spaces and the vertebral column. *See* Table of Arteries—truncus costocervicalis.
linguofacial t. The common trunk by which the lingual and facial arteries frequently arise from the external carotid artery. *See* Table of Arteries—truncus linguofacialis.
thyrocervical t. The blood supply for the neck, thyroid gland, oesophagus and trachea. *See* Table of Arteries—truncus thyrocervicalis.

trusion Malposition; an obsolete term.

try-in Trial *denture.

tube A hollow cylindrical body open at both ends.
auditory t. A canal connecting the upper pharynx with the middle ear; *also called* Eustachian tube.
auricular t. External auditory *meatus.
pharyngotympanic t. Auditory *tube.

tube, Eustachian Auditory *tube.

tube tooth An artificial tooth having a cylindrical hollow running from the occlusal surface to the cervix.

tubercle 1. A nodule. 2. A rounded eminence on a bone. 3. The lesion produced by the tuberculosis bacillus.
dental t. 1. A small elevation of extra enamel on a tooth crown. 2. *Cusp[1].
genial t. Mental *tubercle.
labial t., t. of the upper lip *Procheilon.
maxillary t. A small, rough prominence at the distal end of the maxillary alveolar process.
mental t. One of two small projections of bone on the inner surface of the mandible on either side of the symphysis menti; *also called* mental spine.
paramolar t. An additional cusp occurring on the mesiobuccal aspect of a second or third molar; it is thought to be a rudimentary paramolar.
pterygoid t. Pterygoid *tuberosity of the mandible.

tubercular 1. Relating to a tubercule or tubercules. 2. Relating to tuberculosis.

tuberculate Having tubercles.

tuberculated Covered with tubercles.

tuberculosis The disease caused by *Mycobacterium*, and more specifically by *M. tuberculosis*; it is characterized by the presence of tubercles, and is usually chronic and granulomatous. It may affect the jaws, lymph nodes, mouth, oral mucosa and temporomandibular joint.

tuberoplasty The surgical reshaping of the maxillary tuberosity.

tuberosity A broad protuberance on a bone.
maxillary t. Maxillary *tubercle.
pterygoid t. of the mandible The roughened area on the inner surface of the ramus and the angle of the mandible; the site of the insertion of the medial pterygoid muscle.

tubule A small tube.
dentinal t. One of the minute tubes in dentine, radiating from the pulp chamber to the amelodentinal junction and the cementodentinal junction.

tufts
enamel t. Bundles of poorly mineralized enamel rods extending into the tooth enamel from the amelodentinal junction.

tularaemia A bacterial infection caused by *Francisella tularensis*, contracted from rodents such as squirrels; oral manifestations include necrotic ulceration of the mucous membrane, extending to the pharynx, and regional lymphadenitis.

tumefaction The state of being or becoming swollen; a swelling.

tumour An abnormal mass of tissue, the growth of which exceeds and is unco-ordinated with that of the normal tissues, and persists in the same excessive manner after cessation of the stimuli which evoked the change (Willis). It may also be used in the more general sense of any localized swelling.
acinic-cell t. A benign epithelial tumour of the salivary glands made up of cells resembling the serous cells of those glands.
adenomatoid odontogenic t. A benign tumour containing odontogenic epithelium with duct-like structures, which may occur in the wall of a large cyst; it is more frequently seen in the maxilla, commonly associated with an unerupted tooth, and occurs usually between the ages of 10 years and 20 years.
brown t. A type of giant-cell granuloma associated with hyperparathyroidism; it has a red-brown colour, and recurs frequently if the systemic disease is not treated.
calcifying epithelial odontogenic t. A locally malignant intraosseous epithelial tumour characterized by the development of intra-epithelial structures which become mineralized; it is most frequently seen in the region of the crown of an unerupted tooth. *Also called* Pindborg's tumour.
melanotic neuro-ectodermal t. of infancy A benign tumour arising from neural crest cells, which may present as a pigmented or non-pigmented epulis, or may be contained within the bone; it is generally seen in the anterior part of the maxilla in infants under 1 year of age.
mixed t. Any tumour containing several different cell types; it may be benign or malignant.
muco-epidermoid t. A potentially malignant epithelial tumour of the salivary gland, containing epidermoid and mucous cells.
odontogenic t. Any tumour derived from odontogenic tissue.

tumour, Warthin's *Adenolymphoma[1].

turbid Cloudy.

turbine handpiece One which incorporates an air-driven rotor.

turgid Swollen, congested.

Turner tooth (J.G. Turner, 1870-1955. English dentist). A permanent tooth that has been damaged in some way during development because of infection or trauma affecting its primary predecessor.

turricephaly *Oxycephaly.

tusk A very large canine or incisor protruding beyond the lips.

twinning *In dentistry,* the development of two separate teeth from one follicle; *gemination[2].

tylosis linguae *Leukoplakia (*linguae*).

tympanic Relating to the tympanum.

tympanic artery Supplies the tympanum and tensor tympani muscle; four branches: anterior (*also called* Glaserian artery), posterior, inferior, superior. *See* Table of Arteries—tympanica.

tympanic nerve Supplies the mucosa of the middle ear and the pharyngotympanic tube; *also called*

Jacobsen's nerve. *See* Table of Nerves—tympanicus.

tympanum The middle ear, the ear-drum.

tyndallization (J. Tyndall, 1820-93. English physicist). A method of sterilizing culture media by exposure to steam at 100°C on three successive days, for about 30 minutes each day.

typodont An artificial, articulated model, containing either artificial or natural teeth, used in teaching various aspects of dentistry.

U

ung. Abbreviation for *unguentum*—an ointment; used in prescription writing.

ula The gingiva.

ulaemorrhagia Bleeding from the gingiva.

ulalgia *Gingivalgia.

ulangiectasis Irritation affecting the gingiva.

ulatrophy Gingival recession.
afunctional u. That occurring in congenital malocclusion.
atrophic u. Ischaemic *ulatrophy.
calcic u. That caused by salivary calculus.
ischaemic u. That caused by a deficient blood supply to the gingiva.
traumatic u. That due to some trauma to the gingiva.

ulcer A localized lesion on the surface of the skin or mucous membrane, with superficial necrosis and tissue loss resulting in the exposure of the deeper tissues in an open sore.
aphthous u. *Aphtha[2].
dental u. An ulcer on the oral mucosa produced by local trauma.
rodent u. A basal-cell carcinoma of superficial origin, arising in the epidermis, and occurring generally on the face or neck; *also called* Krompecher's tumour.
serpiginous u. An ulcer that is constantly spreading in one direction while healing in another.
sublingual u. Any ulcer on the under surface of the tongue, the lingual frenum or the floor of the mouth.
traumatic u. Any ulcer resulting from a traumatic injury.

ulceration The formation of ulcers.

ulcerative Relating to or characterized by ulceration.

ulcerogenic Ulcer-producing.

ulceromembranous Characterized by ulceration accompanied by a membranous exudation.

ulceronecrotic Characterized by ulceration accompanied by necrosis.

ulcerous Relating to or characterized by ulcers.

ulectomy 1. Excision of scar tissue. 2. *Gingivectomy.

ulemorrhagia Bleeding from the gingiva.

uletic Relating to the gingiva.

ulitis Generalized inflammation of the gingiva.

ulo- Prefix signifying 1. *a scar*; 2. *the gingiva*.

ulocace Gingival ulceration.

ulocarcinoma Gingival carcinoma.

uloglossitis Inflammation of both the gingiva and the tongue.

uloncus Any gingival tumour or swelling.

ulorrhagia Bleeding from the gingiva.

ulorrhoea Oozing of blood from the gingiva.

ulotomy 1. Surgical division of scar tissue. 2. Incision of the gingiva.

ulotripsis The nourishing and revitalizing of the gingiva by massage.

ultra- Prefix signifying *excessive* or *beyond*.

umbra Latin for *shadow*. *In radiography* it denotes any area of sharp contrast on an x-ray image.

uncal Relating to an uncus.

unciform Hook-shaped.

uncinate Hooked.

uncus (*pl.* unci) Any hook-shaped structure.

undercut 1. That part of a tooth or cavity that provides, by design or fortuitously, an area of resistance to withdrawal of a clasp or restoration. 2. *In prosthetic dentistry*, that part of the tooth crown below the clasp guide line.

unerupted Relating to a tooth that has not come through the gum, either in the normal course or because it lacks the physiological impetus.

unguentum Latin for *ointment*; used in prescription writing, and abbreviated *ung*.

uni- Prefix signifying *one*.

unicameral Having only one chamber.

unicuspid, unicuspidate Having only one cusp or tubercle.

unilateral Occurring on or relating to one side only.

unit 1. A specific amount, length, etc., used as a standard of measurement. 2. A complete system, the parts all performing one specific function.
dental u. All the mechanical equipment, mobile or fixed, in a dental surgery, which provides the means for patient treatment.
SI u. Any one of the units of measurement or weight adopted in the Système International d'Unités, based on the metric system.

unitubercular *Unicuspid.

uran-, urano- Prefix signifying *palate*.

uraniscochasma Cleft *palate.

uraniscolalia Defective speech caused by a palatal cleft.

uranisconitis Inflammation of the palate.

uraniscoplasty *Palatoplasty.

uraniscorraphy *Palatorraphy.

uraniscus The palate.

uranoplastic Relating to uranoplasty.

uranoplasty Surgical closure of a hard palate cleft.

uranoplegia Palatal paralysis; paralysis affecting the soft palate muscles.

uranorrhaphy *Palatorraphy.

uranoschisis, uranoschism Cleft *palate.

uranostaphyloplasty Repair of a cleft involving both hard and soft palates, by means of plastic surgery.

uranostaphylorrhaphy Closure of a cleft involving both hard and soft palates with sutures.

uranostaphyloschisis Palatal fissure affecting both the hard and soft palates.

uranosteoplasty *Uranoplasty.

utricular nerve Supplies the macula of the utricle. *See* Table of Nerves—utricularis.

utriculoampullary nerve Supplies the utricle and the ampullae of the semicircular ducts. *See* Table of Nerves—utriculoampullaris.

uveal artery A. ciliaris posterior brevis. *See* Table of Arteries.

uveoparotid fever A form of sarcoidosis affecting the parotid gland and characterized by firm, painless swelling accompanied by xerostomia.

uvula 1. *In anatomy,* any fleshy hanging mass. 2. The palatine *uvula.
bifid u. A cleft of the uvula, thought to be an incomplete cleft palate.
cleft u. Bifid *uvula.
palatine u. A small muscular appendage hanging from the posterior border of the soft palate.

uvular Relating to the uvula.

uvular muscle Forms the uvula. *See* Table of Muscles—uvulae.

uvulectomy Surgical excision of the palatine uvula.

uvulitis Inflammation of the uvula.
uvuloptosis A relaxed, dropped position of the palatine uvula.
uvulorraphy *Staphylorraphy.
uvulotomy Surgical removal of the uvula, or of some part of it.

V

vaccine 1. Any material used for preventive inoculation against a specific disease. 2. Lymph obtained from a cowpox vesicle and used in inoculation against smallpox.

vacuum A space from which the air content has been exhausted.

vacuum chamber Air *chamber.

vaginate Within a sheath.

vagus nerve The tenth cranial nerve, supplying the striated muscles and mucosa of the pharynx and larynx. *See* Table of Nerves.

Valentin's ganglion (G.G. Valentin, 1810-83. German physiologist). A pseudo-ganglion occurring at the junction of the posterior and middle branches of the dental nerve.

vallate Having a surrounding wall or rim.

Valleix's aphthae (F.L.I. Valleix, 1807-55. French physician). *Bednar's aphthae.

varicosity A distended vein, superficial, bluish and painless; in the mouth it is most frequently found on the under surface of the tongue, and is common in the elderly.

varnish A solution of resin or resins, which, when painted on thinly, leaves a clear, hard coat over the surface treated.
cavity v. A lining agent, used on the walls of a prepared cavity in a tooth, to improve the seal when placing a restoration.
copal v. A type of cavity varnish containing copal.
mastic v. A type of cavity varnish containing mastic.
periodontal v. A type of varnish applied to the gingiva after periodontal therapy.
rosin v. A type of cavity varnish with rosin as its main ingredient.
sandarac v. A solution of transparent resin in alcohol, used *in dentistry* as a separating fluid and protective coating for plaster casts.
separating v. Any varnish used to coat a plaster mould and prevent adhesion of fresh plaster poured in to produce a model.

vascular Relating to or composed of vessels; used particularly of blood vessels.

vasi-, vaso- Prefix signifying *vessel* or *duct.*

vasoconstrictor A nerve, or some external agent, which causes vascular contraction.

vasodentine Dentine containing blood vessels; found in the teeth of fish.

vasodilator A nerve, or some external agent, which causes vascular dilatation.

vasomotor nerve Any nerve that controls the calibre of blood or lymph vessels; it may be a *vasodilator* or a *vasoconstrictor.*

vault Any arch- or dome-like structure; used *in dentistry* as a term for the roof of the mouth.

Veau's operation (V. Veau, b. 1871. French surgeon). An operation for repair of cleft palate which includes dissection and suturing of the nasal mucosa.

vehicle *In medicine,* any inert substance employed as a medium for the administration of a medicine.

Veillonella (A. Veillon, 1864-1931. French bacteriologist). The type genus of the Veillonellaceae family of anaerobic, Gram-negative diplococci, seen as non-motile, nonsporing spheres; parasitic in the mouth, intestinal tract and respiratory tract in man.

Veillonellaceae (A. Veillon, 1864-1931. French bacteriologist). A family of parasitic, Gram-negative, anaerobic cocci, non-motile and seen characteristically as pairs of cells.

vein One of the blood vessels conveying de-oxygenated blood to the heart.
pulmonary v. One of the short, thick blood vessels conveying oxygenated blood from the lungs to the heart.

velar Relating to a velum.

velopharyngeal Relating to the soft palate and the pharynx.

velosynthesis Repair of a cleft in the soft palate.

velum Any veil-like structure.
artificial v. An appliance used in prosthetic treatment of a cleft of the soft palate.

velum palatinum The soft palate.

veneer A thin covering layer of material which is fused on to the surface of an object. *In dentistry* it is used to cover artificial tooth crowns to match with the natural teeth, or to replace the natural tooth surface if it is damaged or discoloured.

venose Supplied with veins.

venous Relating to a vein or veins.

venous sinus *Sinus[2]. For venous sinuses *see* Table of Veins—sinus.

venter 1. The stomach or abdomen. 2. Any hollow, belly-shaped part, as the belly of a muscle.

ventral 1. Towards the front, as opposed to *dorsal*. 2. Relating to a belly, the abdomen or any other venter.

venule A minute vein.

vermiform Worm-like.

verruca vulgaris The common wart, caused by a virus, and seen most frequently on the fingers; in the mouth, a rare oral variant may affect the lips and the palate, and is often indistinguishable from squamous-cell papilloma.

version The act of turning, as of teeth during orthodontic treatment.

vertebra (*pl.* vertebrae) Any one of the bones of the spinal column.

vertebral Relating to a vertebra or to vertebrae.

vertebral artery Supplies the cerebellum, the cerebrum, spinal cord, meninges and neck muscles. *See* Table of Arteries—vertebralis.

vertebral veins Veins draining from the venous plexus on the vertebral artery. *See* Table of Veins—vertebralis.

vertical muscle of the tongue M. verticalis linguae. *See* Table of Muscles.

verticalis linguae muscle Changes the shape of the tongue; *also called* lingualis verticalis. *See* Table of Muscles.

verticomental Relating to the crown of the head and the chin.

vertigo A sensation of loss of equilibrium in which sufferers feel either that the world is revolving round them or that they are revolving in space.

vesicle 1. A small bladder or sac containing liquid. 2. A blister.

vesiculation The formation of vesicles.

vessel Any tube or canal conveying fluid, especially lymph or blood.

vestibular 1. Relating to a vestibule. 2. *In dentistry*, used to describe the buccal and labial surfaces of the teeth, collectively.

vestibular nerve Supplies ampullae of semicircular ducts, maculae of utricle and saccule, via vestibular ganglion. *See* Table of Nerves—vestibularis.

vestibule A cavity or space serving as the entrance to a canal.

vestibule *of the ear* The oval cavity in the inner ear leading to the cochlea.

vestibule *of the mouth* The space between the lips and cheek and the gums and teeth.

vestibulocochlear nerve The eighth cranial nerve, dividing into N. cochlearis and N. vestibularis. *See* Table of Nerves—vestibulocochlearis.

vestibuloplasty Any surgical process used to deepen the vestibular sulcus; it is performed to facilitate the fitting of a denture, and in periodontal surgery to increase the area of attached gingiva after gingivectomy.

vestige A rudimentary part or remnant which at some stage was fully developed and functional.

vestigial Relating to a vestige; rudimentary.

viability Ability to live after birth.

viable Able to live of itself.

vibration Any rapid to-and-fro movements; oscillation.

vibrator 1. Anything that causes vibration. 2. *In dentistry*, a device used in the making of dentures and casting of inlays, to ensure a good reproduction.

oral v. A prosthetic appliance designed to provide a method of speaking for those patients who, either from operation or paralysis, have no current of air passing through the mouth. It consists of a flexible diaphragm fitted into the palate of an upper denture and vibrated by means of electric batteries, thus creating the necessary current of air.

Vibrio The type genus of the Vibrionaceae family of bacteria, Gram-negative and facultatively anaerobic, seen as short rigid, straight or curved motile rods, found in marine animals; some species are pathogenic to man.

Vibrionaceae A family of microorganisms seen as rigid rods, motile, Gram-negative, facultatively anaerobic; found in fresh or sea water.

vicarious 1. Relating to a normal process occurring in an abnormal position or under abnormal conditions. 2. Acting as a substitute.

vidian canal (V. Vidius [G. Guidi], 1500-69. Italian anatomist and physician). Pterygoid *canal.

vidian nerve, Vidius' nerve (V. Vidius [G. Guidi], 1500-69. Italian anatomist and physician). N. canalis pterygoidei. *See* Table of Nerves.

Vignal's bacillus (G. Vignal, 1852-93. French physiologist). **Leptotrichia buccalis*.

villiform Hair-like, having hair-like projections.

Vincent's angina (J.H. Vincent, 1862-1950. French physician and bacteriologist). Acute ulcerative *tonsillitis.

Vincent's infection (J.H. Vincent, 1862-1950. French physician and bacteriologist). Acute ulcerative *gingivitis.

Vincent's stomatitis (J.H. Vincent, 1862-1950. French physician and bacteriologist). Acute ulcerative *stomatitis.

vinculum A ligament or frenum.

vinculum linguae *Frenulum linguae.

Vinson syndrome (P.P. Vinson, 1890-1959. American surgeon). *See* Plummer-Vinson syndrome.

Virchow's angle (R.L.K. Virchow, 1821-1902. German pathologist). The angle formed at the intersection of a line joining the nasofrontal suture and the most prominent point on the lower edge of the maxillary alveolar process with a line joining the lower border of the orbit to the external auditory meatus.

virulence 1. Malignancy. 2. The infectiousness of a micro-organism.

virulent 1. Toxic, poisonous. 2. Related to or characterized by virulence.

virus A complex organic particle, of submicroscopic dimensions, capable of growth and reproduction only within the cells of the host organism it infects.

viscera The organs in the thoracic, abdominal or pelvic cavity; used particularly of those organs in the abdomen.

visceral Relating to the viscera.

viscid, viscous Sticky, adhesive.

viscosity The property or state of being glutinous or adhesive.

viscus (*pl.* viscera) Any one of the organs of the body cavities, especially those of the abdomen; usually used in the plural.

vital Living; relating to life or necessary for life.

vitality The state of being alive.

vitalometer A name given to an apparatus used to test for the vitality of tooth pulp.

vitreodentine Vitreous *dentine.

vitreous Relating to glass, glassy.

vitrodentine Vitreous *dentine.

vocal muscle Shortens the vocal cords. *See* Table of Muscles—vocalis.

Vogt's angle (K. Vogt, 1817-95. German physiologist). The angle formed between the nasobasilar and the alveolonasal lines.

vomer The flat bone forming the posterior and lower portion of the nasal septum.

vomerine Relating to the vomer.

vomit 1. To cast up from the stomach through the mouth. 2. The substance so cast up.

vomiting The forcible expulsion of the contents of the stomach upwards through the mouth.

vomitus *Vomit[2].

von Ebner's fibrils, glands, lines *See under* Ebner.

von Korff's fibres *See under* Korff.

von Recklinghausen's disease (F.D. von Recklinghausen, 1833-1910. German pathologist). *Neurofibromatosis.

vulcanite A thermohardening material produced by heating raw rubber with sulphur; the degree of hardness depends on the amount of sulphur used.

vulcanization The process of making vulcanite.

vulcanize To treat rubber with sulphur so as to render it flexible or hard.

W

Waldeyer's ring (H.W.G. Waldeyer, 1836-1921. German anatomist, embryologist and pathologist). A circular band of lymphoid tissue, made up of the lingual, palatine, tubal and pharyngeal tonsils, surrounding the opening to the larynx and pharynx.

Walker appliance *Crozat appliance.

wall *of a cavity* One of the walls that form the outline of a tooth cavity; named after the tooth surface towards which it faces: *i.e.* mesial, distal, buccal, lingual, pulpal, axial, gingival, occlusal, incisal, labial.
subpulpal w. The floor of any prepared cavity that has been extended into the pulp chamber.

wall-tooth A molar *tooth; obsolete term.

Walther's duct (A.F. Walther, 1688-1746. German anatomist). The duct of the sublingual salivary gland.

wandering *of the teeth* The vertical or horizontal displacement of teeth due to destruction of the periodontal ligament.

wang tooth A molar *tooth; obsolete term.

Wardill's operation (W.E.M. Wardill, 1895-1961. English surgeon). Operation for the repair of cleft palate by dividing the long mucoperiosteal flaps obliquely and rotating and sliding them to obtain greater length of the soft palate without loss of continuity.

warp To change in shape, becoming twisted or bulging; used of the effect on material such as plaster or vulcanite left exposed to the air for too long.

wart *Verruca vulgaris.

Warthin's tumour (A.S. Warthin, 1866-1931. American pathologist). *Adenolymphoma[1].

watchmaker's broach A tapered broach, sharp-angled and having four or five sides, used to enlarge root canals.

water fluoridation The adjustment of the level of fluoride ion in the drinking water supply to an optimum concentration of 1 p.p.m., to reduce the incidence of dental caries in a community. Usually achieved by the addition of small quantities of sodium fluoride in areas where the naturally occurring concentration is below the optimum.

wax A plastic substance obtained from plants or from deposits of insects. That used for dental impressions is generally beeswax.

wax carver A specially designed type of carver with a blunt blade used for fashioning wax, and capable of being heated for this use.

waxing up The construction and contouring of a wax base plate for an artificial denture, and the temporary attachment of teeth to it with wax.

weal A reddish, raised and circumscribed lesion on the skin, generally caused by a blow or a bite.

Weber's artery (M.I. Weber, 1795-1875. German anatomist). The external auditory artery.

Weber's glands (E.H. Weber, 1795-1878. German anatomist). The lateral lingual glands.

Weil's basal layer (L.A. Weil, 1849-95. German dentist). Subodontoblastic *layer.

Weisbach's angle (A.W. Weisbach, 1837-1914. Austrian anthropologist). The angle formed at the alveolar point by lines from the basion and the mid-point of the frontal suture.

Welcker's angle (H. Welcker, 1822-98. German anatomist and anthropologist). The sphenoid angle of the parietal bone.

Weston crown (H. Weston, fl. 1883. American dentist). A porcelain pivot crown attached to the tooth by means of a flat post riveted to the crown before insertion.

whartonitis Inflammation of the submandibular duct (Wharton's duct).

Wharton's duct (T. Wharton, 1614-73. English anatomist). Submandibular *duct.

wheal *See* weal.

wheel A solid round disc or a hollow round frame capable of revolving on a central axis. Wheels of different sizes and materials are used *in dentistry* in the handpiece of a dental engine for polishing or cutting, and these are usually named by the materials of which they are made or with which they are covered.

Willis gauge An instrument used to measure vertical dimensions of the face.

Willis's circle (T. Willis, 1621-75. English anatomist and physician). *Circulus arteriorus cerebri.

Wilson's curve *See* curve of Wilson.

window crown An acrylic-veneer gold crown, covering all but the labial or buccal surface of a tooth, and frequently used as a bridge abutment.

wing *In anatomy,* any structure or part, often paired, resembling a bird's wing.

Winter's elevator (G.B. Winter, contemporary American oral surgeon). An elevator for removing lower third molars.

wire 1. Fine, flexible metal rods or metal thread used in surgery and in dentistry. 2. To immobilize fractures by means of wire. 3. *In orthodontics*, to apply wire to the teeth in the correction of malocclusion.

arch w. See archwire.

expansion w. An orthodontic appliance of wire, conforming to the dental arch, and used for anchorage in the movement of teeth.

orthodontic w. *Archwire.

wiring 1. The application of wires in the immobilization of fractures. 2. *Wire[3].

anterior nasal aperture w. Piriform aperture *wiring.

circumferential w. A method of immobilization of a jaw fracture in an edentulous mandible where the vulcanite or other splint is held in place by wires passed over the bone and through the soft tissues.

continuous loop w. A method of reduction and fixation of jaw fractures by looping a single length of wire over both mandibular and maxillary teeth, and attaching the loops to an intermaxillary elastic.

direct interdental w. Immobilization of a jaw fracture by twisting wires round suitable teeth in both the upper and lower jaws and then joining the twisted ends of opposing upper and lower wires to help maintain the occlusion.

interdental w. Immobilization of a jaw fracture by means of wires passed round several teeth on each side of the fracture.

interdental eyelet w. A form of direct wiring in which the wires are doubled to form an eyelet and a tail; these are fastened round two teeth at a time and then linked between the jaws with connecting wires or rubber bands.

intermaxillary w. Any form of wiring used for immobilizing jaw fractures that links the upper to the lower jaw.

perialveolar w. Immobilization of a jaw fracture by wires passed through the alveolar bone; used in edentulous patients or those with no suitable teeth to support a splint.

piriform aperture w. Stabilization of a jaw fracture using wires passed through the piriform aperture.

pyriform fossa w. Piriform aperture *wiring.

wisdom tooth A third molar *tooth.

wolf jaw Bilateral cleft extending through the palate, jaw and lip.

Wolinella (M.J. Wolin, contemporary American bacteriologist). A genus of the family Bacteroidaceae, rod-shaped bacteria, Gram-negative, anaerobic and motile, found in the human oral cavity and in cattle.

W. recta A species found in human infected root canals, periodontal pockets and gingival tissue.

Wood crown A porcelain crown baked to a platinum cap.

working side The side towards which the mandible is moving during lateral movement.

wormian bones (O. Worm, 1588-1654. Danish anatomist). Small bones in the sutures of the skull.

wound Any injury to the tissues or organs caused by cut, stab or tear, usually going deeper than the outer skin or integument.

X

X-bite *Crossbite.

X plate An orthodontic screw-adjusted appliance used to retract protrusive incisors and prevent excessive overbite.

x-ray Radiant energy of short wavelength, penetrating solid masses impervious to ordinary light rays, and by means of which photographs may be taken of internal body structures.

xanth-, xantho- Prefix signifying *yellow*.

xanthodont, xanthodontous Having yellow teeth.

xanthoma A localized deposit of fatty tissue or serum lipids, seen as a yellow or orange elevation on the skin or mucous membranes, most often occurring on the eyelids.
verruciform x. A rare verrucous or papillary lesion of the oral mucosa, usually occurring on the mandibular alveolar ridge, characterized by a whitish surface, with shallow, regular corrugations.

xeno- Prefix signifying *foreign*.

xenograft A graft derived from a donor of a different species.

xero- Prefix signifying *dry*.

xerocheilia Inflammation of the lips marked by excessive dryness.

xerostomia Dryness of the mouth, due to failure of salivary secretion; *also called* Zagari's disease.

xylitol A sugar derivative of xylose, used as an artificial sweetener.

Z

Zn Chemical symbol for zinc.

Zagari's disease (G. Zagari, 1863-1946. Italian physician). *Xerostomia.

zinc A bluish-white, crystalline, lustrous metal, chemical symbol Zn. Malleable and ductile at moderately high temperatures, brittle at over 200°C.

Zinn's artery (J.G. Zinn, 1727-59. German anatomist). Central artery of the retina. *See* Table of Arteries—centralis retinae.

Zinn's circle (J.G. Zinn, 1727-59. German anatomist). *Circulus vasculosus nervi optici.

zona 1. *In anatomy,* a band or band-like section with specific boundaries or specific characteristics. 2. *Herpes zoster.

zone *In anatomy,* a band or band-like section with specific boundaries or specific characteristics; *also called* zona.

apical z. The narrow band over the apices of the tooth roots.

cervical z. The cervical third of the area of enamel covering the crown of a tooth from the cementoenamel junction.

contact area z. The area of contact between adjacent teeth; the middle third of the area of enamel covering the crown of a tooth.

coronal z. The enamel area covering the crown of a tooth, from the cementoenamel junction.

dentofacial z. The lower part of the face, the area covering the teeth and jaws.

neutral z. The area between the tongue and the cheeks or lips, within which the muscles exert equal and opposing forces on the teeth.

occlusal z. The area of enamel on the tooth crown nearest to the occlusal surface; the occlusal third of the coronal zone.

zoo- Prefix signifying *animal.*

zoster *Herpes zoster.

zygion The most lateral point on the surface of the zygoma; one of a pair of craniometric landmarks.

zygoma Zygomatic process of the *temporal bone.

zygomatic Relating to the zygomatic bone.

zygomatic bone The cheek bone - os zygomaticum; *also called* the malar bone.

zygomatic muscle The *greater* zygomatic muscle raises the corner of the mouth. *See* Table of Muscles—zygomaticus major. The *lesser* zygomatic muscle is part of M. levator labii superioris; *also called* M. distortor oris. *See* Table of Muscles—zygomaticus minor.

zygomatic nerve Supplies the skin over the zygomatic bone and the temporal region. *See* Table of Nerves—zygomaticus.

zygomatico- Prefix signifying *zygomatic bone.*

zygomaticofacial Relating to the zygomatic bone and the face.

zygomaticofacial nerve Supplies the skin over the zygomatic bone. *See* Table of Nerves—zygomaticofacialis.

zygomaticomaxillary *Zygomaxillary.

zygomatico-orbital artery Supplies the orbicularis oculi muscle. *See* Table of Arteries—zygomatico-orbitalis.

zygomaticotemporal nerve Supplies the skin over the anterior portion of the temporal region. *See* Table of Nerves—zygomaticotemporalis.

zygomaxillare A point at the lower end of the zygomatic suture, a craniometric landmark.

zygomaxillary Relating to the zygomatic bone, zygomatic arch or zygomatic process and the maxilla.

TABLE OF ARTERIES OF THE HEAD AND NECK

ARTERY	ORIGIN	PARTS SUPPLIED
alveolaris inferior [*dentalis inferior*]	Maxillary	Mandibular teeth, floor of mouth, buccal mucous membrane.
alveolaris superior anterior [*dentalis superior anterior*]	Infra-orbital	Maxillary incisors and canines.
alveolaris superior posterior [*dentalis superior posterior*]	Maxillary	Antral mucous membrane, maxillary molars and premolars.
angularis	Facial	Inferior portion of orbicularis palpebrum, lacrimal sac.
auditiva interna	*Labyrinthi.	
auditory	*Labyrinthi.	
auricularis (*inconstant*)	Branch of occipital	Concha.
auricularis anterior	Branch of superficial	Lateral aspect of pinna, temporal external auditory meatus.
auricularis posterior	External carotid	Digastric and other muscles, parotid gland, middle ear, mastoid cells, auricle.
auricularis profunda	Maxillary	Skin of external auditory meatus and tympanic membrane.
basilaris	Subclavian	Cerebellum and cerebrum.
buccalis [*buccinator*]	Maxillary	Buccal mucous membrane, skin of cheek, buccinator muscle.
buccinator	*Buccalis.	
canalis pterygoidei	Maxillary	Levator and tensor veli palatini muscles, pharyngotympanic tube, upper portion of pharynx.
caroticotympanica	Branch of internal carotid	Tympanic cavity.
carotis communis	*right*: Brachiocephalic *left*: Aortic arch	Divides into internal trunk; and external carotid arteries.

ARTERY	ORIGIN	PARTS SUPPLIED
carotis externa	Common carotid	Meninges, neck, thyroid gland, tongue, tonsils, side of head, face, skin, middle ear.
carotis interna	Common carotid	Parts of brain, orbit, forehead, nose.
centralis retinae	Ophthalmic	Retina.
cerebelli inferior anterior	Basilar	Lower anterior surface of cerebellum.
cerebelli inferior posterior	Vertebral	Medulla, vermiform process, cerebellar cortex.
cerebelli superior	Basilar	Outer rim of cerebellum, superior vermiform process.
cerebri anterior	Internal carotid	Corpus callosum, frontal lobe, optic and olfactory tracts.
cerebri media	Internal carotid	Basal ganglia, island of Reil, frontal, parietal and temporal lobes.
cerebri posterior	Basilar	Temporal and occipital lobes.
cervicalis ascendens	Inferior thyroid	Neck muscles, spinal cord and vertebrae.
cervicalis profunda	Costocervical trunk	Deep muscles at back of neck.
cervicalis superficialis	Variable superficial branch of transversa cervicis.	
choroidea	*Choroidea anterior.	
choroidea anterior [*choroidea*]	Internal carotid	Choroid plexus of lateral ventricle, corpus fibriatum, hippocampus major.
ciliaris anterior	Muscular	Perforating sclera and anastomosing with posterior ciliary.
ciliaris posterior brevis [*uveal*]	Ophthalmic	Choroid and ciliary processes of the eye.
ciliaris posterior longa	Ophthalmic	From sclerotic and choroid to iris.
communicans anterior	Anterior cerebral	Forms part of circle of Willis.
communicans posterior	Internal carotid	Uncinate gyrus, thalamus; forms part of circle of Willis.

ARTERY	ORIGIN	PARTS SUPPLIED
conjunctivalis anterior	Muscular	Conjunctiva.
conjunctivalis posterior	Medial palpebral	Conjunctiva, lacrimal caruncle.
cricothyroidea	Branch of superior thyroid	Cricothyroid muscle.
dentalis	1. Branch of alveolar; 2. *Alveolaris, British terminology.	Maxillary or mandibular teeth
dorsalis linguae	Branch of lingual	Pillars of fauces, tonsils, dorsum of tongue.
dorsalis nasi [*nasi externa*]	Ophthalmic	Skin of dorsum of nose.
episcleralis	Muscular	Joins greater arterial circle of iris.
ethmoidalis anterior	Ophthalmic	Dura mater, frontal sinuses, anterior ethmoid cells, nose, facial skin.
ethmoidalis posterior	Ophthalmic	Dura mater, posterior ethmoid cells, nose.
facialis [*maxillaris externa*]	External carotid	Pharynx, soft palate, tonsil, submandibular gland, part of orbit and lacrimal sac.
Glaserian	*Tympanica anterior.	
gustatoria	*Lingualis.	
hyoidea	*Infrahyoidea, *suprahyoidea.	
infrahyoidea	Branch of superior thyroid	Thyrohyoid muscle and membrane.
infraorbitalis	Maxillary	Upper lip, side of nose, lower eyelid and lacrimal sac.
innominate	*Truncus brachiocephalicus.	
labialis inferior	Facial	Lower lip.
labialis superior	Facial	Upper lip, nasal septum.
labyrinthi [*auditiva interna; auditory*]	Inferior anterior cerebellar	Internal ear.
lacrimalis	Ophthalmic	Cheek, eyelids, eye muscle, lacrimal gland.
laryngea inferior	Inferior thyroid	Larynx.
laryngea superior	Superior thyroid	Laryngeal muscles and mucous membrane.
lingualis [*gustatoria*]	External carotid	Sublingual gland, tongue, tonsil, epiglottis.

ARTERY	ORIGIN	PARTS SUPPLIED
masseterica	Maxillary	Deep surface of masseter muscle.
mastoidea	Branch of occipital	Dura mater, lateral sinuses, mastoid cells.
maxillaris [*maxillaris interna*]	External carotid	Meninges, muscles of cheek, palate, nose, mandibular alveolar process and teeth, ear.
maxillaris externa	*Facialis.	
maxillaris interna	*Maxillaris.	
meningea	Branch of vertebral	Dura mater of posterior cranial fossa.
meningea accessoria	*Pterygomeningea.	
meningea anterior	Anterior ethmoid	Dura mater of middle cranial fossa.
meningea media	Maxillary	Dura mater and cranium.
meningea posterior	Ascending pharyngeal	Dura mater.
mentalis	Branch of inferior alveolar	Lower lip and chin.
muscularis	Ophthalmic	Muscles of the eye.
nasalis posterior lateralis	Sphenopalatine	Nasal cavity and adjacent sinuses.
nasi externa	*Dorsalis nasi.	
nasopalatina	*Sphenopalatina.	
occipitalis	External carotid	Neck and scalp muscles.
ophthalmica	Internal carotid	Eyeball, eye muscle, nose, ethmoid sinuses.
palatina ascendens	Facial	Palate, tonsils, upper portion of pharynx.
palatina descendens	Maxillary	Hard and soft palates.
palatina major	Descending palatine	Hard palate.
palatina minor	Descending palatine	Soft palate.
palpebralis inferior	Medial palpebral	Caruncle, conjunctiva, lacrimal sac, lower eyelid.
palpebralis lateralis	Lacrimal	Eyelids, conjunctiva.
palpebralis medialis	Ophthalmic	Conjunctiva, lacrimal sac, eyelid.
palpebralis superior	Medial palpebral	Upper eyelid.
parotidea	1. Branch of superficial temporal; 2. Branch of posterior auricular	Parotid gland.
petrosa	Branch of middle meningeal	Tympanic cavity.

ARTERY	ORIGIN	PARTS SUPPLIED
pharyngea	Branch of ascending pharyngeal	Pharynx.
pharyngea ascendens	External carotid	Membranes of brain, neck muscles and nerves, pharynx, soft palate, tympanum.
pontis	Basilar	Pons.
profunda linguae [*ranine*]	Lingual	Lower surface of tongue.
pterygoidea	Branch of posterior temporal	Pterygoid muscles.
pterygomeningea [*meningea accessoria*]	Maxillary	Trigeminal ganglion.
ranine	*Profunda linguae.	
septalis posterior	Branch of sphenopalatine	Nasal mucous membrane.
sphenopalatina [*nasopalatina*]	Maxillary	Lateral nasal wall and septum.
sternocleidomastoidea	1. Branch of occipital; 2. Branch of superior thyroid	Sternocleidomastoid muscle.
stylomastoidea	Posterior auricular	Middle ear.
subclavia	*right*: Brachiocephalic *left*: Aortic arch	Upper limb, spinal cord, trunk; neck, brain, meninges.
sublingualis	Lingual	Lower jaw muscles, floor of mouth, side of tongue, sublingual gland.
submentalis	Facial	Tissues below jaw.
suprahyoidea	Branch of lingual	Muscles above hyoid bone.
supraorbitalis	Ophthalmic	Forehead.
supratrochlearis	Ophthalmic	Anteromedial part of forehead.
temporalis media	Superficial temporal	Temporal fascia.
temporalis profunda anterior	Maxillary	Zygomatic bone, greater wing of sphenoid, temporal muscles.
temporalis profunda posterior	Maxillary	Temporal muscles.
temporalis superficialis	External carotid	Temporal fascia.
thyroidea ima (*inconstant*)	Brachiocephalic trunk	Thyroid gland.

ARTERY	ORIGIN	PARTS SUPPLIED
thyroidea inferior	Subclavian	Neck muscles, oesophagus, larynx, thyroid gland.
thyroidea superior	External carotid	Thyroid gland, larynx, sternocleidomastoid and infrahyoid muscles.
tonsillaris	Branch of facial	Base of tongue and faucial tonsil.
trachealis	Branch of inferior thyroid	Trachea.
transversa cervicis [*transversa colli*]	Subclavian or thyrocervical trunk	Root of neck and muscles of scapula.
transversa colli	*Transversa cervicis.	
transversa faciei [*transversa facialis*]	Superficial temporal	Masseter muscle, parotid gland, facial skin.
truncus brachiocephalicus [*innominate*]	Aortic arch	Right upper limb, right side of head and neck.
truncus costocervicalis	Subclavian	Deep muscles of neck and back, 1st & 2nd intercostal spaces, vertebral column.
truncus linguofacialis	The common trunk by which the lingual and facial arteries frequently arise from the external carotid artery.	
truncus thyrocervicalis	Subclavian	Neck, thyroid gland, oesophagus, trachea.
tympanica anterior [*Glaserian*]	Maxillary	Tympanum.
tympanica inferior	Ascending pharyngeal	Tympanum.
tympanica posterior	Posterior auricular	Tympanic membranes.
tympanica superior	Middle meningeal	Tensor tympani muscle.
uveal	*Ciliaris posterior brevis.	
vertebralis	Subclavian	Cerebellum, cerebrum, spinal cord, meninges, neck muscles.
zygomatico-orbitalis	Superficial temporal	Orbicularis oculi.

TABLE OF MUSCLES OF

MUSCLE	ORIGIN
abducens oris	*Levator anguli oris.
alveololabialis	*Buccinator.
alveolomaxillary	*Buccinator.
aponeurosis epicranialis	*Galea aponeurotica.
aryepiglotticus	Inconstant fascicle of oblique arytenoid, from the apex of the arytenoid cartilage
arytenoideus obliquus	Dorsal aspect of muscular process of arytenoid cartilage
arytenoideus transversus	Dorsal aspect of arytenoid cartilage
auricularis anterior	Lateral part of galea aponeurotica
auricularis posterior	Lateral part of mastoid process
auricularis superior	Lateral part of galea aponeurotica
buccinator [*alveololabialis; alveolomaxillary*]	Maxillary alveolar process, buccinator ridge on mandible, and pterygomandibular ligament
buccopharyngeus	Part of constrictor pharyngis superior.
caninus	*Levator anguli oris.
cephalopharyngeus	*Constrictor pharyngis superior.
ceratopharyngeus	Part of constrictor pharyngis medius.
chondroglossus	Lesser horn of hyoid bone
chondropharyngeus	Part of constrictor pharyngis medius.
ciliaris	Sphincter of ciliary body and scleral spur
complexus	*Semispinalis capitis.
compressor naris	*Nasalis, pars transversa.
constrictor pharyngis inferior	Lateral surface of ala of thyroid cartilage, tendinous arch to cricoid cartilage, side of cricoid cartilage
constrictor pharyngis medius	Lower part of stylohyoid ligament, and both horns of hyoid bone
constrictor pharyngis superior [*cephalopharyngeus*]	Posterior border and hamulus of medial pterygoid plate, pterygomandibular raphe, upper end of mylohyoid line, and side of tongue
corrugator supercilii	Superciliary arch on frontal bone
cricoarytenoideus lateralis	Lateral part of cricoid cartilage
cricoarytenoideus posterior	Posterior surface of cricoid cartilage

INSERTION	NERVE SUPPLY	FUNCTION
Lateral margin of epiglottis.		
Apex of opposing arytenoid cartilage	Recurrent laryngeal	Closes inlet of larynx.
Opposing arytenoid cartilage	Recurrent laryngeal	Approximates arytenoid cartilages.
Anterior part of helix of auricle	Facial	Draws forward auricle.
Cranial surface of auricle	Facial	Draws back auricle.
Cranial surface of auricle	Facial	Raises auricle.
Orbicularis oris, at angle of mouth	Buccal branch of facial	Closes lips, compresses cheeks.
Tongue	Hypoglossal	Draws back and depresses tongue.
Ciliary processes	Oculomotor and ciliary ganglion	Accommodation of vision.
Posterior median raphe of pharyngeal wall	Pharyngeal plexus	Constriction of pharynx.
Posterior median raphe of pharyngeal wall	Pharyngeal plexus	Constriction of pharynx.
Pharyngeal tubercle, posterior median raphe of pharyngeal wall	Pharyngeal plexus	Constriction of pharynx.
Skin of eyebrow	Facial	Draws eyebrow down and wrinkles forehead, as in frowning.
Muscular process of arytenoid cartilage	Recurrent laryngeal	Narrows glottis.
Muscular process of arytenoid cartilage	Recurrent laryngeal	Opens glottis.

MUSCLE	ORIGIN
cricopharyngeus	Part of constrictor pharyngis inferior.
cricothyroideus	Front and side of cricoid cartilage
depressor alae nasi	*Depressor septi.
depressor anguli oris [*triangularis*]	Mandible
depressor labii inferioris [*mentolabialis; quadratus labii inferioris*]	Mandible
depressor septi [*depressor alae nasi*]	Maxilla
depressor supercilii	Fibres from orbital part of orbicularis oculi
digastricus, *anterior belly*	Digastric fossa on base of mandible
digastricus, *posterior belly*	Mastoid notch
dilator naris [*dilatator naris*]	*Nasalis, pars alaris.
distortor oris	*Zygomaticus minor.
epicranius	Muscular cover of scalp; it includes the
frontalis (*anterior belly of occipitofrontalis*)	Galea aponeurotica
galea aponeurotica [*aponeurosis epicranialis*]	The aponeurosis connecting the separate parts
genioglossus	Inner surface of mandible near symphysis
geniohyoideus	Inner surface of mandible near symphysis
glossopalatinus	*Palatoglossus.
glossopharyngeus	Part of constrictor pharyngis superior.
hyoglossus	Hyoid bone
levator anguli oris [*abducens oris; caninus*]	Maxillary canine fossa
levator labii superioris [*quadratus labii superioris*]	Inferior margin of orbit
levator labii superioris alaeque nasi	Nasal process of maxilla
levator menti	*Mentalis.
levator palati	*Levator veli palatini.
levator palpebrae superioris	Roof of orbit

INSERTION	NERVE SUPPLY	FUNCTION
Lamina of thyroid cartilage	Superior laryngeal	Tenses vocal folds.
Skin at angle of mouth	Facial	Pulls down angle of mouth.
Skin about the mouth	Facial	Pulls down lower lip.
Nasal septum	Facial	Assists in widening nostril.
Eyebrow		Depresses eyebrow.
Lesser horn of hyoid bone	Mylohyoid branch of inferior alveolar	Raises and stabilizes hyoid bone.
Lesser horn of hyoid bone	Facial	Raises and stabilizes hyoid bone.

temporoparietal and occipitofrontal muscles and the galea aponeurotica.

INSERTION	NERVE SUPPLY	FUNCTION
Skin of forehead	Facial	Raises eyebrows and draws scalp forward.

of the occipitofrontal muscle.

INSERTION	NERVE SUPPLY	FUNCTION
Hyoid bone, and under side of tongue	Hypoglossal	Raises hyoid bone, retracts and protrudes tongue.
Anterior surface of hyoid bone above the mylohyoid attachment	1st cervical, via hypoglossal	Raises and draws forward hyoid bone with jaw fixed.
Base and sides of tongue	Hypoglossal	Draws down sides of tongue.
Angle of mouth	Facial	Raises angle of mouth.
Orbicularis oris	Facial	Raises upper lip.
Orbicularis oris and ala	Facial	Dilates nostril and raises upper lip.
Skin of upper eyelid	Oculomotor	Raises upper eyelid.

MUSCLE	ORIGIN
levator veli palatini [*levator palati*]	Apex of petrous portion of temporal bone and cartilage of pharyngotympanic tube
lingualis inferior	*Longitudinalis inferior.
lingualis superior	*Longitudinalis superior.
lingualis transversus	*Transversus linguae.
lingualis verticalis	*Verticalis linguae.
longissimus capitis [*trachelomastoideus*]	Articular processes of lower cervical and transverse processes of upper thoracic vertebrae
longissimus cervicis [*transversus colli*]	Transverse process of upper thoracic vertebrae
longitudinalis inferior [*lingualis inferior*]	Root of tongue
longitudinalis superior [*lingualis superior*]	Root of tongue
longus capitis	Transverse processes of 3rd, 4th, 5th and 6th cervical vertebrae
longus cervicis	*Longus colli.
longus colli [*longus cervicis*]	Lower cervical and upper thoracic vertebrae
masseter	Zygomatic arch
mentalis [*levator menti*]	Incisive fossa of mandible
mentolabialis	*Depressor labii inferioris.
mylohyoideus	Mylohyoid line of mandible
mylopharyngeus	Part of constrictor pharyngis superior.
nasalis, *pars alaris*	Maxilla
nasalis, *pars transversa*	Maxilla
obliquus auriculae (*vestigial*)	Helix
obliquus capitis inferior	Spine of axis
obliquus capitis superior	Lateral mass of atlas
obliquus inferior	Middle of floor of orbit

INSERTION	NERVE SUPPLY	FUNCTION
Aponeurosis of soft palate	Accessory, via pharyngeal plexus	Raises soft palate.
Mastoid process of temporal bone	Posterior branches of spinal	Extends vertebral column.
Transverse processes of cervical vertebrae	Posterior branches of spinal	Extends spinal column.
Tip of tongue	Hypoglossal	Changes shape of tongue.
Tip of tongue	Hypoglossal	Changes shape of tongue.
Inferior surface of basilar portion of occipital bone	1st and 2nd cervical	Controls movements of head and neck.
Anterior tubercles of cervical vertebrae and atlas	Anterior branches of cervical	Flexes vertebral column.
Lateral surface of ramus of mandible	Mandibular branch of trigeminal	Raises mandible.
Skin of chin	Facial	Protrudes lower lip and wrinkles skin of chin.
Hyoid bone	Mylohyoid branch of inferior alveolar	Assists in raising hyoid bone and depressing mandible during swallowing.
Bridge of nose	Facial	Assists in widening nostrils.
Into nasal cartilage by aponeurosis	Facial	Compresses nostrils.
Antihelix	Facial.	
Transverse process of atlas	Posterior branch of 1st cervical	Aids in lateral movements and extension of head.
Between superior and inferior nuchal lines of occipital bone	Posterior branch of 1st cervical	Aids in lateral movements and extension of head.
Sclera	Oculomotor	Elevates and abducts eyeball.

MUSCLE	ORIGIN
obliquus superior	Edge of optic foramen
occipitalis (*posterior belly of occipitofrontalis*)	Superior nuchal line of occipital bone
occipitofrontalis	The scalp muscle; consisting of 4 bellies: aponeurosis. *See* frontalis and occipitalis
omohyoideus, *inferior belly*	Superior border of scapula and suprascapular ligament
omohyoideus, *superior belly*	Intermediate tendon to *inferior* belly
orbicularis oculi	Sphincter of palpebral fissure
orbicularis oris	Sphincter of mouth
orbitalis (*vestigial*)	Bridges the inferior orbital fissure
palatoglossus [*glossopalatinus*]	Soft palate
palatopharyngeus [*pharyngopalatinus*]	Soft palate and pharyngotympanic tube
pharyngopalatinus	*Palatopharyngeus.
platysma	Fascia of pectoralis major and deltoid muscles
procerus	Skin over nose
pterygoideus	*Pterygoideus lateralis.
pterygoideus externus	*Pterygoideus lateralis.
pterygoideus lateralis [*pterygoideus; pterygoideus externus*]	*upper head*: Infratemporal crest and infratemporal surface of greater wing of sphenoid *lower head*: Lateral surface of lateral pterygoid plate
pterygoideus medialis	*deep head*: Medial surface of lateral pterygoid plate and posterior surface of pyramid of palatine bone *superficial head*: Lateral surface of pyramid of palatine bone and adjacent part of maxillary tuberosity

INSERTION	NERVE SUPPLY	FUNCTION
Sclera	Trochlear	Depresses and abducts eyeball.
Galea aponeurotica	Facial	Draws back scalp.

2 frontal (*frontalis*) and 2 occipital (*occipitalis*), connected by the epicranial muscles.

INSERTION	NERVE SUPPLY	FUNCTION
Intermediate tendon to *superior* belly	Ansa cervicalis	Depresses hyoid bone and tightens deep cervical fascia in lower part of neck.
Lower border of hyoid bone beside sternohyoid	Superior branch of ansa cervicalis	Depresses hyoid bone and tightens deep cervical fascia in lower part of neck.
	Facial	Closes eyelids.
	Facial	Purses lips and puckers up mouth.
	Sympathetic.	
Tongue	Accessory	Raises tongue and constricts anterior fauces.
Aponeurosis of pharynx	Accessory, via pharyngeal plexus	Aids in swallowing.
Skin about chin, oblique line of mandible, and skin and muscles at angle of mouth	Cervical branch of facial	Raises skin from underlying structures and, with risorius, retracts angle of mouth.
Skin of forehead	Facial	Wrinkles skin over nose.
Anterior part of capsule of mandibular joint, anterior border of articular disc and pterygoid fovea on anterior surface of neck of mandible	Mandibular	Draws articular disc down and forward to the articular eminence.
Deep surface of mandible between angle and groove for mylohyoid nerve	Mandibular	With masseter and temporalis muscles closes mouth; with lateral pterygoid protrudes mandible.

MUSCLE	ORIGIN
pterygopharyngeus	Part of constrictor pharyngis superior.
quadratus labii inferioris	*Depressor labii inferioris.
quadratus labii superioris	*Levator labii superioris.
quadratus menti	*Depressor labii inferioris.
rectus capitis anterior	Lateral mass of atlas
rectus capitis lateralis	Transverse process of atlas
rectus capitis posterior major	Spine of axis
rectus capitis posterior minor	Posterior tubercle of atlas
rectus inferior	Lower margin of optic foramen
rectus lateralis	Lateral margin of optic foramen
rectus medialis	Median margin of optic foramen
rectus superior	Upper edge of optic foramen
risorius	Fascia over masseter and parotid gland
salpingopharyngeus	Part of palatopharyngeus, arising from pharyngotympanic tube.
semispinalis capitis [*complexus*]	4th cervical to 5th thoracic vertebrae
semispinalis cervicis [*semispinalis colli*]	Transverse processes of lower cervical and upper thoracic vertebrae
semispinalis colli	*Semispinalis cervicis.
spinalis capitis (*inconstant*)	Spinous processes of lower cervical and upper thoracic vertebrae
spinalis cervicis (*inconstant*) [*spinalis colli*]	Spinous processes of lower cervical and upper thoracic vertebrae
spinalis colli	*Spinalis cervicis.
splenius capitis	Spinous processes of lowest cervical and upper thoracic vertebrae and nuchal ligament
splenius cervicis [*splenius colli*]	Spinous processes of lowest cervical and upper thoracic vertebrae and nuchal ligament
splenius colli	*Splenius cervicis.
stapedius	Pyramid of tympanum
sternocleidomastoideus [*sternomastoideus*]	Clavicle and manubrium sterni
sternohyoideus	Clavicle and manubrium sterni
sternomastoideus	*Sternocleidomastoideus.

INSERTION	NERVE SUPPLY	FUNCTION
Basilar portion of occipital bone	1st cervical	Aids in support and movement of head.
Jugular process of occipital bone	1st cervical	Aids in support and movement of head.
Occipital bone	1st cervical	Draws head back and rotates it.
Occipital bone	1st cervical	Draws head back and rotates it.
Sclera	Oculomotor	Depresses and adducts eyeball.
Sclera	Abducens	Abducts eyeball.
Sclera	Oculomotor	Adducts eyeball.
Sclera	Oculomotor	Elevates and adducts eyeball.
Skin of angle of mouth	Facial	Draws angle of mouth sideways, as in grinning.
Occipital bone, between superior and inferior nuchal lines	Posterior branches of spinal	Extends head.
Spinous processes of lower cervical and upper thoracic vertebrae	Posterior branches of spinal	Extends vertebral column and rotates it.
Occipital bone	Posterior branches of spinal	Extends head.
Spinous processes of 2nd, 3rd and 4th cervical vertebrae	Posterior branches of spinal	Extends vertebral column.
Mastoid process and superior nuchal line	Posterior branches of spinal	Extends head.
Transverse processes of upper cervical vertebrae	Posterior branches of spinal	Extends spinal column.
Neck of stapes	Facial	Retracts stapes.
Mastoid process	Accessory	Flexes head and turns it to the opposite side.
Hyoid bone	Ansa cervicalis	Depresses hyoid bone.

MUSCLE	ORIGIN
sternothyroideus	Manubrium sterni and 1st costal cartilage
styloglossus	Styloid process of temporal bone
stylohyoideus	Styloid process of temporal bone
stylopharyngeus	Styloid process of temporal bone
temporalis	Temporal fossa
temporoparietalis	Temporal fascia over ear
tensor palati	*Tensor veli palatini.
tensor tympani	Cartilage of pharyngotympanic tube
tensor veli palatini [*tensor palati*]	Scaphoid fossa of sphenoid bone and cartilage of pharyngotympanic tube
thyroarytenoideus	Lamina of thyroid cartilage
thyroepiglotticus	Lamina of thyroid cartilage
thyrohyoideus	Oblique line of thyroid cartilage
thyropharyngeus	Part of constrictor pharyngis inferior.
trachelomastoideus	*Longissimus capitis.
transversus colli	*Longissimus cervicis.
transversus linguae [*lingualis transversus*]	Median lingual raphe
transversus menti	Superficial fibres of depressor anguli oris.
trapezius	Inion, superior nuchal line, cervical and thoracic spines and supraspinous ligament
triangularis	*Depressor anguli oris.
uvulae	Posterior nasal spine
verticalis linguae [*lingualis verticalis*]	Dorsum of tongue
vocalis	Thyroid cartilage
zygomaticus major	Zygomatic bone
zygomaticus minor [*distortor oris*]	Part of levator labii superioris.

INSERTION	NERVE SUPPLY	FUNCTION
Oblique line of lamina of thyroid cartilage	Ansa cervicalis	Depresses thyroid cartilage and larynx.
Side of tongue	Hypoglossal	Raises tongue.
Hyoid bone	Facial	Raises tongue and hyoid bone, and draws them back.
Lamina of thyroid cartilage and side of pharynx	Glossopharyngeal	Raises and opens pharynx.
Medial surface, apex and anterior border of coronoid process, and anterior border of ramus of mandible	Deep temporal branches of anterior division of mandibular	Retracts protruded mandible and closes mouth.
Galea aponeurotica	Temporal branches of facial	Tightens scalp.
Manubrium mallei	Mandibular	Tenses tympanic membrane.
Aponeurosis of soft palate	Mandibular	Tightens soft palate and opens pharyngotympanic tube.
Muscular process of arytenoid cartilage	Recurrent laryngeal	Closes larynx and relaxes vocal cords.
Epiglottis	Recurrent laryngeal	Closes larynx.
Lower border of great horn of hyoid bone	1st cervical via hypoglossal	Depresses hyoid bone or raises larynx.
Dorsum and sides of tongue	Hypoglossal	Changes shape of tongue.
Posterior border and upper surface of clavicle, spine and acromion of scapula	Accessory, and anterior branches of cervical	Raises shoulder and draws back scapula.
Aponeurosis of soft palate	Accessory, via pharyngeal plexus.	
Sides and base of tongue	Hypoglossal	Changes shape of tongue.
Vocal process of arytenoid cartilage	Recurrent laryngeal	Shortens vocal cords.
Skin about face	Facial	Raises corner of mouth.

TABLE OF NERVES OF

NERVE	ORIGIN
abducens (m) (*6th cranial*)	Brain stem, lower border of pons
accessorius (m) (*11th cranial*)	*bulbar*: Lateral aspect of medulla oblongata *spinal*: Upper segments of cervical cord
acusticus	*Vestibulocochlearis.
alveolaris inferior (m and s) [*dentalis inferior*]	Mandibular
alveolaris superior anterior (s) [*dentalis superior anterior*]	Infraorbital
alveolaris superior medius (s) [*dentalis superior medius*]	Infraorbital
alveolaris superior posterior (s) [*dentalis superior posterior*]	Maxillary
ampullaris anterior (s)	Vestibular ganglion of vestibulocochlear
ampullaris lateralis (s)	Vestibular ganglion of vestibulocochlear
ampullaris posterior (s)	Vestibular ganglion of vestibulocochlear
ansa cervicalis, *radix anterior* (m) [*ansa hypoglossi; descendens hypoglossi; ansa cervicalis, radix inferior*]	Cervical plexus
ansa cervicalis, *radix posterior* (m) [*descendens cervicalis; ansa cervicalis, radix superior*]	Cervical plexus
ansa hypoglossi	*Ansa cervicalis.
auditorius	*Vestibulocochlearis.
auricularis (s)	Branch of vagus
auricularis anterior (s)	Auriculotemporal
auricularis magnus (m)	Cervical plexus
auricularis posterior (s)	Facial
auriculotemporalis (s)	Mandibular
buccalis (m) [*buccinator*]	Facial
buccalis (s) [*buccinator*]	Mandibular
buccinator	*Buccalis.
canalis pterygoidei (m and s)	Union of N. petrosus major and N. petrosus profundus
caroticotympanicus (s) [*petrosus profundus minor*]	Tympanic plexus of glossopharyngeal
caroticus externus (m)	Superior cervical ganglion
caroticus internus (m)	Superior cervical ganglion

DISTRIBUTION

Lateral rectus muscle of eye.
Striated muscles of pharynx and larynx.

Sternocleidomastoid and trapezius muscles.

Teeth and gingivae of lower jaw, mylohyoid and anterior belly of digastric muscles.
Mucosa of nasal floor, maxillary incisors and canines and their associated gingivae.
Maxillary premolars and associated gingivae.

Maxillary molars, gingivae and buccal mucosa; mucosa of maxillary sinus.

Ampulla of anterior semicircular duct.

Ampulla of lateral semicircular duct.

Ampulla of posterior semicircular duct.

Omohyoid, sternohyoid and sternothyroid muscles.

Omohyoid, sternohyoid and sternothyroid muscles.

Skin of auricle and external auditory meatus.
Skin of frontal part of pinna.
Occipitalis muscle and intrinsic muscles of auricle.
Skin over angle of mandible and of adjacent part of auricle.
Skin over temple and scalp.
Buccinator muscle.
Skin and mucous membrane of cheek.

Lacrimal gland and glands of nose and palate, via pterygopalatine ganglion.

Tympanic region and parotid gland.

Filaments to glands and smooth muscles of head, via external carotid plexus.
Filaments to glands and smooth muscles of head, via internal carotid plexus.

NERVE	ORIGIN
cervicales (m):	
1st anterior and posterior	1st segment of cervical cord
2nd anterior and posterior	2nd segment of cervical cord
3rd anterior and posterior	3rd segment of cervical cord
4th anterior	4th segment of cervical cord
4th-8th posterior	4th-8th segment of cervical cord
5th-8th anterior	5th-8th segment of cervical cord
chorda tympani (m and s)	Intermedius
ciliaris brevis (m)	Ciliary ganglion
ciliaris longus (s)	Nasociliary
cochlearis (s)	Brain stem, inferior border of pons; part of vestibulocochlearis
craniales 1st = olfactorius 2nd = opticus 3rd = oculomotorius 4th = trochlearis 9th = glossopharyngeus 10th = vagus 11th = accessorius 12th = hypoglossus	
cutaneous colli	*Transversus colli.
dentalis inferior (s)	1. Branches of inferior alveolar; 2. *Alveolaris inferior.
dentalis superior (s)	Branches of superior alveolar
dentalis superior anterior	*Alveolaris superior anterior.
dentalis superior medius	*Alveolaris superior medius.
dentalis superior posterior	*Alveolaris superior posterior.
descendens cervicalis [*descendens cervicis*]	*Ansa cervicalis, radix posterior.
descendens hypoglossi	*Ansa cervicalis, radix anterior.
ethmoidalis anterior (s)	Nasociliary
ethmoidalis posterior (s)	Nasociliary
facialis (m and s) (*7th cranial*) [*intermediofacialis*]	Brain stem, lower border of pons
frontalis (s)	Ophthalmic
gingivalis inferior (s)	Branches of inferior alveolar
gingivalis superior (s)	Branches of superior alveolar
glossopalatinus	*Intermedius.
glossopharyngeus (m and s) (*9th cranial*)	Medulla oblongata, lateral aspect
hypoglossus (m) (*12th cranial*)	Medulla oblongata
infraorbitalis (s)	Maxillary
infratrochlearis (s)	Nasociliary
intermediofacialis	*Facialis.
intermedius (m and s) [*glossopalatinus*]	Part of facial
jugularis	Communicating branch to vagus from superior cervical ganglion.

DISTRIBUTION

Neck muscles.
Neck muscles and skin of neck.
Deep muscles and skin of neck.
Back and neck muscles, skin of neck, diaphragm.
Deep muscles of upper part of back and of neck, skin on upper part of back.
Muscles and skin of arms.
(m): Submandibular and sublingual glands via lingual nerve and submandibular ganglion.
(s): Taste buds on anterior two-thirds of tongue, via lingual nerve.
Eyeball, ciliary muscle and constrictor pupillae.
Eyeball.
Spiral organ of cochlea.

5th = trigeminus 6th = abducens 7th = facialis 8th = vestibulocochlearis

Mandibular teeth.

Maxillary teeth.

Mucosa of nasal cavity and anterior ethmoidal sinus, and skin of nose.
Mucosa of posterior ethmoidal and of sphenoidal sinuses.
Muscles of facial expression, posterior belly of digastric muscle, stapedius and stylohyoid.
Skin of scalp, forehead and upper eyelids.
Mandibular gingivae.
Maxillary gingivae.

(m): Stylopharyngeus and parotid gland.
(s): Mucosa of posterior third of tongue and taste buds.
Muscles of tongue.
Lower eyelid, skin and mucosa of nose, upper lip and maxillary teeth.
Skin of bridge of nose.

(m): Nasal, palatal, sublingual and submandibular glands.
(s): Taste buds of anterior two-thirds of tongue.

NERVE	ORIGIN
labialis (s) [*labialis inferior*]	Branch of mental
labialis superior (s)	Branch of infraorbital
lacrimalis (s)	Ophthalmic
laryngealis externus (m) [*laryngeus externus*]	Branch of superior laryngeal
laryngealis internus (s) [*laryngeus internus*]	Branch of superior laryngeal
laryngealis recurrens (m and s) [*laryngeus recurrens; recurrens*]	Vagus
laryngealis superior (m and s) [*laryngeus superior*]	Vagus
laryngeus (other than l. inferior)	*See* laryngealis.
laryngeus inferior (m and s)	*Pharyngealis.
lingualis (s)	Mandibular
malar	*Zygomaticofacialis.
mandibularis (m and s)	Trigeminal
massetericus (m and s)	Mandibular
maxillaris (s)	Trigeminal
meatus acustici externi (s)	Auriculotemporal
meningeus (s)	Branches of vagus, maxillary and mandibular
meningeus medius (s)	Branch of maxillary
mentalis (s)	Mandibular
musculi tensoris tympani (m)	Mandibular, via otic ganglion
musculi tensoris veli palatini (m)	Mandibular, via otic ganglion
mylohyoideus (m)	Inferior alveolar
nasalis externus (s)	Branch of nasociliary
nasalis internus (s)	Branch of nasociliary
nasalis lateralis (s)	Branch of nasociliary
nasalis medialis (s) [*nasalis medius*]	Branch of nasociliary
nasalis posterior inferior lateralis	*Nasalis posterior superior medialis.
nasalis posterior superior lateralis (s) [*sphenopalatinus brevis*]	Branch from pterygopalatine ganglion
nasalis posterior superior medialis (s) [*nasalis posterior inferior lateralis; nasalis posterior superior medius*]	Branch from pterygopalatine ganglion
nasociliaris (s)	Ophthalmic
nasopalatinus (s) [*sphenopalatinus longus*]	Pterygopalatine ganglion

DISTRIBUTION

Skin of lower lip.
Skin of cheek and upper lip.
Skin about lateral commissure of eye.
Cricothyroid.

Larynx above vocal cords.

(m): Constrictor pharyngis inferior and intrinsic laryngeal muscles.
(s): Larynx below vocal cords.
(m): Cricothyroid (N. laryngealis externus).
(s): Larynx above vocal cords (N. laryngealis internus).

Mucosa of anterior two-thirds of tongue and of floor of mouth.

(m): Mylohyoid, anterior belly of digastric, tensor tympani, tensor veli palatini, and muscles of mastication.
(s): Mucosa of cheek, floor of mouth, anterior two-third of tongue, skin of lower part of face, mandibular teeth, meninges.
Masseter muscle and temporomandibular joint.
Meninges, skin of upper part of face, mucosa of nose, cheeks and palate, maxillary teeth.
Skin lining external auditory meatus, and tympanic membrane.
Meninges.

Meninges.
Skin of chin, lower lip and gingiva.
M. tensor tympani.
M. tensor veli palatini.
Mylohyoid and anterior belly of diagstric muscles.
Skin of nose.
Nasal mucosa.
Nasal mucosa.
Mucosa of nasal septum.

Mucosa of superior and middle nasal conchae.

Mucosa of superior and middle nasal conchae.

Eyeball, skin and mucosa of eyelid, nose, and ethmoidal and sphenoidal air sinuses.
Mucosa of hard palate and nose.

NERVE	ORIGIN
occipitalis major (s)	Posterior branch of 2nd cervical
occipitalis minor (s)	Cervical plexus
occipitalis tertius (s)	Posterior branch of 3rd cervical
oculomotorius (m) (*3rd cranial*)	Brain stem
olfactorius (s) (*1st cranial*)	Olfactory bulb
ophthalmicus (s)	Trigeminal
opticus (s) (*2nd cranial*)	Optic tracts
orbitalis (s)	Branch from pterygopalatine ganglion
palatinus anterior	*Palatinus major.
palatinus major (s) [*palatinus anterior*]	Maxillary, via pterygopalatine ganglion
palatinus medius	*Palatinus minor.
palatinus minor (s) [*palatinus medius* and *palatinus posterior*]	Maxillary, via pterygopalatine ganglion
palatinus posterior	*Palatinus minor.
palpebralis (s) [*palpebris*]	Branch of infratrochlear
palpebralis inferior (s) [*palpebris inferior*]	Branch of superior alveolar
palpebris	*Palpebralis.
palpebris inferior	*Palpebralis inferior.
petrosus major (m and s)	Intermedius, via pterygopalatine ganglion
petrosus minor (m)	Glossopharyngeus
petrosus profundus (s)	Intermedius, via pterygopalatine ganglion
petrosus profundus minor	*Caroticotympanicus.
pharyngealis (m) [*pharyngeus*]	Branch of vagus
pharyngealis (s) [*pharyngeus*]	Glossopharyngeal
pharyngealis (m and s) [*laryngeus inferior*]	Branch of recurrent laryngeal
pharyngeus	*See* pharyngealis.
pterygoideus lateralis (m)	Mandibular
pterygoideus medialis (m)	Mandibular
pterygopalatinus (s) [*sphenopalatinus*]	Joins maxillary nerve to pterygopalatine ganglion.
recurrens	*Laryngealis recurrens.
saccularis (s)	Vestibulocochlearis
sphenopalatinus	*Pterygopalatinus.
sphenopalatinus brevis	*Nasalis posterior superior lateralis.
sphenopalatinus longus	*Nasopalatinus.
stapedius (m)	Facial
statoacusticus	*Vestibulocochlearis.
sublingualis (s)	Lingual
suboccipitalis (m)	1st cervical
supraorbitalis (s)	Frontal
supratrochlearis (s)	Frontal

DISTRIBUTION

Skin over posterior portion of scalp.
Skin over posterior portion of scalp and posterior aspect of auricle.
Skin over posterior aspect of neck and scalp.
Muscles of eye and upper eyelid.
Olfactory mucosa.
Skin of anterior portion of scalp and forehead, orbit and eyeball, meninges, mucosa of nose, frontal, ethmoidal and sphenoidal air sinuses.
Retina.
Orbit.

Mucosa of palate.

Mucosa of palate and uvula.

Upper eyelid.
Lower eyelid.

Palatal mucosa and glands.

Parotid gland, via otic ganglion and auriculotemporal nerve.
Palate, via pterygoid canal.

Pharyngeal muscles.
Pharyngeal mucosa.
(m): intrinsic laryngeal muscles.
(s): larynx below vocal chords.

Lateral pterygoid muscle.
Medial pterygoid muscle, tensor tympani, tensor veli palatini.

Filaments to macula sacculi.

Stapedius muscle.

Area of sublingual gland.
Semispinalis capitis muscle and muscles of occipital triangle.
Mucosa of frontal sinus, skin of forehead and upper eyelid.
Skin of centre of forehead, bridge of nose and upper eyelid.

NERVE	ORIGIN
temporalis profundus (m)	Mandibular
tentorius (s)	Branch of ophthalmic
terminalis (s)	Medial olfactory tract
transversus colli (s) [*cutaneous colli*]	Cervical plexus
trigeminus (m and s) (*5th cranial*)	Brain stem at inferolateral surface of pons
trochlearis (m) (*4th cranial*)	Dorsal surface of midbrain
tympanicus (s)	Inferior ganglion of glossopharygeal
utricularis (s)	Vestibular
utriculoampullaris (s)	Vestibular
vagus (m and s) (*10th cranial*)	Post-olivary sulcus of medulla oblongata
vestibularis (s)	Brain stem; part of vestibulocochlearis
vestibulocochlearis (s) (*8th cranial*) [*statoacusticus*]	Divides into *cochlearis and *vestibularis.
zygomaticus (s)	Maxillary
zygomaticofacialis (s) [*malar*]	Branch of zygomatic
zygomaticotemporalis (s)	Branch of zygomatic

DISTRIBUTION

Temporal muscles.
Meninges.
Nasal mucosa.
Skin of anterior triangle of neck.
Divides into *N. ophthalmicus, *N. maxillaris and *N. mandibularis.

Obliquus superior of eyeball.
Mucosa of middle ear and pharyngotympanic tube.
Macula of utricle.
Utricle and ampullae of semicircular ducts.
Branches to striate muscles of larynx and pharynx, skin of external auditory meatus, meninges, laryngeal and pharyngeal mucosa, thoracic and abdominal viscera.
Branches to ampullae of semicircular ducts, maculae of utricle and saccule, via vestibular ganglion.

Skin in temporal region and over zygoma.
Skin over zygoma.
Skin over anterior portion of temporal region.

TABLE OF VEINS OF

This table includes only those veins whose names or courses differ

VEIN	DRAINAGE OR TRIBUTARIES
anonyma	*Brachiocephalica.
basalis	Formed by union of anterior cerebral and
brachiocephalica (*dextra and sinistra*) [*anonyma, innominate*]	Internal jugular and subclavian, vertebral, internal mammary, 1st posterior intercostal, and *sinister*: thoracic duct
cerebri inferior	Lower part of hemisphere, draining into adjacent sinus.
cerebri interna	Thalamostriate and choroid veins
cerebri magna	Internal cerebral veins
cerebri media profunda	Insula
cerebri media superficialis	Lower part of lateral surface of hemisphere
cerebri superioris	Upper portion of medial and lateral surfaces of hemisphere
facialis [*facialis anterior*]	Junction of supratrochlear and supraorbital veins
facialis anterior	*Facialis.
facialis communis	Junction of facial and retromandibular veins
facialis posterior	*Retromandibularis.
faciei profunda	*Profunda faciei.
innominate	*Brachiocephalica.
jugularis anterior	Arises in submental region
jugularis externa	Posterior auricular and branch from retromandibular veins
jugularis interna	Brain, face and neck
nasalis externa	Side of nose
ophthalmica inferior	Tributaries corresponding to branches of ophthalmic artery
ophthalmica superior	Tributaries corresponding to those of ophthalmic artery
palatina externa [*paratonsillar*]	Palatal region
paratonsillar	*Palatina externa.
plexus basilaris	Inferior petrosal sinuses
plexus pharyngeus [*plexus pharyngealis*]	Plexus in lateral wall of pharynx, from which the pharyngeal veins arise.

from the accompanying artery, or that have no accompanying artery.

DESTINATION	LOCATION
deep middle cerebral veins, and joins the great cerebral.	
Superior vena cava	Medial portion of root of neck, to terminate behind 1st right costal cartilage.
Great cerebral	Below splenium of corpus callosum.
Straight sinus	Behind and below splenium of corpus callosum.
Joins anterior cerebral to form basal vein	
Cavernous sinus	Lateral sulcus.
Superior sagittal sinus.	
Joins retromandibular to form common facial, and ends in internal jugular	Front portion of side of face from medial angle of eye.
Internal jugular	Below angle of mandible.
External jugular or subclavian	Lateral to midline of neck.
Subclavian	Side of neck, below and behind angle of mandible.
Brachiocephalic	Side of neck, deep to sternomastoid muscle.
Facial.	
Pterygoid plexus and cavernous sinus	Near floor of orbit.
Cavernous sinus	Near roof of orbit.
Facial.	
Vertebral plexus	Basilar portion of occipital bone.

VEIN	DRAINAGE OR TRIBUTARIES
plexus pterygoideus [*plexus venosus pterygoideus*]	Corresponds to branches of maxillary artery
plexus venosus pterygoideus	*Plexus pterygoideus.
plexus venosus suboccipitalis	Occipital vein
profunda faciei [*faciei profunda; profunda facialis*]	Communicating vein to facial from
retromandibularis [*facialis posterior*]	Superficial temporal and maxillary veins
sinus cavernosus	Superior and inferior ophthalmic veins, cerebral veins, sphenopalatine sinus
sinus intercavernosus	One of two (*anterior* and *posterior*) sinuses fossa.
sinus occipitalis	Variable anastomosing channel between the transverse and sigmoid sinuses
sinus petrosus inferior	Cavernous sinus
sinus petrosus superior	Cavernous sinus
sinus rectus	Formed by union of inferior sagittal sinus and great cerebral vein
sinus sagittalis inferior	Dura mater
sinus sagittalis superior	Superior cerebral, diploe of cranium, dura mater
sinus sigmoideus	Continuous with transverse sinus
sinus sphenoparietalis	Dura mater
sinus transversus	Superior sagittal or straight sinus, cerebral and cerebellar veins, superior petrosal sinus
terminalis	*Thalamostriata superior.
thalamostriata	*Thalamostriata superior.
thalamostriata superior [*terminalis; thalamostriata*]	Caudate nucleus and thalamus
thyroidea inferior	Lower part of thyroid gland, via plexus thyroidea impar
thyroidea media	Lower part of thyroid gland
vertebralis accessoria (*inconstant*)	Venous plexus on vertebral artery
vertebralis anterior	Arises from venous plexus

DESTINATION	LOCATION
Maxillary vein	Between the pterygoid muscles, in the infratemporal fossa.
Vertebral vein	Posterior portion of scalp.
pterygoid plexus, between masseter and buccinator muscles.	
Common facial and external jugular	Parotid gland and side of face by ear.
Divides into superior and inferior petrosal sinuses	At the side of the pituitary fossa.
joining the two cavernous sinuses and forming a ring round the pituitary	
	Cranial attachment of falx cerebelli.
Internal jugular	Inferior petrosal sulcus.
Junction of transverse and sigmoid sinuses	Upper margin of petrous portion of temporal bone.
Transverse sinus	Junction of tentorium cerebelli and falx cerebri.
Joins great cerebral vein to form straight sinus (sinus rectus)	Lower free margin of falx cerebri.
Transverse sinus	Cranial attachment of falx cerebri.
Internal jugular	Mastoid portion of temporal bone.
Cavernous sinus	
Via sigmoid sinus to internal jugular	Groove on occipital bone and postero-inferior angle of parietal bone.
With choroid veins forms internal cerebral	Floor of central part of lateral ventricle.
Left brachiocephalic.	
Internal jugular	Short vein in front of common carotid artery.
Vertebral.	
Vertebral	Cervical transverse processes.

Appendix of Dental Periodicals

This list of dental periodicals gives country of origin and frequency of publication where this is known. Major title changes are indicated by reference to the later name. Minor changes within a title are shown by the use of parentheses: ( ) denotes an earlier title; (—) indicates a word added or changed at a later date.

ABESP boletim. (Associação Brasiliera de Endodontia, secção São Paulo). Brazil. Q.

ADM. Revista de la Asociación Dental Mexicana. *Now called* Revista ADM (Asociación Dental Mexicana).

ALAFO: Revista de la Asociación Latinoamericana de Facultades de Odontología. El Salvador. 2 a year.

AMDI bollettino: organo ufficiale dell'Associazione Medici Dentisti Italiani. Italy. M.

ASDA news. (American Student Dental Association). *Now called* New dentist.

ASDC journal of dentistry for children. USA. Bi-M.

Academia odontologica. Colombia. Q.

Acta clinica odontologica. Colombia. 2 a year.

Acta odontologica pediatrica. Dominican Republic. 2 a year.

Acta odontologica scandinavica. Sweden. Bi-M.

Acta odontologica venezolana. Venezuela. Q.

Acta parodontologica. *Now in* Schweizerische Monatsschrift für Zahnmedizin.

Acta stomatologica belgica. Belgium. Q.

Acta stomatologica hellenica. Stomatologika chronika. *Now called* Hellenika stomatologika chronika: Hellenic stomatological review.

Acta stomatologica Patavina. Italy.

Actualités odonto-stomatologiques. France. Q.

Advances in dental research. (Supplement to Journal of dental research). USA. Irr.

Advances in orthodontics. *Now called* Update in orthodontics.

Advances in periodontics. *Now called* Update in periodontics.

Aichi Gakuin dental science. Japan. A.

Aichi-Gakuin journal of dental science. [Aichi Gakuin Daigaku Shigakkai Shi]. Japan. Q.

Alam Tub Al-Asnan. *See* Arab dental.

Alexandria dental journal. [Magallat Al-Iskandiriyyah Li-Tibb Al-Asnan]. Egypt. Q.

Alumni bulletin—Indiana University School of Dentistry (—School of Dentistry, Indiana University). USA.

American journal of dentistry. USA. Bi-M.

American journal of orthodontics (— and dentofacial orthopedics). USA. M.

Anais da Faculdade de farmacia e odontologia da Universidade de São Paolo. *Continued in* Revista de odontologia da UNESP.
Anais da Faculdade nacional de odontologia (da Universidade do Brasil). Brazil. A.
Anais da Faculdade de odontologia da Universidade Federal de Pernambuco. Brazil. A.
Anais da Faculdade de odontologia da Universidade Federal do Rio de Janeiro. Brazil. A.
Anais da Faculdade de odontologia da Universidade do Parana. Brazil.
Anais da Faculdade de odontologia da Universidade do Recife. *Now called* Anais da Faculdade de odontologia da Universidade Federal de Pernambuco.
Anales argentinos de odontología. Argentina. Q.
Anales españoles de odontoestomatología. Spain. Bi-M.
Anales de la Facultad de odontología, Universidad de la Republica Oriental del Uruguay. Uruguay. Irr.
Anesthesia and pain control in dentistry. USA. Q.
Anesthesia progress: journal of the American Dental Society of Anesthesiology. USA. 4 a year.
Angle orthodontist. USA. Bi-M.
Anglo-Continental Dental Society journal. *See* Journal of the Anglo-Continental Dental Society.
Annales odonto-stomatologiques. France. Bi-M.
Annales d'oto-laryngologie et de chirurgie cervico-faciale. France. Bi-M.
Annali di stomatologia. Italy. M.
Annals of the (—Royal) Australian College of Dental Surgeons. *Now called* Annals of the Royal Australasian College of Dental Surgeons.
Annals of dentistry. USA. 2 a year.
Annals of the Royal Australasian College of Dental Surgeons. Australia. 2-3 a year.
Année odonto-stomatologique et maxillo-faciale. France. A.
Annuaire dentaire. France. A.
Annual publications-Nippon Dental University. Japan. A.
Annual publications, Royal Dental School, Malmö, Sweden (—School of Dentistry, University of Lund). Sweden. A.
Annual report on advanced dental education. USA. A.
Anuario da Faculdade de farmacia e odontologia de Natal. Brazil. A.
Apex: the journal of the UCH Dental Society. Great Britain. Bi-M.
Apollonia. Australia. A.
Apollonia. Sweden.
Arab dental. [Alam Tub Al-Asnan]. Germany. Q. (*Text in Arabic*).
Archives of oral biology. Great Britain. M.
Archivio italiano di biologia oral. *Supplement to* Rassegna trimestriale di odontoiatria.
Archivio stomatologico. Italy. Q.
Argentina odontológica. Argentina. Q.
Arkansas dental journal. *Now called* Arkansas dentistry.
Arkansas dentistry. Official publication of the Arkansas State Dental Association. USA. Q

Arquivos do Centro de Estudos da Faculdade de odontologia (—curso de odontologia) da UFMG (Universidade Federal de Minas Gerais). Brazil. 2 a year.

Ars curandi em odontologia. Brazil.

Art dentaire liberal. France. M.

Der Artikulator: Zeitschrift der kritische Zahnmedizin. Germany. Q.

Assistance et le prothèsiste dentaire. France. Bi-M.

Australian dental journal. Australia. Bi-M.

Australian journal of dentistry. *Now in* Australian dental journal.

Australian orthodontic journal. Australia. 2 a year.

Australian prosthodontic journal. Australia. A.

Australian Society of Prosthodontists bulletin. *Now called* Australian prosthodontic journal.

BZB: Bayerisches Zahnärzteblatt. Germany. M.

Bahia odontologica. Brazil.

Baurú odontologico. Brazil.

Bayerisches Zahnärzteblatt. *Now called* BZB: Bayerisches Zahnärzteblatt.

Baylor dental journal. USA. 2 a year.

Belgisch blad voor tandheelkunde. *See* Journal dentaire belge: Belgisch blad voor tandheelkunde.

Belgisch tijdschrift voor tandheelkunde. (Revue belge de médecine dentaire). Belgium. Q.

Berichte aus der Bonner Universitätsklinik und Poliklinik für Mund-, Zahn- und Kieferkrankheiten. Germany. A.

Bibliografia brasileira de odontologia. Brazil.

Boletim da Associação brasileira de odontologia. Brazil. Bi-M.

Boletim. Curso de odontolgia de Santa Maria. Centro de Estudos Antonio Pimenta: Universidade Federal de Santa Maria. Brazil. 2 a year.

Boletim da equipe de odontologia sanitaria. Brazil. Q.

Boletim da Faculdade de farmacia e odontologia de Ribeirão Preto. *Continued as* Revista da Faculdade de odontologia (—farmacia e odontologia) de Ribeirão Preto.

Boletim de materiais dentarios. Brazil. 2 a year.

Boletim do servico de odontologia sanitaria (da Secretaria da Saude do Rio Grande do Sul). *Now called* Boletim da equipe de odontologia sanitaria.

Boletín. Academia de estomatología del Peru. Peru. Q.

Boletín de la Asociación dental del Estado de Puebla. Mexico.

Boletín de la Asociación odontológica argentina. *Continued in* Revista odontológica.

Boletín de la Catedrá de protesis estomatológica. Spain.

Boletín del Circulo argentino de odontología. Argentina. *See also* Revista del Circulo argentino de odontología.

Boletín del Circulo odontológico de Rosario. Brazil. *See also* Revista del Circulo odontológico de Rosario.

Boletín del Colegio estomatólogico de Guatemala. *Continued as* Revista del Colegio estomatológico de Guatemala.

Boletín del Colegio estomatológico de La Habana. Cuba.

Boletín: Confederación odontológica inter-americana. Mexico.

Boletín dental argentino. *Now called* Boletín odontológico.
Boletín dental chileno. Chile. Bi-M.
Boletín dental uruguayo. Uruguay. M.
Boletín de la dirección general de odontología. Argentina.
Boletín de la Escuela de odontología. Universidad central de Ecuador. Ecuador.
Boletín de la Escuela de odontología de la Universidad Nacional. *Now called* Boletín de odontología.
Boletín de la Facultad de odontología. Argentina.
Boletín de información dental. *Continued as* Revista de actualidad estomatológica española.
Boletín de odontología. Colombia. Bi-M.
Boletín odontológico. Argentina.
Boletín odontológico. Bolivia.
Boletín de la Sociedad dental de Guatemala. Guatemala.
Bollettino AMDI: Organo ufficiale dell'Associazione Medici Dentisti Italiani. *Now called* AMDI bollettino.
Bollettino metallografico e di odonto-stomatologia. Italy. Q.
Bollettino odonto-implantologico. Italy.
Bollettino della Societa italiana di odontoiatria infantile. Italy.
Brazilian dental journal. Brazil.
British dental journal. Great Britain. 2 a month.
British dental surgery assistant. Great Britain. Q.
British journal of oral (—and maxillofacial) surgery. Great Britain. Bi-M.
British journal of orthodontics. Great Britain. Q.
British Society of Dental (—Dental and Maxillofacial) Radiology newsletter (—proceedings). Great Britain. A.
Bulletin de l'Academie de chirurgie dentaire. France.
Bulletin de l'Academie dentaire. *Now called* Bulletin de l'Academie de chirurgie dentaire.
Bulletin. Academy of Dentistry for the Handicapped. USA.
Bulletin of the Academy of General Dentistry. *Continued as* Journal of the Academy of General Dentistry.
Bulletin of the Alabama Dental Association. *Now called* Journal of the Alabama Dental Association.
Bulletin of the American Association of Public Health Dentists. USA. Q.
Bulletin des chirurgiens-dentistes independants. *Now in* Revue d'odonto-stomatologie.
Bulletin—Cincinnatti Dental Society. USA.
Bulletin dentaire. *See* Dental bulletin. (Bulletin dentaire).
Bulletin of dental education. USA. M.
Bulletin of the Dental Guidance Council for Cerebral Palsy. *Now called* Journal of the Dental Guidance Council on the Handicapped.
Bulletin du groupement international pour la recherche scientifique en stomatologie (— et odontologie). Belgium. Q.
Bulletin of the history of dentistry. USA. 3 a year.
Bulletin of the Illinois Dental Hygienists' Association. USA. 3 a year.
Bulletin of the Iranian Dental Association. Iran. M.
Bulletin of the Josai Dental University. *Now called* Journal of Meikai University School of Dentistry.

Bulletin of Kanagawa Dental College. Japan. 2 a year.
Bulletin of the Manitoba Dental Association. Canada. Q.
Bulletin of the Massachusetts Dental Hygienists' Association. USA.
Bulletin of the Michigan (State) Dental Hygienists' Association. USA. Q.
Bulletin of the National Dental Association. *Continued as* Quarterly of the National Dental Association.
Bulletin national. Fédération Nationale Independante des Syndicats des personnels des Cabinets et Laboratoires Dentaires. France. Bi-M.
Bulletin: National Medical and Dental Association and National Advocates Society. USA.
Bulletin of the New Jersey College of Medicine and Dentistry. USA.
Bulletin of the New York State Dental Society of Anesthesiology. USA. 2 a year.
Bulletin of the New York State Society of Dentistry for Children. USA. 2 a year.
Bulletin of Nippon Dental College (—University), General Education. [Nippon Shika Daigaku Shingaku Katei Kiyo]. Japan. A.
Bulletin officiel du Conseil national de l'ordre (—de l'ordre national) des chirurgiens-dentistes. France. Q.
Bulletin of the Oklahoma State Dental Society. *Now called* Journal of the Oklahoma State Dental Association.
Bulletin, Pacific Coast Society of Orthodontists. USA. Q.
Bulletin of the Philadelphia County Dental Society. USA. 6 a year.
Bulletin de la Société française de prothèse maxillo- faciale. *See* Revue française de prothèse maxillo-faciale. (Bulletin de la Société française de prothèse maxillo-faciale).
Bulletin of stomatology, Kyoto University. Japan. Q.
Bulletin of Tokyo Dental College. [Tokyo Shika Daigaku Obun Kiyo]. Japan. Q.
Bulletin of Tokyo Medical and Dental University. [Tokyo Ika Shika Daigaku Kiyo]. Japan. Q.
Bulletin trimestriel de la Société d'odonto-stomatologie de l'Ouest. France. Q.
Bulletin of the Virginia State Dental Association. *Now called* Virginia dental journal.
Bulletin: Washington State Dental Association. *Continued as* Washington State dental journal.
Bur. USA. 2 a year.

CDA journal. (California Dental Association). USA.
CDS review. (Chicago Dental Society). *Now called* Chicago Dental Society review.
CENT: Centro de estudios de recursos odontológicos para el niño. Venezuela.
CERON: Centro de estudios de recursos odontológicos para el niño. *See* CENT: Centro de estudios de recursos odontológicos para el niño.
Cahiers d'odonto-stomatologie de Touraine. France.
Cahiers de prothèse: revue trimestrielle de prothèse odontologique. France. Q.
Cahiers de stomatologie et de chirurgie maxillo-faciale. France. Bi-M.
Calcified tissue abstracts. USA. Q.
Calcified tissue international. USA. M.

Calcified tissue research. *Now called* Calcified tissue international.
Canadian Dental Association journal: journal de l'Association Dentaire Canadienne. Canada. M.
Canadian dental hygienist. Hygieniste dentaire du Canada. *Now called* Probe (Canadian Dental Hygienists' Association).
Canadian Forces Dental Services quarterly (—bulletin). Canada. Q.
Caries research: journal of the European Organization for Caries Research (ORCA). Switzerland. Bi-M.
Centro America Odontológica. El Salvador. Q.
Ceska stomatologie: casopis stomatologickych spolecnosti. Czech Republic. Bi-M.
Ceskoslovenska stomatologie. *Now called* Ceska stomatologie.
Ceylon dental journal. Sri Lanka. A.
Chicago Dental Society review. USA. M.
Chinese journal of stomatology. [Zhonghua Konqiangke zazhi]. China. Q.
Chirurgien-dentiste de France. France. W.
Chirurgien-dentiste liberal. France. Bi-M.
Christian Medical Dental Society journal. USA.
Ciencia arte docencia odontologia. Uruguay. 2 a year.
Cincinnati Dental Society Bulletin. USA. M.
Cleft palate - craniofacial journal. USA. Bi-M.
Cleft palate journal. *Now called* Cleft palate - craniofacial journal.
Clinic-odontologia. France. Bi-M.
Clinica odontoiatria. *Now in* Annali di stomatologia.
Clinica odonto-protesia. Italy. **Q.**
Clinical dental briefings. USA. M.
Clinical oral implants research. Denmark. Q.
Clinical preventive dentistry. USA. Bi-M.
Community dental health. Great Britain. Q.
Community dentistry and oral epidemiology. Denmark. Bi-M.
Compendium of continuing education in dentistry. USA. 12 a year.
Conector: organo oficial del Instituto de Implant-odontología. Argentina. Q.
Contact point. USA. Q.
Cooperador dental. Argentina. Irr.
Critical reviews in oral biology and medicine. USA. Q.
Current advances in oral and maxillofacial surgery. USA. Every 3 years.
Current opinion in cosmetic dentistry. USA. A.
Current opinion in dentistry. *Continued as* Current opinion in cosmetic dentistry, Current opinion in orthodontics and pedodontics, *and* Current opinion in periodontology.
Current opinion in orthodontics and pedodontics. USA. A.
Current opinion in periodontology. USA. A.
Czasopismo Stomatologiczne. Poland. M.

DDZ—Das Deutsche Zahnärzteblatt. *Now in* ZWR.
DE: journal of dental engineering. Japan. Q.
Dalhousie dental journal. Canada. A.
Dens. *Now in* Infodont.
Dens. (Faculdade de odontologia, Universidade Federal do Parana). Brazil.

Dens sapiens. Denmark. 10 a year.
Dental abstracts. USA. M.
Dental anaesthesia and sedation. Journal of the Australian Society for the Advancement of Anaesthesia and Sedation in Dentistry. Australia. 3 a year.
Dental annual. Great Britain. A.
Dental asepsis review. USA. M.
Dental assistant (—journal). (American Dental Assistants Association). USA. Q.
Dental assisting. USA. Bi-M.
Dental bulletin. (Australian Dental Association). Australia. 10 a year.
Dental bulletin. (Bulletin dentaire). Canada.
Dental bulletin of Osaka University. *Now called* Journal of Osaka University School of Dentistry.
Dental cadmos. Italy. Fortnightly.
Dental clinics of North America. USA. Q.
Dental concepts. USA.
Dental corps international. Germany. 2 a year.
Dental cosmos. *Now in* Journal of the American Dental Association.
Dental currents. USA. 2 a month.
Dental Dienst. Germany. M.
Dental digest. *Now in* Quintessence international/dental digest: journal of practical dentistry.
Dental Echo. Germany. 9 a year.
Dental economics (—oral hygiene). USA. M.
Dental health. Great Britain. Bi-M.
Dental historian: newsletter of the Lindsay Club. Great Britain. 2 a year.
Dental hygiene. *Now called* Journal of dental hygiene. (American Dental Hygienists' Association).
Dental hygienist: journal of the Northern California State Dental Hygienists' Association. USA. Q.
Dental implantology update. USA. M.
Dental journal. S. Korea. M.
Dental journal: journal dentaire. *Now called* Canadian Dental Association journal: journal de l'Association Dentaire Canadienne.
Dental journal of Australia. *Now in* Australian dental journal.
Dental journal of Iwate Medical University. [Iwate Ika Daigaku Shigaku Zasshi]. Japan. 3 a year.
Dental journal of Malaysia (— and Singapore). Malaysia. 2 a year.
Dental journal of Nihon University. *Now called* Journal of Nihon University School of Dentistry.
Dental-Labor. Germany. M.
Dental Laboratorie Bladet. Denmark. 4 a year.
Dental laboratory. Great Britain. M.
Dental laboratory age. *Now called* Dental laboratory world.
Dental laboratory review. USA. M.
Dental laboratory world. USA. M.
Dental laboratory yearbook and directory. Great Britain. A.
Dental magazine and Oral topics. *Now in* British dental journal.
Dental management. USA. M.

Dental material. Italy. 10 a year.
Dental materials. USA and Denmark. Bi-M.
Dental materials journal. (Japanese Society for Dental Materials and Devices). **[Nihon Shika Riko Gakkai].** Japan. 2 a year.
Dental medicine: journal of the Israel Dental Association. [Refuat Hape Vehashinaim]. Israel. Q.
Dental mirror: journal of Philippine dentistry. Philippines. 2 a year.
Dental office. USA. M.
Dental outlook. Australia. Q.
Dental outlook. [Shikai Tenbo]. Japan. M.
Dental practice. Great Britain. 2 a month.
Dental practitioner and Dental record. *Now in* Journal of dentistry.
Dental press. *Now called* Rivista italiana degli odontotecnici - Dental press.
Dental protesis. Spain. Bi-M.
Dental radiography and photography. USA. 3 a year.
Dental record. *Continued in* Dental practitioner and Dental record.
Dental reporter. Australia. M.
Dental review. Hong Kong. Bi-M.
Dental-Revue. Austria. M.
Dental spectrum. USA.
Dental student. USA. M.
Dental survey. USA. M.
Dental teamwork. USA. Bi-M.
Dental technician. Great Britain. M.
Dental therapeutics newsletter. USA.
Dental therapy journal. Australia. A.
Dental update. Great Britain. 10 a year.
Dental world. USA. Bi-M.
Dentaletter. Canada. 10 a year.
Dentalhygiene. Switzerland. 5 a year.
Dentalpractice. USA. M.
Denteksa. South Africa. Q.
Dentiste de France. *Now called* Chirurgien-dentiste de France.
Dentistische Reform. *Continued as* Zahnärztliche Reform.
Dentistische Rundschau. *Now called* Zahnärztliche Praxis.
Dentistry (—year). (American Student Dental Association). USA. Q.
Dentistry in Japan. Japan. A.
Dentistry today. USA. 9 a year.
Dento-maxillo-facial radiology: journal of the International Association of Dento-maxillo-facial Radiology. Sweden. USA. Q.
Das Deutsche Zahnärzteblatt. *See* DDZ—Das Deutsche Zahnärzteblatt.
Deutsche zahnärztliche Wochenschrift. *Continued in* Zahnärztliche Zeitschrift.
Deutsche zahnärztliche Zeitschrift. Germany. M.
Deutsche Zahn-, Mund- und Kieferheilkunde mit Zentralblatt. Germany. 8 a year.
Deutsche Zahn-, Mund- und Kieferheilkunde mit Zentralblatt für die gesamte Zahn-, Mund- und Kieferheilkunde. *Continued as* Zahn-, Mund- und Kieferheilkunde mit Zentralblatt (*and now called* Deutsche Zahn-, Mund- und Kieferheilkunde mit Zentralblatt).

Deutsche Zeitschrift für biologische Zahnmedizin. Germany. Q.
Deutsche Zeitschrift für Mund-, Kiefer-, und Gesichts-Chirurgie. Germany. Bi-M.
Dialog: Fairleigh Dickinson University School of Dentistry. USA.
Diastema. South Africa.
Divulgación cultural odontológica. Spain.
Dundee dental journal. Great Britain.

Edinburgh Dental Hospital gazette. Great Britain. 3 a year.
Educación dental. Peru. 2 a year.
Education directions for dental auxiliaries. USA. 4 a year.
Egyptian dental journal. Egypt. Q.
Endo: revue française d'endodontie. France. Q.
Endodoncía. Spain. Q.
Endodontic bibliography. USA.
Endodontic report. USA.
Endodontics and dental traumatology. Denmark. Bi-M.
Endodontie: die Zeitschrift für die Praxis. Germany. Q.
Especialidades odontologicas. Brazil. M.
Esthetic dentistry update. USA. Bi-M.
Estodont/press. Spain.
Estomatología. Mexico. 2 a year.
Estomatologia e cultura. Brazil. 2 a year.
European journal of oral sciences. Denmark. Bi-M.
European journal of orthodontics. Great Britain. Bi-M.
European journal of prosthodontics and restorative dentistry. Great Britain. Bi-M.
European Orthodontic Society reports. *Continued as* Transactions of the European Orthodontic Society.

Facial orthopedics and temporomandibular arthrology. USA. Bi-M.
Facial plastic surgery. USA. Q.
Farmacodonto. Brazil.
Farmacodontologia. Brazil.
Finska Tandlälarsällskapet Forhandlingar. *See* Suomen Hammaslääkäriseuran Toimituksia. (*Now called* Proceedings of the Finnish Dental Society).
Florida dental journal. USA. Q.
Fluoridation reporter. USA.
Fluoride: official quarterly journal of International Society for Fluoride Research. *Now called* Journal of the International Society for Fluoride Research.
Fogorvosi szemle. [Dental review]. Hungary. M.
Folia odontologica. Switzerland. Q.
Folia odontologica practica. [Rinshu Shika]. Japan. Q.
Folia stomatologica. Yugoslavia. Q.
Fortnightly review of the Chicago Dental Society. *Now called* CDS review.
Fortschritte der Kieferorthopaedie. Germany. Bi-M.
Fortschritte der Kiefer- und Gesichts-Chirurgie. Germany. Biennial.
Fortschritte der zahnärztliche Implantologie. *Now called* Zeitschrift für zahnärztliche Implantologie.

Freie Zahnarzt: Monatsschrift deutscher Zahnärzte. Germany. M.
Frontiers of oral physiology. Switzerland. Irr.
Functional orthodontist (—a journal of functional jaw orthopedics). USA. Bi-M.

Gaceta dental. Spain. M.
Gaceta odontológica. Venezuela. Bi-M.
General dentistry. USA. Bi-M.
Georgetown dental journal. USA. 2 a year.
Gerodontics. Denmark.
Gerodontology. USA. 3 a year.
Giornale di anesthesia stomatologica. Italy. Q.
Giornale di stomatologia et di ortognatodonzia. Italy. Q.
Giornale di stomatologia delle Venezia. Italy. Bi-M.
Glasgow dental journal. Great Britain. 2 a year.

Hawaii dental journal. Hawaii. M.
Hellenic dental journal: the journal of the Society of Hellenic Dentistry. Greece. 2 a year.
Hellenic stomatological annals. *Now called* Hellenic stomatological review. *See* Hellenika stomatologika chronika.
Hellenika stomatologika chronika: Hellenic stomatological review. Greece. Q.
Helvetica odontologica acta. *Now in* Schweizerische Monatsschrift für Zahnmedizin.
Heraldo dental. Colombia.
Hygie: Revue française de médecine, d'hygiene et de santé bucco-dentaire. France. Q.

Illinois dental journal. USA. Bi-M.
Implant dentistry. USA. Q.
Implantologie. Germany. Q.
Index to dental literature. USA. Q.
Index to orthodontic literature of the world. Spain. A.
Indian dental journal. *Continued as* Journal of the All-India Dental Association.
Indice de la literatura dental en castellano. Argentina. A.
Indonesian dental journal. *Now called* Journal of the Indonesian Dental Association.
Infodont. Denmark. 6-8 a year.
Información dental. Spain. Bi-M.
Information dentaire. France. W.
Informationen aus Orthodontie und Kieferorthopaedie (—mit Beitragen aus der internationalen Literatur). Germany. Q.
International dental journal. Great Britain. Bi-M.
International dental review. *Now called* Dental review.
International dentistry. Egypt. M.
International endodontic journal. Great Britain. Bi-M.
International journal of adult orthodontics and orthognathic surgery. USA. 4 a year.
International journal of forensic dentistry. Great Britain. Q.

International journal of the Japanese Society of Pediatric Dentistry. *See* Pediatric dental journal.
International journal of oral implantology. USA. 2 a year.
International journal of oral and maxillofacial implants. USA. Bi-M.
International journal of oral myology. *Now called* International journal of orofacial myology.
International journal of oral (— and maxillofacial) surgery. Denmark. Bi-M.
International journal of orofacial myology. USA. M.
International journal of orthodontia. *Continued as* American journal of orthodontics *and* Oral surgery, oral medicine, oral pathology.
International journal of orthodontics. USA. Q.
International journal of paediatric dentistry. Great Britain. Q.
International journal of periodontics and restorative dentistry. USA. Bi-M.
International journal of prosthodontics. USA. Bi-M.
Internationales Journal für Paradontologie und restaurative Zahnheilkunde. *German edition of* International journal of periodontics and restorative dentistry.
Iowa dental bulletin (—journal). USA. Q.
Ipse odontologico. Brazil. Bi-M.
Iraqui dental journal. Iraq.
Irish dental journal. *Now called* Journal of the Irish Dental Association.
Irish dental review. *Now in* Journal of the Irish Dental Association.
Israel journal of dental medicine. Israel. 2-3 a year.

JAO: jornal das auxiliares odontologicas. Brazil.
JDQ: journal dentaire du Québec. Canada. M.
Japanese dental journal. *Now called* Dentistry in Japan.
Japanese journal of conservative dentistry. [Nippon Shika Hozongaku Zasshi]. Japan. 3 a year.
Japanese journal of dental health. *Now called* Journal of dental health.
Japanese journal of oral biology. Japan.
Japanese journal of oral (— and maxillofacial) surgery. [Nihon Kohku Geka Gakkai Zasshi]. Japan. Bi-M.
Japanese journal of pediatric dentistry. [Shoni Shikagaku Zasshi]. Japan. Q.
Japanese journal of pedodontics. *Now called* Japanese journal of pediatric dentistry.
Jordan dental journal. Jordan.
Jornal das auxiliares odontologicas. *Now called* JAO: jornal das auxiliares odontologicas.
Jornal de estomatologia. Portugal. 2 a year.
Jornal odontologico. Brazil. M.
Journal of the Academy of General Dentistry. *Now called* General dentistry.
Journal (of the) Alabama Dental Association. USA. Q.
Journal of the All-India Dental Association. *Now called* Journal of the Indian Dental Association.
Journal of the Allied Dental Societies. *Now called* Journal of dental research.
Journal (of the) American Academy of Gold-Foil Operators. *Now called* Operative dentistry.
Journal of the American College of Dentists. USA. 2 a year.

Journal of the American Dental Association. USA. M.
Journal of the American Dental Hygienists' Association. *Continued as* Dental hygiene.
Journal of the American Dental Society of Anesthesiology. *Now called* Anesthesia progress.
Journal of the American Society of Forensic Odontology. *Now called* International journal of forensic dentistry.
Journal of the American Society for Geriatric Dentistry. *Now called* Special care in dentistry.
Journal of the American Society of Psychosomatic Dentistry (—and Medicine). USA. Q.
Journal of the American Society for the Study of Orthodontics. USA. 2 a year.
Journal of the Anglo-Continental Dental Society. *Continued as* Restorative dentistry: journal of the Anglo-Continental Dental Society.
Journal de l'Association Dentaire Canadienne. *See* Canadian Dental Association journal.
Journal of the Baltimore College of Dental Surgery. USA. 2 a year.
Journal of the Bergen County Dental Society. USA. M.
Journal de biologie buccale. France. Q.
Journal of the British Dental Association. *Now called* British dental journal.
Journal of the British Dental Students Association. Great Britain. A.
Journal of the British Endodontic Society. *Now called* International endodontic journal.
Journal of the California (State) Dental Association (and Nevada State Dental Association). USA. 4 a year.
Journal of the Canadian Dental Association. (Journal de l'Association Dentaire Canadienne). *Continued as* Dental journal: journal dentaire.
Journal of the Charles H. Tweed International Foundation. USA. Q.
Journal of clinical dentistry. USA. 4 a year.
Journal of clinical orthodontics. USA. M.
Journal of clinical pediatric dentistry. USA. Q.
Journal of clinical periodontology. Denmark. 10 a year.
Journal of the Colorado (State) Dental Association. USA. Q.
Journal (of the) Connecticut State Dental Association. USA. Q.
Journal de la Corps dentaire. France.
Journal of craniofacial genetics and developmental biology. USA. Q.
Journal of craniofacial surgery. USA. Q.
Journal of craniomandibular disorders: facial and oral pain. USA. Q.
Journal of cranio-mandibular practice. USA. Q.
Journal of craniomaxillofacial surgery. (European Association for Cranio-Maxillo-Facial Surgery). Great Britain. Bi-M.
Journal dentaire belge: belgisch blad voor tandheelkunde. *Continued as* Revue belge de médecine dentaire.
Journal dentaire du Québec. *Now called* JDQ: journal dentaire du Québec.
Journal of the Dental Association of South Africa. Tydskrif van die Tandheelkundige Vereniging van Suid Afrika. South Africa. M.
Journal of the Dental Association of Thailand. Thailand. Bi-M.
Journal of the dental auxiliaries. China.
Journal of the Dental Auxiliaries Federation of Malaya. Malaysia.

Journal of dental education. USA. M.
Journal of the Dental Faculty of Istanbul. Turkey.
Journal of the Dental Guidance Council on the Handicapped. USA. 3 a year.
Journal of dental health. [Koku Eisei Gakkai Zasshi]. Japan. Q.
Journal of dental hygiene. Japan. M.
Journal of dental hygiene. (American Dental Hygienists' Association). USA. 9 a year.
Journal of dental medicine. *Now called* Journal of oral medicine.
Journal of dental practice administration. USA. Q.
Journal of dental research. USA. M.
Journal of the Dental School, National University of Iran. *Now called* Journal of the Faculty of Dentistry, Shaheed Beheshti University.
Journal of dental science. China. Q.
Journal of dental technics. [Shika Giko]. Japan. M.
Journal of dentistry. Great Britain. Bi-M.
Journal of dentistry for children. *Now called* ASDC journal of dentistry for children.
Journal of dentistry for the handicapped. *Now in* Special care in dentistry.
Journal of the District of Columbia Dental Society. USA. Q.
Journal of endodontics. USA. M.
Journal of esthetic dentistry. Canada. Bi-M.
Journal of the Faculty of Dentistry, Shaheed Beheshti University. Iran. Q.
Journal of the Florida State Dental Society. *Now called* Florida dental journal.
Journal of forensic odonto-stomatology. Australia. 2 a year.
Journal français d'oto-rhino-laryngologie, audiphonologie et chirurgie maxillo-faciale. France.
Journal of general orthodontics. USA. Q.
Journal of the Georgia Dental Association. USA. Q.
Journal - Gifu Dental Society. Japan. 2 a year.
Journal of gnathology. USA. 2 a year.
Journal of Hacettepe Faculty of Dentistry. [Hacettepe dis Hekimligi Fakultesi Dergisi]. Turkey. Q.
Journal of the Hawaii (State) Dental Association. *Now called* Hawaii dental journal.
Journal of Hiroshima University Dental Society. [Hiroshima Daigaku Shigaku Zasshi]. Japan. 2 a year.
Journal of the Hokkaido Dental Association. Japan.
Journal of hospital dental practice. USA. Q.
Journal of the Indian Academy of Dentistry. India. 2 a year.
Journal of the Indian Dental Association. India. M.
Journal of the Indian Orthodontic Society. India. Q.
Journal of the Indian Society of Pedodontics and Preventive Dentistry. India. Q.
Journal (of the)/Indiana (State) Dental Association. USA. Bi-M.
Journal of the Indonesian Dental Association. Indonesia.
Journal of the International Association of Dentistry for Children. *Now in* International journal of paediatric dentistry.
Journal of the International Society for Fluoride Research. USA. Q.

Journal of the International Society of Forensic Odonto-Stomatology. *Now in* International journal of forensic dentistry.
Journal of the Iranian Dental Association. *Now called* Majda (Iranian Dental Association).
Journal of the Irish Dental Association. Eire. Q.
Journal of the Japan Dental Association. [Nippon Shika Ishikai Zasshi]. Japan. M.
Journal of Japan Orthodontic Society. [Nippon Kyosei Shika Gakkai Zasshi]. Japan. Q.
Journal of the Japan Prosthodontic Society. Japan. Bi-M.
Journal of the Japan Research Society of Dental Materials and Appliances. Japan.
Journal of the Japan Society for Dental Apparatus and Materials. *Now in* Journal of the Japanese Society for Dental Materials and Devices.
Journal of the Japanese Association (—Society) of Periodontology. [Nippon Shishubyo Gakkai Kaishi]. Japan. Q.
Journal of Japanese Dental Society of Anesthesiology. [Nihon Shika Masui Gakkai Zasshi]. Japan. 3 a year.
Journal of the Japanese Society for Dental Materials and Devices. [Shika Zairyo Kikai]. Japan. Bi-M.
Journal of the Japanese Stomatological Society. [Nippon Kokuka Gakkai Zasshi]. *Now called* Journal of the Stomatological Society.
Journal of Kanagawa Odontological Society. [Kanagawa Shigaku]. Japan. Q.
Journal of the Kansas (State) Dental Association. USA. Q.
Journal of the Kentucky (State) Dental Association. *Now called* Kentucky dental journal.
Journal of the Korea Research Society for Dental Materials. Korea. Q.
Journal of the Korean Dental Association. [Taehan Chikkwi Uisa Hyophoe Chi]. Korea. M.
Journal Kyushu Dental Society. Japan. Bi-M.
Journal of the Louisiana (State) Dental Association. USA. Q.
Journal of the Macomb Dental Society. USA.
Journal of Marmara University Dental Faculty. Turkey. Q.
Journal of the Maryland State Dental Association. USA. Q.
Journal of the Massachusetts Dental Society. USA. Q.
Journal of Matsumoto Dental College Society. [Matsumoto Shigaku]. Japan. 3 a year.
Journal of maxillofacial surgery. Germany. Bi-M.
Journal of Meikai University School of Dentistry. Japan. 3 a year.
Journal of the Michigan (State) Dental Association (—Society). USA. 8 a year.
Journal of the Mississippi Dental Association. *Now called* Mississippi Dental Association journal.
Journal of the Missouri (State) Dental Association. *Now called* Missouri dental journal.
Journal of the National Dental Association. *Now called* Journal of the American Dental Association.
Journal of the Nebraska (State) Dental Association. USA. Q.
Journal of the New Hampshire Dental Society. USA.
Journal of the New Jersey (State) Dental Association. USA. Q.

Oral implantology. *See* Journal of oral implantology.
Oral and maxillofacial surgery clinics of North America. USA. Q.
Oral microbiology and immunology. Denmark. Bi-M.
Oral radiology. [Shika Hoshasen]. Japan. 2 a year.
Oral surgery. Japan.
Oral surgery - oral diagnosis. Finland. A.
Oral surgery, oral medicine, oral pathology. USA. M.
Oral therapeutics and pharmacology. (Japanese Society of Oral Therapeutics and Pharmacology). Japan. 3 a year.
Orale Implantologie. Germany. 2 a year.
Oralprophylaxe. Germany. Q.
Oregon State dental journal. *Now called* Journal of the Oregon Dental Association.
Orthodontic bulletin. USA.
Orthodontic review. USA. Q.
Orthodontics and dental traumatology. Denmark & USA. Bi-M.
Orthodontie française. France. A.
The Orthodontist. *Now in* British journal of orthodontics.
Ortodoncia. Argentina. 2 a year.
Ortodoncia clinica. Argentina. 2 a year.
Ortodontia. Brazil. 3 a year.
Ortopedia maxilar. Argentina. Q.

Pain control in dentistry. USA. 2 a year.
Pakistan dental review. Pakistan. Q.
Pakistan oral and dental journal. Pakistan.
Paradentium: Zeitschrift für die Grenzegebieten der Medizin und Odontologie. Germany.
Paradentología. Argentina. 2 a year.
Paraiba odontologica. Brazil. Q.
Parodontologia e stomatologia (nuova). Italy. Q.
Parodontologie. Germany. Q.
Pediatric dental journal: international journal of Japanese Society of Pediatric Dentistry. Japan. A.
Pediatric dentistry. USA. Bi-M.
Pediatric dentistry today. USA. Bi-M.
Pedodontie française. France.
Penn dental journal. USA. 2 a year.
Pennsylvania dental journal. USA. Bi-M.
Periodicals digest in dentistry. USA. Bi-M.
Periodoncia: revista oficial de la Sociedad Española de Periodoncia (SEPA). Spain. Q.
Periodontal abstracts: journal of the Western Society of Periodontology. *Now called* Journal of the Western Society of Periodontology: periodontal abstracts.
Periodontal case reports. USA. 2 a year.
Periodontal clinical investigations. USA. 2 a year.
Periodontics. *Now in* Journal of periodontology.
Periodontology. Australia. 2 a year.

Periodontology today. USA. 2 a year.
Periodontology 2000. Denmark. 3 a year.
Pernambuco odontologico. Brazil. Q.
Pharmacology and therapeutics in dentistry. USA. Q.
Philippines medical-dental journal. Philippines. M.
Plomjo. Germany. Bi-M.
Plugger: Iowa dental assistants journal. USA.
Postçepy stomatologii. Poland. A.
Postgraduate dentist: Middle East. Great Britain. Q.
Practica odontologica. Mexico. M.
Practical periodontics and aesthetic dentistry. USA. 9 a year.
Practice in prosthodontics. [Hotetsu rinsho]. Japan. Bi-M.
Prakticke zubni lekarstvi. Czech Republic. 10 a year.
Praktische Kieferorthopaedie. Germany. Q.
Pratique odonto-stomatologique. Switzerland.
Preventive dentistry bulletin. USA.
Prevenzione e assistenza dentale. Italy. Bi-M.
Prevenzione stomatologica. *Now called* Prevenzione e assistenza dentale.
Probe. Great Britain. M.
Probe. (Canadian Dental Hygienists' Association). Canada. Q.
Proceedings of the American Society for the Advancement of Anesthesia in Dentistry. *Now called* Pain control in dentistry.
Proceedings of the British Paedodontic Society. *Continued in* Journal of paediatric dentistry.
Proceedings of the British Society of Dental and Maxillofacial Radiology. Great Britain. A.
Proceedings of the British Society of Periodontology. Great Britain. A.
Proceedings of the British Society for the Study of Prosthetic Dentistry. Great Britain. A.
Proceedings of the European Prosthodontic Association. Great Britain. A.
Proceedings of the Finnish Dental Society. Finland. Bi-M.
Proceedings of the Institute of Maxillofacial Technology. Great Britain. A.
Proceedings of the International Conference on Oral Surgery. Denmark.
Proceedings of the Royal Society of Medicine—Section of Odontology. *Now called* Journal of the Royal Society of Medicine—Odontology Section.
Profesion dental. Spain.
Promotion dentaire. France. Q.
Protese dentaria. Brazil.
Protesista dental. Argentina.
Protetyka stomatologiczna. Poland. Bi-M.
Punjab dental journal. India. Q.

QDT. USA. A.
QDT yearbook. *Now called* QDT.
Quarterly dental review. *Now in* Journal of dentistry.
Quarterly of the National Dental Association. *Now called* National Dental Association journal.
Queensland dental journal. *Now in* Australian dental journal.
Quintessence of dental technology. *Continued as* QDT yearbook.

Quintessence international. USA. M.
Quintessence international/dental digest: journal of practical dentistry. *Now called* Quintessence international.
Quintessence tecnica. Spain. M. Spanish translation of Quintessenz der Zahntechnik.
Quintessencia. Brazil. M.
Quintessencia de protese de laboratorio. Brazil. Bi-M.
Quintessenz: die Monatszeitschrift für den praktizierenden Zahnarzt. Germany. M.
Quintessenz journal: Zeitschrift für die Zahnarzthelferin. Germany. M.
Quintessenz der zahnärztlichen Literatur. Germany. M.
Quintessenz der Zahntechnik. Germany. M.
Quintessenza: rivista mensile de odontostomatologia pratica. Italy. M.

RFPD actualités - revue française des prothèsistes dentaires. France. 10 a year.
Radiodoncia. Argentina.
Rassegna internazionale di stomatologia pratica. *Now called* Odontostomatologia e implantoprotesi.
Rassegna della letteratura odontoiatrica. Italy. 3 a year.
Rassegna di odontoiatria. Italy. Q.
Rassegna di odontotecnica. Italy. Bi-M.
Rassegna trimestriale di odontoiatria. Italy. Q.
Realités cliniques: revue européenne d'odontologie. France. Irr.
Refuat Hape Vehashinaim. *Now called* Dental medicine: journal of the Israel Dental Association.
Refuat Hashinaim. *Continued as* Refuat Hape Vehashinaim.
Reseñas odontológicas. Paraguay.
Restorative dentistry: journal of the Anglo-Continental Dental Society. *Now called* European journal of prosthodontics and restorative dentistry.
Resúmenes de la Facultad de odontología. Cuba.
Review of dentistry for children. *Continued as* Journal of dentistry for children.
Revista ADM. (Asociación Dental Mexicana). Mexico. Bi-M.
Revista de ALAFO: Asociación Latinoamericana de Facultades de Odontología. *Now called* ALAFO: Revista de la Asociación Latinoamericana de Facultades de Odontología.
Revista de actualidad estomatológica (española). *Now called* Revista de actualidad odonto-estomatológica española.
Revista de actualidad odonto-estomatológica española. Spain. 10 a year.
Revista de la Agrupación odontológica argentina. Argentina. Q.
Revista de la Agrupación odontológica de la Capital federal. *Now called* Revista de la Agrupación odontológica argentina.
Revista argentina para la defusion de la anestesia general en odontología. Argentina. Bi-M.
Revista de la Asociación Dental Mexicana. *See* Revista ADM. (Asociación Dental Mexicana).
Revista (de la) Asociación odontólogica argentina. *Continued in* Revista odontológica.
Revista de la Asociación odontológica de Costa Rica. *Now called* Revista odontológica de Costa Rica.

Revista de la Asociación odontológica del Cuba. Cuba.
Revista de la Asociación odontológica del Peru. Peru. Q.
Revista de la Asociación odontológica uruguaya. Uruguay.
Revista de la Associação brasileira de odontologia. Brazil.
Revista de la Associação paulista de cirurgioes dentistas. Brazil. Bi-M.
Revista del Ateneo de la Catedrá de tecnica de operatoría dental. Argentina.
Revista bahiana de odontologia. Brazil. Bi-M.
Revista brasileira de odontologia. Brazil. Bi-M.
Revista catarinense de odontologia. (Associação brasileira de odontologia, secção Santa Catarina). Brazil. 2 a year.
Revista Centro América Odontológica. *Now called* Centro America Odontológica.
Revista de chirurgie, oncologie, radiologie, ORI, oftalmologie, stomatologie. Seriia stomatologie. Rumania. 4 a year.
Revista del Circulo argentino de odontología. Argentina. Q.
Revista del Circulo odontológico de Córdoba. Argentina. 3 a year.
Revista del Circulo odontológico correntino. Argentina.
Revista del Circulo odontológico del Oeste. Argentina. Q.
Revista del Circulo odontológico de Rosario. Argentina. Q.
Revista del Circulo odontológico santafesino. Argentina.
Revista del Circulo odontológico de Tucumán. Argentina. Bi-M.
Revista o cirurgião dentista. Brazil.
Revista del Colegio estomatológico de Guatemala. *Now called* Revista guatemalteca de estomatología.
Revista cubana de estomatología. Cuba. 2 a year.
Revista cubana de ortodoncia. Cuba. 2 a year.
Revista dental. Dominican Republic. Q.
Revista dental. El Salvador. Q.
Revista dental de Chile. Chile. Bi-M.
Revista dental de Puerto Rico. Puerto Rico.
Revista española de cirugía oral y maxilofacial. Publicación oficial de la Sociedad Española de Cirugía Oral y Maxilofacial. Spain. Q.
Revista española de endodoncia. Spain. Q.
Revista española de estomatología. Spain. Bi-M.
Revista española de ortodoncia. Spain. Q.
Revista española de parodoncía. Spain. Bi-M.
Revista estomatológica de Cuba. Cuba. M.
Revista estomatológica de La Habana. Cuba.
Revista da Faculdade de farmacia e odontologia de Araraquara. *Now in* Revista de odontologia da UNESP.
Revista da Faculdade de odontologia de Aracatuba. *Now in* Revista de odontologia da UNESP.
Revista da Faculdade de odontologia de Bauru. Brazil. Q.
Revista da Faculdade de odontologia de Pelotas. Brazil. M.
Revista da Faculdade de odontologia Porto Alegre. Brazil. 2 a year.
Revista da Faculdade de odontologia (—farmacia e odontologia) de Ribeirão Preto - USP. *Now in* Revista de odontologia da Universidade de São Paulo.
Revista. Faculdade de odontologia de São Jose dos Campos. *Now in* Revista de odontologia da UNESP.

Revista da Faculdade de odontologia da Universidade federal da Bahia. El Salvador.
Revista da Faculdade de odontologia (da Universidade) de Pernambuco. Brazil. 2 a year.
Revista da Faculdade de odontologia, Universidade de São Paulo. *Now in* Revista de odontologia da Universidade de São Paulo.
Revista de la Facultad de odontología de Buenos Aires. Argentina. 2 a year.
Revista de la Facultad de odontología, Universidad de Buenos Aires. Argentina.
Revista de la Facultad de odontología, Universidad de Los Andes. Venezuela. 2 a year.
Revista de la Facultad de odontología, Universidad Nacional de Cordoba. Argentina. Q.
Revista de la Facultad de odontología, Universidad Nacional de Tucumán. Argentina.
Revista de farmacia e odontologia. *Now called* Especialidades odontologicas.
Revista de la Federación odontológica argentina. Argentina. Q.
Revista de la Federación odontológica colombiana. Colombia. 4 a year.
Revista de la Federación odontológica ecuatoriana. Ecuador.
Revista gaucha de odontologia. Brazil. Q.
Revista gautemalteca de estomatología. Guatemala. 3 a year.
Revista ibero-americana de ortodoncia. Spain. 3 a year.
Revista internacional de periodoncia y odontología restauradora. *Spanish edition of* International journal of periodontics and restorative dentistry.
Revista latino-americana de periodoncia. Argentina.
Revista mineira de odontologia. Brazil.
Revista nacional de endodoncia. *Now called* Acta clinica odontologica.
Revista naval de odontologia. Brazil. Q.
Revista odonto ciencia. Faculdade de odontologia, Pontificia Universidade Catolica do Rio Grande do Sul. Brazil. 2 a year.
Revista odonto-estomatologia. Brazil. Q.
Revista odontología. Colombia. 3 a year.
Revista de odontologia de Metodista. Brazil. 2 a year.
Revista de odontologia da UNESP (Universidade Estadual Paulista). Brazil. 2 a year.
Revista de odontologia da Universidade Federal da Santa Catarina. Brazil.
Revista de odontologia da Universidade de São Paulo. Brazil. Q.
Revista odontológica. *Now called* Revista. Universidad nacional de Cordoba Facultad de odontología.
Revista odontológica del Circulo de odontológos del Paraguay. Paraguay. Q.
Revista odontológica de Concepcion. Chile. Q.
Revista odontológica de Costa Rica. Costa Rica.
Revista odontológica ecuatoriana. Ecuador. Q.
Revista odontológica de Merida. *Now called* Revista de la Facultad de odontología, Universidad de Los Andes.
Revista odontológica de Mexico. Mexico.
Revista odontologica de Paraiba. Brazil. Q.
Revista odontológica de Puerto Rico. Puerto Rico.
Revista passofundense de odontologia. Brazil.
Revista paulista de odontologia. Brazil.

Revista pernambucana de odontologia. Brazil. Bi-M.
Revista portuguesa de estomatologia e cirurgia maxilo-facial. Portugal. Q.
Revista regional de Aracatuba. Associação Paulista de Cirurgioes Dentistas. Brazil.
Revista seara odontologica brasileira. Brazil. M.
Revista do Sindicato dos odontologistas do Rio de Janeiro. Brazil. Q.
Revista Sociedad colombiana de ortodoncia. Colombia. Q.
Revista de la Sociedad de estudios de ortodoncia Tweed de México. Mexico. 2 a year.
Revista de la Sociedad odontológica de Atlantico. Colombia.
Revista da Sociedade portuguesa de estomatologia. *Now called* Revista portuguesa de estomatologia e cirurgia maxilo-facial.
Revista da União odontologica brasileira. *Now called* Revista da Associação brasileira de odontologia.
Revista. Universidad nacional de Cordoba Facultad de Odontología. Argentina. Q.
Revue belge de médecine dentaire. *Now called* Belgisch tijdschrift voor tandheelkunde.
Revue belge d'odontologie. Belgium.
Revue belge de science dentaire. *Continued as* Revue belge de médecine dentaire.
Revue belge de stomatologie. *Continued in* Acta stomatologica belgica *and* Revue belge de science dentaire.
Revue du Cercle odontologique douaisien. France.
Revue dentaire de France. *Now in* Revue d'odonto-stomatologie.
Revue dentaire libanaise. (Lebanese dental journal). Lebanon. Q.
Revue dentaire de Syrie. Syria.
Revue française d'endodontie. *Now called* Endo: revue française d'endodontie.
Revue française d'odonto-stomatologie. *Now in* Revue d'odonto-stomatologie.
Revue française de la prothèse dentaire (—des prothèsistes dentaires). *Now called* RFPD actualités - revue française des prothèsistes dentaires.
Revue française de prothèse maxillo-faciale. (Bulletin de la Société française de prothèse maxillo-faciale). France.
Revue d'histoire de l'art dentaire. France.
Revue de l'Institut d'odonto-stomatologie d'Alger. Algeria. Q.
Revue internationale de parodontie et dentisterie restauratrice. *French edition of* International journal of periodontics and restorative dentistry.
Revue mensuelle suisse d'odonto-stomatologie. *See* Schweizerische Monatsschrift für Zahnheilkunde: Revue mensuelle suisse d'odonto-stomatologie: Rivista mensile svizzera di odontologia e stomatologia.
Revue d'odonto-implantologie. France. Q.
Revue odontologique. *Now in* Revue d'odonto-stomatologie.
Revue d'odonto-stomatologie. France. Bi-M.
Revue d'odonto-stomatologie du Midi de la France. France. Bi-M.
Revue odonto-stomatologique du Nord-Est. France. A.
Revue d'orthopédie dento-faciale. France. Q.
Revue de stomatologie (—et de chirurgie maxillo-faciale). France. Bi-M.
Revue stomato-odontologique du Nord de la France. France. Q.
Rheinisches Zahnarztblatt. Germany. 24 a year.
Rhode Island dental journal. USA. Q.

Riogrande odontologico. Brazil. Bi-M.
Rivista internationale di parodontologia e odontoiatria ricostruttiva. *Italian edition of* International journal of periodontics and restorative dentistry.
Rivista italiana di odontoiatria infantile. Organo ufficiale della Società italiana di odontoiatria infantile. Italy. Q.
Rivista italiana degli odontotecnici. *Continued as* Dental press.
Rivista italiana degli odontotecnici - Dental press. Italy. 9 a year.
Rivista italiana di stomatologia. Italy. M.
Rivista mensile svizzera di odontologia e stomatologia. *See* Schweizerische Monatsschrift für Zahnheilkunde: Revue mensuelle suisse d'odonto-stomatologie: Rivista mensile svizzera di odontologia e stomatologia.
Rivista di odontoiatria degli Amici de Brugg. Italy. Q.
Rivista di odontostomatologia e implantoprotesi. *See* Odontostomatologia e implantoprotesi.

SAAD digest: Society for the Advancement of Anaesthesia in Dentistry. Great Britain. Q.
SOLAIAT: Sociedad odontológico Latino-Americano de implantes aloplásticos y transplantes. Venezuela.
SSO: Schweizerische Monatsschrift für Zahnheilkunde. *Continued as* Schweizerische Monatsschrift für Zahnheilkunde: Revue mensuelle suisse d'odonto-stomatologie: Rivista mensile svizzera di odontologia e stomatologia.
Salud bucal. Argentina.
Saudi dental journal. Saudi Arabia. 3 a year.
Scandinavian journal of dental research. *Now called* European journal of oral sciences.
Schweizerische Monatsschrift für Zahnheilkunde: Revue mensuelle suisse d'odonto-stomatologie: Rivista mensile svizzera di odontologia e stomatologia. *Now in* Schweizerische Monatsschrift für Zahnmedizin.
Schweizerische Monatsschrift für Zahnmedizin. Switzerland. M.
Selecciones odontológicas. Argentina.
Selecoes odontologicas. Brazil.
Selecta dentalia. Sweden.
Selezione odontoiatrica. Italy. Q.
Singapore dental journal. Singapore. 2 a year.
Sintese odontologica. Brazil. Q.
Sociedad española de ortodoncia: actas. Spain.
Société odonto-stomatologique du Nord-Est: revue annuelle. *Now called* Revue odonto-stomatologique du Nord-Est.
South Australian dental therapy journal. Australia. Irr.
South Carolina dental journal. USA. M.
Special care in dentistry. USA. Bi-M.
Stom. Rivista di stomatologia infantile. Italy.
Stoma. Greece.
Stoma: cadernos de estomatologia, cirugia maxilo-facial e medicina dentaria. Portugal. Q.
Stoma. Zeitschrift für die wissenschaftliche Zahn- Mund- und Kieferheilkunde. *Now in* ZWR.

Stomatologia. Greece. Bi-M.
Stomatologia. Italy. Q.
Stomatologia. Rumania. Bi-M.
Stomatologia mediterranea: SM. Rivista trimestrale di odontoiatria e chirurgia maxilo-faciale. Italy. Q.
Stomatologica. Italy. Q.
Stomatologicke zpravy. Czech Republic. Q.
Stomatologija. Bulgaria. Bi-M.
Stomatologija. Russia. Q.
Stomatologija. Ukraine. A.
Stomatologika chronika. *See* Acta stomatologica hellenica.
Stomatoloski vjesnik. Stomatological review. Rumania. Bi-M.
Sumarios de odontologia. Brazil. Bi-M.
Suomen Hammaslääkäriseuran Toimituksia. Finska Tandläkarsällskapets Forhandlingar. *Now called* Proceedings of the Finnish Dental Society.
Surgical update. (American Association of Oral and Maxillofacial Surgeons). USA. 3 a year.
Svensk tandläkare-Tidskrift. *Now in* Swedish dental journal.
Sveriges Tandläkarförbunds Tidning. *Now called* Tandläkartidningen.
Swedish dental journal. Sweden. Bi-M.
Swiss dent. Switzerland. M.

Tandhygienistbladet. Sweden. Bi-M.
Tandlaegebladet (—: Danish dental journal). Denmark. 18 a year.
Tandläkartidningen. Sweden. 18 a year.
Tandtechnisch takblad. Netherlands.
Tandteknikern. Sweden. M.
Technicien belge en prothèse dentaire. Belgium. Q.
Technique dentaire. *See* Zahntechnik: La technique dentaire: L'odontotecnica.
Temas odontológicas. Colombia. Q.
Temple dental review and Garretsonian. USA.
Texas Dental Assistants' Association bulletin. USA. Q.
Texas dental journal. USA. M.
Thüringer Zahnärzteblatt. Germany. M.
Tidens tann. Norway.
Tidskrift foer odontologisk pedagogik. Sweden. 3 a year.
Tidsskrift for (praktiserende) Tandlaeger. Denmark. 10 a year.
Tijdschrift voor Tandheelkunde. *Now called* Nederlands Tijdschrift voor Tandheelkunde.
Transactions of the American Dental Association. USA. A.
Transactions of the British Society for the Study of Orthodontics. *Now in* British journal of orthodontics.
Transactions of the Canadian Dental Association. Canada. A.
Transactions of the European Orthodontic Society. *Now in* European journal of orthodontics.
Transactions. Hawaii Dental Association. USA. A.
Transactions of the National Dental Association. *Now called* Transactions of the American Dental Association.

Transactions of the Odontological Society of Great Britain. *Continued as* Proceedings of the Royal Society of Medicine—Section of Odontology.
Transactions of the Royal Schools of Dentistry, Stockholm and Umea. Sweden.
Trends and techniques in the contemporary dental laboratory. USA. Bi-M.
Tribuna odontológica. Argentina. Q.
Tribuna odontologica do sindicato dos odontologistas do Estado da Guanabara. Brazil.
Tropical dental journal. *See* Odonto-stomatologie tropicale: tropical dental journal.
Tsurumi University dental journal. [Tsurumi Shigaku]. Japan. Q.
Türk odontoloji bülteni. Turkey.
Tydskrif van die Tandheelkundige Vereniging van Suid Afrika. *See* Journal of the Dental Association of South Africa.

University of Toronto dental journal. Canada. 3 a year.
Update in clinical dentistry. USA. A.
Update in oral surgery. USA. A.
Update in orthodontics. USA. A.
Update in pediatric dentistry. USA. A.
Update in periodontics. USA. A.
Uttar Pradesh State dental journal. India.

Venezuela odontológica. Venezuela. Bi-M.
Vida odontologica. Portugal.
Virginia dental journal. USA. Q.
Voix buccale. France. Bi-M.
Voix dentaire. France. M.

WDA journal. (Wisconsin Dental Association). USA. 6 a year.
WSDA news. (Washington State Dental Association). USA. M.
Washington State Dental Association newsletter. *Now in* WSDA news.
Washington State dental journal. *Now in* WSDA news.
Washington University dental journal. USA.
West Virginia dental journal. USA. Q.
World news on maxillofacial radiology. (International Association of Maxillofacial Radiology). *Now called* Dento-maxillo-facial radiology.

Yearbook of dentistry. USA. A.

ZMF, ZMV (Zahnmedizinische Fachhelferin, Zahnmedizinische Verwaltungshelferin). Germany. 4 a year.
ZWR das deutsche Zahnärzteblatt. (Zahnärztliche Welt. Zahnärztliche Rundschau. Zahnärztliche Reform. Das deutsche Zahnärzteblatt. Stoma). Germany. M.
Zahnärzteblatt Baden-Wurttemberg. Germany. M.
Zahnärzteblatt Sachsen. Germany. M.
Zahnärztliche Fortbildung. Germany.
Zahnärztliche Mitteilungen. Germany. 24 a year.
Zahnärztliche Praxis. Germany. M.

Zahnärztliche Reform. *Now in* ZWR.
Zahnärztliche Rundschau. *Now in* ZWR.
Zahnärztliche Welt. *Now in* ZWR.
Zahnärztliche Zeitschrift. *Continued as* Zahnärztliche Rundschau.
Zahnärztlicher Anzeiger. Germany. 26 a year.
Zahnärztlicher Gesundheitsdienst. Germany. Biennial.
Zahnärztlicher Informations-Dienst. Germany.
Zahnarzt. Germany. M.
Zahnarzt Journal. Germany. Q.
Zahnmedizinische Fachhelferin: ZMF. *Now in* ZMF, ZMV.
Zahn-, Mund und Kieferheilkunde mit Zentralblatt. *Now called* Deutsche Zahn-Mund- und Kieferheilkunde mit Zentralblatt.
Zahntechnik: La technique dentaire: L'odontotecnica. Switzerland. Bi-M.
Zahntechnik: Zeitschrift für Theorie und Praxis der stomatologischen Technik. Germany. Bi-M.
Zahntechniker: Le mécanicien dentiste. Switzerland. Bi-M.
Zeitschrift für Dentistik und Zahntechnik. Austria. M.
Zeitschrift für Stomatologie. Austria. 10 a year.
Zeitschrift für zahnärztliche Implantologie. Germany. Q.
Zentralblatt für die gesamte Zahn-, Mund- und Kieferheilkunde. *See* Zahn-, Mund- und Kieferheilkunde mit Zentralblatt (für die gesamte Zahn-, Mund und Kieferheilkunde).
Zhonghua Konqiangke zazhi. *See* Chinese journal of stomatology.
Zobozdravstveni vestnik. Slovenia. Bi-M.

List of Japanese journals by their transliterated titles, with the English equivalent.

Aichi Gakuin Daigaku Shigakkai Shi. Aichi-Gakuin journal of dental science.
Hiroshima Daigaku Shigaku Zasshi. Journal of Hiroshima University Dental Society.
Hotetsu rinsho. Practice in prosthodontics.
Iwate-Ika Daigaku Shigaku Zasshi. Dental journal of Iwate Medical University.
Josai Shika Daigakai Kiyo. Bulletin of the Josai Dental University. *Now called* Journal of Meikai University School of Dentistry.
Kanagawa Shigaku. Journal of Kanagawa Odontological Society.
Koku Eisei Gakkai Zasshi. Journal of dental health.
Kokubyo Gakkai Zasshi. Journal of the Stomatological Society, Japan.
Matsumoto Shigaku. Journal of Matsumoto Dental College Society.
Nichidai Koko Kagaku. Nihon University journal of oral science.
Nichidai Shigaku. Nihon University dental journal.
Nihon Daigaku Shigakubu Obun Zasshi. Journal of Nihon University School of Dentistry.
Nihon Kohku Geka Gakkai Zasshi. Japanese journal of oral (and maxillofacial) surgery.
Nihon Shika Masui Gakkai Zasshi. Journal of Japanese Dental Society of Anesthesiology.
Nihon Shika Riko Gakkai. Dental materials journal.
Nippon Kokuka Gakkai Zasshi. Journal of the Japanese Stomatological Society. *Now called* Kokubyo Gakkai Zasshi. Journal of the Stomatological Society.
Nippon Kyosei Shika Gakkai Zasshi. Journal of Japan Orthodontic Society.
Nippon Shika Daigaku Shingaku Katei Kiyo. Bulletin of Nippon Dental College (University), General Education.
Nippon Shika Hozongaku Zasshi. Japanese journal of conservative dentistry.
Nippon Shisubyo Gakkai Kaishi. Journal of the Japanese Association (Society) of Peridontology.
Osaka Daigaku Shigaku Zasshi. Journal of the Osaka University Dental Society.
Rinshu Shika. Folia odontologica practica.
Shigaku. Odontology: journal of Nippon Dental College (University).
Shika Gakuho. Journal of Tokyo Dental College Society.
Shika Giko. Journal of dental technics.
Shika Hoshasen. Oral radiology.
Shika Igaku. Journal of Osaka Odontological Society.
Shika Zairyo Kikai. Journal of the Japanese Society for Dental Materials and Devices.
Shikai Tenbo. Dental outlook.
Shiyo. Journal of the Tokyo Dental Association.
Shoni Shikagaku Zasshi. Japanese journal of pediatric dentistry.
Tokyo Ika Shika Daigaku Kiyo. Bulletin of Tokyo Medical and Dental University.
Tokyo Shika Daigaku Obun Kiyo. Bulletin of Tokyo Dental College.
Tsurumi Shigaku. Tsumuri University dental journal.